Development of Quality of Life Theory and Its Instruments

Alex C. Michalos

Development of Quality of Life Theory and Its Instruments

The Selected Works of Alex C. Michalos

Springer

Alex C. Michalos
University of Northern British Columbia
Prince George, BC
Canada

ISBN 978-3-319-51148-1   ISBN 978-3-319-51149-8 (eBook)
DOI 10.1007/978-3-319-51149-8

Library of Congress Control Number: 2017934321

Printed on acid-free paper

This Springer imprint is published by Springer Nature
The registered company is Springer International Publishing AG
The registered company address is: Gewerbestrasse 11, 6330 Cham, Switzerland

Other Books by Alex C. Michalos

North American Social Report, 5 volumes
Global Report on Student Well-Being, 4 volumes
Essays on the Quality of Life
Ancient Views on the Quality of Life
Militarism and the Quality of Life
Foundations of Decision Making
Trade Barriers to the Public Good
Good Taxes
A Pragmatic Approach to Business Ethics
Principles of Logic
Improving Your Reasoning
The Popper-Carnap Controversy

For Deborah, with love

Acknowledgements

Most of the previously published papers in this set of four volumes (and most of my books) appeared in a publication of Springer, Kluwer, Reidel or Nijhoff, a chain of publishers that I have had the opportunity to work with since the 1960s. Since the original source of each paper in the collection is given on its first page in this collection, there is no need to repeat all these sources and express my thanks for permission to reprint them in each occurrence. I am happy to express here my gratitude for the lot and for the many years of our pleasant and productive work together.

In each of the volumes in this set, I will acknowledge permission to reprint each of the previously published papers appearing in scholarly journals, books or newspapers apart from the chain of publishers listed above. In this third volume, I would like to thank the Italian Society for Economics, Demography and Statistics for Chap. 9. Michalos, A.C. (2003). Identifying the horse, the cart and their proper order in sustainable development. *Revista Italiana de Economia Demografica e Statistica*, 52: 151–162; Organization for Economic Co-operation and Development (OECD) for Chap. 10. Michalos, A.C. (2008). Connecting communities with community indicators. In *OECD Statistics, Knowledge and Policy 2007: Measuring and Fostering the Progress of Societies*, (pp. 133–146). Paris: OECD.

In the Appendix of each volume I included some photographs and pictures to provide a somewhat different kind of historical context to my narrative. What I have been able to contribute over the past 50 years or so has been influenced by many more people than I have been able to picture here, but when I reflect on what I have done, most of the people pictured here are very much a part of the story. Most of the photographs and pictures are from my family albums, but some have come from friends and a couple of newspapers. I would like to express my thanks to the following for allowing me to reprint their items: Wolfgang Glatzer for photographs in How Good Policies and Business Ethics Enhance Good Quality of Life, numbered v2.1 (short for photo #1, volume 2), in Development of the Quality of Life Theory and its Instruments (v3.3, v3.5, and v3.6), and in Connecting the

Quality of Life Theory to Health, Well-Being and Education (v4.1); to Ferran Casas for photographs v2.6, v3.1, v3.2 and v3.4; to Filomena Maggino for v4.4, v4.5 and v4.6; to Anna L.D. Lau and Robert A. Cummins for v4.3, v4.8 and v4.9, to Valerie Moller for v3.7 and v3.8; to Joanna Kit-Chun Lam for v3.11; to Daniel T.L. Shek for v4.2; to the Cleveland Plain Dealer for Philosophical Foundations of Quality of Life (v1.4), and to the Detroit Free Press for v1.7.

Contents

Overview of the "The Selected Works of Alex C. Michalos"

Philosophical Foundations of Quality of Life

How Good Policies and Business Ethics Enhance Good Quality of Life

Connecting the Quality of Life Theory to Health, Well-Being and Education

Introduction to "Selected Works of Alex C. Michalos"

Biographical Notes

The central aim of this set of volumes was to describe and explain the context and connections among a subset of papers and books produced over the past 50 years. Rather than a mere reproduction of work already published, this will be an attempt to disclose the productive processes in their various historic contexts that led to the various research projects and publications. In Michalos (2003), I published a collection called *Essays on the Quality of Life* containing 20 articles focused on the quality of life, 3 of which appear in other volumes of this set because they seemed to be so central to the array of issues in the 70 articles in these volumes. For completeness, I mention articles from the earlier collection and books that are directly relevant to the themes in these volumes.

Some years ago (these days it seems that most things begin with "some years ago", unfortunately), in a debate about the existence of God, a member of the audience put the question to us "Why would God want to watch re-runs?". The question made sense from the point of view of one of the debaters, since God was supposed to know everything that is going to happen before it happens. As the atheist in the debate, I could only say that I have no idea why, although a lot of people seem to enjoy them.

While I also enjoy some re-runs, I would not find much joy in re-binding some old papers for a new audience. I do, however, find the idea of describing the historical context in which similar research questions more or less simultaneously appeared to people in diverse parts of the globe and were addressed first individually and then collectively. Here, the historical context includes some of my own biographical material. This is offered as a kind of second-best effort substituting for an autobiography that I have never had the courage to write, notwithstanding having thought about it many times.

My father ended his formal education in the sixth grade and my mother ended hers in the eighth grade. As far as I have been able to discern, in 1917, when he was about 17, my father, Charles K. Michalos, emigrated from the island of Chios,

Greece, to work in the steel mills of Gary, Indiana. He arrived with a pocket-sized Greek–English dictionary, learned to speak English with a heavy Greek accent, moved from the mills to driving a Nabisco bread and pastry truck for another 17 years, bought a small hamburger joint, then a somewhat bigger one and finally something more like a diner on Euclid Avenue in Cleveland, Ohio. Its claim to fame was the fact that many of the Cleveland Browns ate there, which was quite a big deal in 1947 when the Browns were the All American Football Conference champions and I was one of their biggest junior high school fans. My father died in January 1951, at about 51. We were never sure, because he was never sure, how old he was. I was daddy's boy and his loss was a great loss to me.

My mother, Josephine Pucci, was born in Akron, Ohio, one of eight children of immigrants from Palermo, Sicily. She worked at the May Company department store, sang in the chorus of the Cleveland Opera Company, married my father in 1931, produced my brother in 1932 and me in 1935, and provided the mom part of our mom-and-pop diner. Unlike my dad, she was not a particularly happy person, but she lived to be 93 years old, dying in June 1998. Like my dad, and the rest of us I guess, she did the best she could with what she had.

I was generally an above average but not outstanding primary and secondary school student. In secondary school and the first half of university, I was more interested in sports and girls than scholarship, though I enjoyed mathematics and history. I went to what was then Western Reserve University (now Case-Western Reserve University) in 1953, majoring in history with minors in philosophy and religion. When I read Plato's *Republic*, I felt as if he was talking directly to me. It had never occurred to me to ask what a good life might be, but the more I thought about it, the more I *had* to think about it.

I grew up in a very mixed religious family. The story my mother told was that her family were Catholics until the local priest did something that led my grandfather to tell him to go to hell and he took the whole gene pool into a more friendly Baptist church. My father seemed to practice the religion of washing his car on Sundays, but he thought his sons had to be baptized Greek Orthodox in order to preserve something or other that was important to him. So, we were. However, because our house was one block away from a small Quaker church, my brother, Chuck Michalos, and I were sent off together as soon as we were old enough to find our way there and back. I have a gold medal showing that I accumulated three years of Sundays without missing Quaker Sunday school.

Given this background, when I began to think seriously about a good life, I thought I should make my peace with God if there were one. So, besides studying philosophy, I studied the history of religions. Then, I went to graduate school at the University of Chicago. Because I was what one would have called a doubter, I wanted to study religion in a school of believers, assuming that if anyone could convince me that I was wrong, they could. At least they would be inclined to try. So, in 1957 I enrolled in the Divinity School, which seemed to have the most diverse faculty, including visiting experts in Buddhism, which especially interested me.

I also married in the summer of 1957, a marriage that lasted about 23 years and produced Cyndi (1960), Ted (1961) and Stephanie (1963). In 1985, I married the love of my life, Deborah Poff, a lucky break for both of us at the time and ever since.

While studying the history of religions, I took courses in philosophy and it seemed to me that philosophers had more precise and decisive methods of pursuing the truth than theologians. The University of Chicago had a wonderfully flexible approach to higher education, allowing students to pursue more than one degree at a time. To get a Bachelor of Divinity degree, a student was required to pass 7 comprehensive examinations and have a year internship in some relevant field of practice. I took some courses designed to prepare one to take the exams and some courses in philosophy that I found interesting. At the 1961 convocation, I received a B.D. and an M.A. in philosophy and then proceeded to pursue a Ph.D. in philosophy of science. I completed the latter in 1965 with a dissertation on a dispute between Rudolf Carnap and Karl Popper on the nature and use of probability theory in the assessment of scientific theories (Michalos 1971).

Many of the most salient and important features of the following 50 years of research and other activities may be regarded as relatively natural developments of these earlier initiatives. In a memorable essay on the best teacher he ever had, Nathan Keyfitz (2003) said that scholars should replace the metaphor of providing building blocks for a relatively durable corporate body of knowledge with that of providing biodegradable nutrition out of which new knowledge would grow. In a sense, today's nutrient is tomorrow's fertilizer. What I did until 1965 provided the ingredients for what followed, just as the latter will feed what comes afterwards. Most importantly, I think my general approach has been informed by a pragmatic and philosophic interest in a holistic, comprehensive understanding of any particular object of investigation. I will try to explain this approach in the next few paragraphs.

Broadly speaking, there are two ways to define "*philosophy*". From a *functional* point of view, philosophy may be identified as critical thinking about anything at all, from asphalt to zebras. From a *content* point of view, philosophy may be identified as a body of knowledge answering three questions. What is it? What good is it? How do you know?

Answering the question "What is it?" gives one a discussion of the nature or being of something. In short, it gives one an *ontology*, a word derived from the Greek "on" meaning nature or being, and logos, meaning discourse (among other things). Descriptions of the nature of things, ontologies, have at least two aspects. Everything has, after all, a form, structure, morphology or anatomy on the one hand, and a function, activity or physiology on the other. A duck, smile or football game, for examples, can be described at a minimum by describing their structural parts and how the parts function. What Isaac Newton might have referred to as natural philosophy and we now would call natural science is close to what philosophers would call ontology.

Answering the question "What good is it?" gives one a discussion of the value, worth or goodness in some sense of something. In short, it gives one an *axiology*, a word derived from the Greek "axios" meaning worthy or valuable, and logos. Of the variety of kinds of value that may be described, it is most useful to distinguish intrinsic from instrumental value. *Intrinsic value* refers to the worth or goodness of a thing in itself, its value as an end in itself rather than as a means to something else. *Instrumental value* refers to the worth or goodness of a thing as a means to something else, not as a thing in itself. Standard examples include things such as eating an apple or throwing a ball at a target having instrumental value insofar as the former produces nutrition and the latter scores points, which in this context have intrinsic value.

Since practically anything might be a useful means to something else for someone in some circumstances for some purposes, practically anything can have instrumental value. However, some people believe that all alleged sorts of intrinsic value may be reduced to a single one. For example, they would argue that the nutrition obtained from eating an apple is really only instrumentally valuable as a means to good health, which is itself instrumentally valuable for a life of pleasure, happiness or satisfaction. Those who believe that there is finally only one intrinsically valuable thing such as pleasure, happiness or satisfaction may be called monists with respect to the ultimate nature (ontological status) of value, while those who believe that there are many intrinsically valuable things may be called *pluralists*.

For a monist, then, it may be said that ontologically distinct things such as music, cheese and justice have different degrees of some sort of value such as pleasure, happiness or satisfaction, while for a pluralist, such ontologically distinct things have ontologically distinct values (music value, cheese value and justice value) regardless of how much pleasure, happiness or satisfaction these things produce. From an ontological point of view, then, a monist would have a numerically smaller number of ontologically distinct things in his or her world (e.g. music, cheese, justice and some degree of pleasure, happiness or satisfaction generated by the other three), while a pluralist's world would have music, cheese, justice plus music value, cheese value and justice value.

For a monist, the task of measuring the total value of something, a person, event, object, attitude, belief, proposition, action or life itself, is in principle straightforward. One simply needs to measure the degree of intrinsic value generated by that thing in terms of or operationalized as pleasure, happiness or satisfaction. For pluralists, the task of measuring the total value of something is not at all straightforward because there may be no way to compare ontologically distinct values like the value of music versus the value of cheese or justice. There does not appear to be any common measure, scale or instrument available to answer questions such as "How much is music worth compared to the value of justice or cheese?" or "What is the value of this piece of music in terms of the value of justice or cheese?"

Given the severe comparability problems faced by all value pluralists, it is not surprising that the most frequently studied theories of economists and decision theorists, namely preference theory, choice theory, utility theory and game theory, and one of the most popular ethical theories studied by philosophers, utilitarianism, assume value monism of some sort. As we will see in many of the papers in this collection and many more cited in those papers, scholars have invented a great variety of methods for living in and managing a world apparently containing a plurality of values. In particular, I will describe my own efforts over about 50 years, which have been interesting but largely unsuccessful.

Answering the question "How do you know?" gives a discussion of one's knowledge of something. In short, it gives one an *epistemology*, a word derived from the Greek "episteme" meaning knowledge and logos, hence, a theory of knowledge. Strictly speaking, one ought, prudentially and morally, to have a fairly clear answer to the epistemological question before one attempts to answer the ontological and axiological questions. Since a philosopher aims to obtain a body of knowledge about the nature and value of things to be used in the practice of living a good life, a patently necessary condition of achieving that aim is clarity with respect to knowledge itself and its production. That is why the earliest essays in these 4 volumes concern epistemological issues.

Comments on the Articles

All of the papers in this set of volumes are arranged partly in chronological order and partly by their logical connections. Each volume has its own major themes and within those themes, articles have been selected and arranged to provide some idea of the time at which they appeared and its relation to my own and others' research agendas around that time.

Following this introduction, Chap. 1 is a short article from the *Encyclopedia of Quality of Life and Well-Being Research* (2014) summarizing my fundamental assumption about the nature of quality of life or human well-being. It is based on the common sense view of most people that there is a difference between a Fool's Paradise and the real thing, a Real Paradise as we might say with some exaggeration. In a Real Paradise, conditions would be good, all things considered, as assessed by any relatively dispassionate, objective and unbiased observer and they would warrant and get the appreciation (satisfaction) of any particular participant in those conditions. On the contrary, in a Fool's Paradise, there is satisfaction with insufficient or mistaken warrant, proceeding perhaps from formal or informal fallacies (Michalos 1969), or both.

The most important explorations in Chap. 2 concerned tests of two competing explanatory models of happiness and global as well as domain satisfaction. In what I called the "Michigan model" satisfaction and happiness were posited as the result of the perceived gap between what respondents have and want to have (goal-achievement gap), and the latter gap is a result of two other perceived gaps, between what respondents have and the best they ever had before (have-best previously achieved) and what they have and what they believe average folks their age have (have-others have, social comparison). In the competing model, satisfaction and happiness were posited as the result of three equally important perceived gaps, goal-achievement, have-best previously achieved and have-others have. I showed that in every case, for the global and domain assessments, the Michigan model performed better than its competitor.

The robust results that I described in the previous paragraph made it difficult for me to see the more important results right before my eyes. Although the goal-achievement gap mediated the association between satisfaction and happiness on the one hand and the have-best previously achieved gap and social comparison gap on the other, it was also the case that the latter two gaps had direct influence on satisfaction and happiness. I had forced a choice between only direct and only indirect effects for my predictors, while the evidence showed that the predictors had both direct and indirect effects. Once that became clear to me, the general structure of multiple discrepancies theory (MDT) appeared to me. The first relatively complete statement of the theory in roughly axiomatic form is presented and tested in Chap. 3, from Michalos (1985). For a sample of nearly 700 university undergraduates, MDT was able to account for 49% of the variance in happiness scores, 53% of the variance in life satisfaction scores and 50% or more in 7 out of 12 domain satisfaction scores.

Chapter 4 is a note written to explain my views about being a feminist and the role of feminist philosophy in development studies.

Given the success of MDT on university students in Canada, from the fall of 1984 to the fall of 1986 I undertook a much more ambitious test of the theory on 18,000 undergraduates in 39 countries, using a questionnaire translated from English to 19 other languages. I had the help of 68 scholars in 76 universities. Chapter 5 is a brief overview of the four-volume *Global Report on Student Well-Being* (1991a, b, 1993a, b) that resulted from the international surveys. "On average, MDT explained about 55% of the variation in reported satisfaction and happiness scores, reaching as high as 71% for living partner satisfaction and as low as 41% for overall happiness with life". For 12 domains of living and life as a whole, the most influential predictors of satisfaction and happiness were the goal-achievement and social comparison gaps. Social comparison was most important for male respondents and goal-achievement was most important for females.

The first issue of *Social Indicators Research*, Volume 34 (1995) contained 6 articles making use of the global student data set by diverse authors, and Chap. 6 is my brief response to them from the same issue. I was, of course, quite pleased that the data we collected were put to additional good use by very able scholars. Among the 6 articles, using data from 1354 US undergraduates, Lance et al. (1995) produced "the most extensive direct test ever made of three familiar alternative models of the relationships between domain satisfaction and satisfaction with life as a whole". They showed that a model in which the causal arrows run in both directions from domain satisfaction to life satisfaction and from the latter to domain satisfaction (bidirectional model) performed better than either the traditional bottom-up model (from domain satisfaction to global satisfaction) or a top-down model (from global satisfaction to domain satisfaction). In a later paper, using a sample from 32 of the 39 countries in my global student data set, Mallard et al. (1997) showed that "globally" a bidirectional model best describes domain-life satisfaction relationships. This paper is reprinted in Connecting the Quality of Life Theory to Health, Well-Being and Education of this set.

The University of Northern British Columbia was established in 1990 and its main campus in Prince George was officially opened in 1994 by Queen Elizabeth II with 1500 students. I joined the university in the fall term of 1994, and in the summer of that year, I undertook the first community quality of life survey the city had ever had. Chapter 7 summarizes results of that survey. My aim was to establish a baseline of information about the city that might at some later time form the "before" part of a "before and after" investigation of the impact of a new university on a small city. My questionnaire included items on people's use of public services, spending preferences for taxes, satisfaction with a variety of aspects of their community and their lives, and questions about the best and worst things in their lives, and "things they would change first to improve the quality of their lives". The three most frequently mentioned things to change involved first, beautifying the central city; second, reducing crime; and third, eliminating air pollution. Over several years repeating this change question, these three issues regularly appeared at the top in some order. On crime-related issues, see Michalos and Zumbo (2000), and Michalos (2002), reprinted in Michalos (2003).

In 1998, my colleague, Bruno Zumbo, and I established the Institute for Social Research and Evaluation at the university. It was a collaborative initiative of the City of Prince George, Northern Interior Regional Health Board, Human Resources Development Canada, Regional District of Fraser Fort George, Prince George United Way and UNBC. Over my time in Prince George, 1994–2009, the Institute produced at least two surveys every year, one for the city and others for other cities and other clients. Michalos (2003) contains several published reports from the Institute and Michalos (2005a) contains reports on 30 surveys taken from 1994 to 2004, some published and some not. Working with our funding partners and others, we helped create a culture of evidence-based policy making in our City Council. We evaluated the regional employment assistance programme for Service Canada, renal services in our hospitals, the system of walking trails in the city, amenities in the region's provincial parks, services of the Royal Canadian Mounted Police, city services of all sorts, options for new gambling casinos, arts-related activities identified by the local Arts Council, routine aspects of the quality of UNBC's student services and the quality of student lives, and a wide variety of health, well-being and overall quality of life issues for the community.

Table 1 lists average happiness scores, satisfaction scores for 11 domains, overall life satisfaction and satisfaction scores for the overall quality of life taken from 13 Prince George community surveys over 14 years from 1994 to 2008. We have no good way to measure the impact of the new university on these scores, but examining the first and last columns, one finds that only two domains had changes greater than 0.02 from the first to the last survey. Average satisfaction with one's own health decreased from 5.6 to 5.1 and average satisfaction with one's financial security increased from 4.7 to 6.0. Across the whole period, average satisfaction with one's living partner and family received the highest scores in every survey.

Table 1 Prince George mean satisfaction* and happiness** scores, 1994–2008

Life domains	1994 June N = 501	1997 July N = 715	1997 Nov. N = 737	1998 Nov. N = 723	1999 Dec. N = 743	2000 April N = 554	2000 Nov. N = 430	2001 May N = 698	2003 Nov. N = 618	2004 Nov. N = 387	2005 Nov. N = 519	2007 April N = 411	2008 May N = 657
Your house	5.8	5.4	5.5	5.8	5.6	5.8	5.7	5.6	5.6	5.7	5.6	5.6	5.6
Neighbourhood	5.7	5.4	5.3	5.9	5.3	5.6	5.6	5.5	5.6	5.5	5.7	5.5	5.7
Family relations	5.9	5.9	6.0	5.7	5.6	6.0	5.9	5.9	5.9	5.8	5.8	5.9	5.8
Living partner	6.1	6.1	6.3	5.9	6.0	6.3	6.4	6.2	6.1	6.1	6.2	6.2	6.2
Job	5.4	5.4	5.4	5.1	5.3	5.4	5.5	5.2	5.2	5.3	5.3	5.6	5.3
Friendships	5.8	5.9	5.8	5.6	5.8	5.9	5.8	5.8	5.6	5.7	5.6	5.8	5.6
Health	5.6	5.6	5.4	5.3	5.3	5.5	5.6	5.4	5.2	5.4	5.2	5.3	5.1
Spiritual fulfil	5.4	5.4	5.3	5.0	5.2	5.4	5.5	5.2	5.3	5.2	5.3	5.3	5.3
Finance security	4.7	4.8	4.6	4.3	4.0	4.8	4.6	4.6	4.5	4.8	4.7	5.2	6.0
Recreation	5.0	4.9	4.9	4.7	4.9	5.1	5.0	5.1	5.0	5.1	4.8	5.1	5.0
Self-esteem	5.5	5.6	5.5	5.2	5.4	5.6	5.7	5.5	5.4	5.5	5.4	5.7	5.6
Life satisfaction	5.6	5.8	5.8	5.5	5.6	5.9	5.7	5.7	5.6	5.7	5.6	5.8	5.6
Quality of life	5.7	5.6	5.6	5.5	5.3	5.7	5.6	5.7	5.4	5.6	5.5	5.6	5.6
Your happiness	5.6	5.6	5.5	5.6	5.4	6.0	5.5	5.8	5.7	5.9	5.7	5.9	5.8

Source Surveys by the Institute for Social Research and Evaluation, University of Northern British Columbia

*Based on 7-point Likert scale running from ‘very dissatisfied = 1’ to ‘very satisfied = 7’

**Based on 7-point Likert scale running from ‘very unhappy = 1’ to ‘very happy = 7’

Chapter 8 is a report of our community survey in Jasper, Alberta. Jasper is a town inside Jasper National Park, “one of Canada’s most beautiful and famous park areas”. Our survey contained an unusually large number of domain satisfaction items that allowed us to create 15 indexes, 8 of which had Cronbach’s alpha ranging from 0.79 to 0.91. When we regressed our 3 global indicators (happiness, life satisfaction and satisfaction with the quality of life) on the 15 indexes plus some singular items, we found that our index of personal worth was the most influential predictor for each of the 3 global indicators. This index was an average score on satisfaction with one’s own self-esteem and what one is accomplishing in life, $\alpha = 0.79$.

As we approached the third millennium, we thought it would be interesting and useful to researchers if we took the pulse of British Columbians regarding their expectations and attitudes towards the future. Chapter 9 is a report of two independent surveys of the province taken in October and November of 1999 based on a rough division of what is called the “lower mainland” versus “the north”, using the town of Hundred Mile House as the dividing line. Among other things, the questionnaire had a list of “42 events and states of affairs that might occur in the next one hundred years, and respondents were asked to indicate whether they thought ‘it would be good (or bad) if it happened’ and then if they thought it was ‘probably going to happen (or not)’”. For about half of the items, northerners and southerners gave very similar responses, e.g. “fairly large majorities” thought “it would be bad to change our political geography by merging with the United States…or breaking up the country in any way”. On the other hand, “Ninety percent of northerners but 62% of southerners thought it would be good if there were tax breaks for northern residents”, although only “26% of northerners and 38% of southerners thought it would happen”. In response to our question about what to change to improve the quality of their lives, northerners and southerners mentioned the same top three things in the same order, namely issues related to employment and financial security, then health and third educational opportunities.

Chapter 10 is based on a presentation that was to be made at a conference of the Italian Society of Interdisciplinary Studies in Bari, Italy, May 2003. A back injury prevented me from participating. The thesis of the paper arose in response to a comment made by the British Columbia Minister of Sustainable Resource Management at the 2003 Annual General Meeting of the Fraser Basin Council. The Council is responsible for managing a huge natural resource, the Fraser River, and I attended the meeting as a member of the Fraser Basin Council Sustainability Indicators Advisory Committee. I was shocked to hear his apparent assumption that what we were supposed to be sustaining was “*economic development*” rather than “social well-being supported by a vibrant economy and sustained by a healthy environment”. The bottom line of my somewhat drawn-out argument in the paper is that because market value does not correlate well with what people might need or what they might deserve as a matter of fair or just treatment, it is wrong to determine what morally ought to be done (including what ought to be sustained) by what its commercial or market value happens to be. I still think that the case for this thesis is compelling.

As early as 1970, the Organization for Economic Co-operation and Development (OECD) declared that "…'[economic] growth is not an end in itself, but rather an instrument for creating better conditions of life,' from which it followed the notion that quality of life should be given operational content so that policies, including economic policies, could be geared towards it" (Verwayen 1980, p. 237). Nearly 30 years later, the second OECD World Forum on "Statistics, Knowledge and Policy" was held in Istanbul, Turkey, producing, among other things, the Istanbul Declaration in 2007. Chapter 11 is my contribution to the Forum. I made the case for increasing use of (1) multi-levelled statistical analysis in order to give proper weight to the great variety of interactions among the different "nests" in which human beings live, from their own homes to families, friends, neighbourhoods, cities, provinces, and so on, and (2) theories that include human agency (attitudes, motives, intentions, feelings, thoughts, beliefs and knowledge). As complex as our social scientific analyses have increasingly become, human beings and their living conditions are still far more complex than our statistical and conceptual machinery can accommodate.

Chapter 12 is a modest attempt to test the assumption that "27 of the most frequently used measures to assess aspects of the quality of people's lives…are sensitive to the changes in the circumstances of one's life measured by self-perceptions of change and by self-assessments of the net balance of salient positive and negative events one has experienced in some specified period of time". We surveyed a panel of British Columbia residents at three points in time, February 2005, 2006 and 2007, and found that "The success rate of the assumption using self-perceptions of change (61.7%) was much higher than the success rate using a net balance of experienced events (37.3%)".

The impact of arts-related activities on the perceived quality of life is one of the most under-investigated areas in the field of quality of life research, surpassed only by the impact of food and sexual activity. In forty years of editing *Social Indicators Research*, I saw no studies submitted on the importance of food and sexual activity in all their aspects (social, economic, health, psychological, political) for the quality of life. Studies of arts-related activities could be counted on at best a finger or two beyond one hand. So, there is a great deal of work to be done in these areas. Chapter 13 is a report of our third study of arts-related activities. It is based on a 2007 province-wide survey and 5 individual, small community surveys in 2006 in British Columbia. We measured time spent by the hour (e.g. listening to music) or by the numbers of events (e.g. attending live theatre performances) and levels of satisfaction obtained for over 67 kinds of arts-related activities, and we regressed perceived quality of life scores measured in seven different ways on the arts-related activities and other frequently used measures. We showed that the different ways of measuring overall perceived quality of life had a variety of associations with different arts-related activities, i.e. the measures were by no means equally sensitive to changes in all kinds of activities and other predictors. From this, we concluded that to avoid being misled by the varied and limited sensitivity of diverse global measures to different predictors, researchers should always use more than one kind of dependent variable.

In February 2008, President of the French Republic, Nicolas Sarkozy, formed a Commission on the Measurement of Economic Performance and Social Progress, chaired by the Nobel Laureat Joseph Stiglitz and including several other former Laureats. The Commission's Report came out in 2009 and received considerable publicity and discussion. Chapter 14 is my contribution to a symposium with 6 scholars held at the Seventeenth World Congress of Sociology in July 2010 at Gothenberg, Sweden, organized by Heinz-Herbert Noll and sponsored by the International Sociological Association. All of the papers were published together in *Social Indicators Research* in 2011. Given the distinguished scholars on the Commission, social indicators/quality of life researchers all had high hopes that it would produce a thorough state-of-the-art Report with good guidelines for future research. Most of us were disappointed. The Report had three parts, the first telling us what we already knew about the limitations of the national income and product accounts, the second telling us quite a bit less than we knew about quality of life research and the third telling us to get someone else to address problems of measuring sustainable development. Maybe our hopes were too high and our criticisms too severe, but all the documents are publicly available and readers can judge for themselves. In May 2013, Stiglitz was asked by the OECD to lead a high-level expert group to continue the work of Commission. The rest of us will continue to hope.

The United Nations Educational, Scientific and Cultural Organization (UNESCO) was the lead agency for the UN Decade of Education for Sustainable Development, 2005–2014, and I was appointed to the UN Monitoring and Evaluation Expert Group to assess the degree to which the aims of the designated decade were achieved. I thought we would not be able to make a rigorous assessment without some standardized baseline measures of what students know and what their attitudes and behaviours are towards sustainable development. Accordingly, with colleagues at Brandon University and the province of Manitoba Ministry of Education and Advanced Learning, we undertook some surveys leading to the construction of such measures. Chapter 15 is a report of our third investigation. We were able to craft a pretty good 20-item Index of Knowledge of Sustainable Development, a 15-item Index of Attitudes Favourable to Sustainable Development and a 16-item index of Behaviours Favourable Toward Sustainable Development, although only about 25% of the variance in the Behaviours scores could be accounted for by scores for Knowledge and Attitudes. In the future, much more work needs to be done on measuring appropriate behaviours.

Chapter 16 is a short farewell note for readers of *Social Indicators Research*. In Michalos (2005b), I published a report on the development of the journal based on a paper presented at the Ninth World Congress of Sociology in Uppsala, Sweden, in 1978. In that paper, I explained how I came to initiate the journal like the Little Red Hen in the children's story, after everyone else I suggested might do it seemed quite happy to leave it to me. It turned out to be one of the most rewarding initiatives I ever had.

The last Chap. 17 in this volume describes some features of what we call the Michalos-Zumbo Well-Being Index. It is a measure of subjective well-being built on 4 single item, 7-response category, Likert-type measures frequently used as dependent variables covering life satisfaction, happiness, overall quality of life and standard of living. Besides the studies cited in the article, its usage can be compared with other familiar measures in Michalos (2003, 2005a, b; Michalos et al. 2005, 2011).

References

Lance, C. E., Mallard, A. G. & Michalos, A. C. (1995). Tests of the causal directions of global-life facet satisfaction relationships. *Social Indicators Research, 34*, 69–92.

Mallard, A. G., Lance, C. E. & Michalos, A. C. (1997). Culture as a moderator of overall life satisfaction-life facet satisfaction relationships. *Social Indicators Research, 40*, 259–284.

Michalos, A. C. (1969). *Principles of logic*. Englewood Cliffs: Prentice-Hall, Inc.

Michalos, A. C. (1971). *The Popper-Carnap controversy*. Hague: Martinus Nijhoff, Inc.

Michalos, A. C. (1985). Multiple discrepancies theory (MDT). *Social Indicators Research, 16*, 347–413.

Michalos, A. C. (1991a). *Global report on student well-being, vol. 1: Life satisfaction and happiness*. Dordrecht: Springer.

Michalos, A. C. (1991b). *Global report on student well-being, vol. 2: Family, friends, living partner and self-esteem*. Dordrecht: Springer.

Michalos, A. C. (1993a). *Global report on student well-being, vol. 3: Employment, finances, housing and transportation*. Dordrecht: Springer.

Michalos, A. C. (1993b). *Global report on student well-being, vol. 4: Religion, education, recreation and health*. Dordrecht: Springer.

Michalos, A. C. (2002). Policing services and the quality of life. *Social Indicators Research, 61*, 1–18.

Michalos, A. C. (2003). *Essays on the quality of life*. Dordrecht: Kluwer Academic Publishers.

Michalos, A. C. (2005a). *Prince George papers on the quality of life, 1994–2004*. Prince George: Institute for Social Research and Evaluation.

Michalos, A. C. (2005b). Social indicators research: A case study of the development of a journal. In A. C. Michalos (Ed.), *Citation classics from social indicators research* (pp. 57–73). Dordrecht: Springer.

Michalos, A. C. (Ed.). (2014). *Encyclopedia of quality of life and well-being research*. Dordrecht: Springer.

Michalos, A. C., Ramsey, D., Eberts, D., & Kahlke, P. M. (2011). Good health is not the same as a good life: Survey results from Brandon, Manitoba. *Social Indicators Research, 107*, 201–234.

Michalos, A. C., Thommasen, H. V., Read, R., Anderson, N., & Zumbo, B. D. (2005). Determinants of health and the quality of life in the Bella Coola Valley. *Social Indicators Research, 72*, 1–50.

Michalos, A. C., & Zumbo, B. D. (2000). Criminal victimization and the quality of life. *Social Indicators Research, 50*, 245–295.

Verwayen, H. (1980). The specification and measurement of quality of life in OECD countries. In A. Szalai & F. M. Andrews (Eds.), *The quality of life* (pp. 235–248). London: SAGE.

Chapter 1
Quality of Life, Two-Variable Theory

Alex C. Michalos

Synonyms

Fool's hell; Fool's paradise

Definition

While the quantity of our lives is notoriously limited to one per person, its quality is as varied as the perspectives or domains from which it is viewed. Viewed from one perspective, a person may be well-off, but from another not at all well-off. This fact of life is familiar to everyone. So, the whole research field of "quality of life" studies might be more accurately called "qualities of life" studies. In any case, the general sense of the phrase "quality of life" is here understood as a ▶ good life all things considered. However, one of the first questions ancient philosophers addressed as early as the fifth century BCE is "What is a good life?" As demonstrated in many essays in this encyclopedia, the question and its proposed answers continue to intrigue us. One general approach is discussed here. What is here called a "two-variable theory" is any theory that holds that the well-being or overall quality of life of a person or ▶ community requires considerations beyond that person's or community's own endorsement, i.e., an individual or community's personal endorsement that their life is good is not sufficient to make it good.

This is reprinted from A.C. Michalos (ed.), Encyclopedia of Quality of Life and Well-Being Research, pp. 5307–5309. DOI: 10.1007/978-94-007-0753-5 © Springer Science+Business Media Dordrecht 2014.

A.C. Michalos (✉)
University of Northern British Columbia, Prince George, BC, Canada
e-mail: michalos@brandonu.ca

A.C. Michalos, *Development of Quality of Life Theory and Its Instruments*,
DOI 10.1007/978-3-319-51149-8_1

Description

In very broad strokes, one may think of the quality of life of an individual or community as a function of two variables, the actual conditions of that life and what an individual or community makes of those conditions. What a person or community makes of those conditions is in turn a function of how the conditions are perceived, what is thought and felt about those conditions, what is done, and finally, what consequences follow from what is done. People's perceptions, thoughts, ▶ feelings, and actions, then, have an impact on their own and others' living conditions. Taking the two main variables together (conditions of life and what people make of them), one can construct four scenarios which, with some exaggeration, may be described as different kinds of paradise and hell:

1. If people's living conditions are good, and people accurately perceive and think about them, feel good, and act appropriately, we may describe that as Real Paradise.
2. If people's living conditions are bad, and people accurately perceive and think about them, feel bad, and act appropriately, we may describe that as Real Hell.
3. If people's living conditions are bad, and people inaccurately perceive and/or think about them, feel good, and act inappropriately, we may describe that as the classical Fool's Paradise.
4. If people's living conditions are good, and people inaccurately perceive and/or think about them, feel bad, and act inappropriately, we may describe that as a Fool's Hell.

Although some complicated epistemological and evaluative material was smuggled into the four scenarios, it may be neglected for present purposes. The most important point to be made here is that the classical notion of a Fool's Paradise, which survives today, requires at least the sort of two-variable model mentioned in the first paragraph. This notion is based on the common sense view that there is a real world, however roughly apprehended and that there are good reasons for believing that some perceptions, thoughts, feelings and actions are more appropriate than others in that sort of world. As the remnants of the works of ancient authors reveal and as one would easily discover by examining the works of contemporary authors, the common sense view of the human condition is not universally appreciated and accepted. While anyone with any democratic sensitivity would grant that each person's assessment of his or her own life should be accorded some privileged status, it is far from obvious that such privilege should override all other considerations. Nevertheless, for some of the ancients and their modern followers, it is apparently supposed that people's personal assessments of the quality of their lives are not only privileged, but ultimately definitive. For example, Diener et al. (2009), p. 10 wrote, "Subjective definitions of well-being are aligned with the interests of the individuals whose wellbeing is being assessed. A life is going well only if the individual who lives this life endorses it as good and evaluates it positively. (That is, an individual's endorsement of his or her life as good is necessary to justify the claim that the individual's life is going well.) In this book, we adopt a subjective definition of well-being." It seems to be supposed, wittingly or not, that however constrained the perceptions, beliefs, and so on of the people living in poor conditions and assessing them as satisfactory, their assessments are paramount. For people holding such populist and somewhat postmodern views, there can be no Fool's Paradise, because there can be no fools foolish enough to misjudge their own satisfaction. For people holding such views, the quality of life, the good life, is completely internalized and determined by each person's own experiences. Then, since each person has privileged access to his or her own experiences, personal reports of those experiences must be equally privileged. On the contrary, the good life that we must want and achieve for all people is not just a life in which people feel good, no matter how terrible their real life conditions are, but one in which they feel good with the best of all reasons, because the objectively measurable conditions of their lives merit a positive assessment by any reasonable person.

The best way to address the problem of what to say when relatively objective conditions are not consistent with subjective assessments is to say that normally or in the *standard case*, objective conditions and subjective assessments are each *necessary* and *jointly* provide a clear *sufficient condition* of a life being bad or good, and being regarded as such with good reasons. Then, if someone's perceptions, assessments and actions are inconsistent with relatively objective conditions as a result of his or her ignorance, disability, disease, substance abuse or some sort of duress, we are reasonably warranted in over-riding their judgments. As well, if what we regard as relatively objective conditions are not as we think they are (which often happens, including disagreements among well-informed people), it would be unreasonable to insist that our claims about them are true and that we must act accordingly. In both kinds of cases, the normal or standard conditions for assuming the necessity of objective conditions and personal assessments are not met. When the normal or standard conditions are not met, we have the possibility of a Fool's Paradise or Fool's Hell. So we must adjust our judgments to fit the cases before us.

Cross-References

▶ Aristotle
▶ Happiness
▶ Life Satisfaction
▶ Plato
▶ Quality of Life, Conceptualization
▶ Well-being, Philosophical Theories of

References

Diener, E., Lucas, R. E., Schimmack, U., & Helliwell, J. F. (2009). *Well-being for public policy*. Oxford: Oxford University Press.

Further Reading

Michalos, A. C. (2003). *Essays on the quality of life*. Dordrecht: Kluwer Academic.
Michalos, A. C. (2004). Social indicators research and health-related quality of life research. *Social Indicators Research, 65*(1), 27–72.
Michalos, A. C. (Ed.). (2005). *Citation classics from social indicators research*. Oxford, England: Springer.
Michalos, A. C. (2010). Stability and sensitivity in perceived quality of life measures: Some panel results. *Social Indicators Research, 98*(3), 403–434.
Michalos, A. C., et al. (2011). The Canadian index of wellbeing: Technical report 1.0. Canadian Index of Wellbeing and University of Waterloo.

Chapter 2
Satisfaction and Happiness

Alex C. Michalos

Introduction

The structure of this paper is as follows. There is a review of some of the anomalies that have been encountered by social indicators researchers section "Anomalies as Prods to Research", and an overview of studies exploring various explanatory hypotheses of the anomalies section "Overview of Previous Research". Plausible next steps are considered in the fourth section "Next Steps". Beginning with section "Method and Sample", I report the results of a small survey undertaken at Guelph to at least prepare the way for others to take the important next steps on a grander scale. The methods and sample are described section "Method and Sample" and some basic statistics are provided section "Means, Standard Deviations and Skews". Substantial intercorrelations among domain satisfaction scores and life as a whole satisfaction and happiness scores are shown section "Intercorrelation". A path model of satisfaction and happiness, called simply the Michigan model, is examined in relation to a dozen domains section "Path Models of Satisfaction". Types of satisfaction are distinguished section "Types of Satisfaction", and there is a brief conclusion section "Conclusion".

Michalos, A.C.: 1980. Satisfaction and Happiness. Soclal Indicators Research, 8, pp. 385–422. 0303-8300/80/0084-0385503.80.

A.C. Michalos (✉)
University of Northern British Columbia, Prince George, BC, Canada
e-mail: michalos@brandonu.ca

A.C. Michalos, *Development of Quality of Life Theory and Its Instruments*,
DOI 10.1007/978-3-319-51149-8_2

Anomalies as Prods to Research

Nobody ever needed social indicators to learn that different people often have different feelings about the same things. That, after all, is what makes a horse race. Nevertheless, it is precisely this commonplace phenomenon that has stimulated much of the current research on so-called subjective or perceptual social indicators. We want to know *why* different people often have different feelings about the same things. If one asks oneself why this question seems so pressing, I think the answer must be because much more often, most of the time, most people feel practically the same way about most things. For very good physical, biological and social reasons most people are more similar than dissimilar to each other. If it were not so, then within any society the habits of communication, entertainment, transportation, eating, working, and so on would be unmanageable. Without plenty of uniformity, we would have plenty of chaos. We expect and in more or less subtle ways we cultivate and construct uniformity. Consequently, non-uniform, unexpected, unplanned phenomena confront us as anomalies. Moreover, perceived anomalies are necessary conditions of scientific research. When nothing is regarded as strange and unaccounted for, nothing is regarded as in need of explanation. The perceived need for an explanation of something is the threshold of scientific investigation, and probably magic, religion and philosophy for that matter (This is basically Kuhn's 1962, 1977 view).

The social indicators movement has generated its own anomalies. For example, although Cantril (1965, p. 194) reported a rank order correlation of 0.67 between his socioeconomic index and people's ratings of their present life on the Self-Anchoring Striving Scale, he also found that

> the rank order correlation between the index and personal economic concerns was 0.01, with national economic concerns, −0.05; and with national social concerns, −0.01 – all indicating a complete lack of any relationship.

(Cantril 1965, p. 201) Campbell (1972) reported that nearly half of the relatively poor white American respondents in a 'large-scale urban survey' described themselves as 'very satisfied' with their housing. Schneider (1975) reported significant differences between American cities when appraised using objective versus subjective indicators. Duncan (1975a) noticed that although there was an increase in the standard of living of respondents in Detroit from 1955 to 1971, there was no increase in the reported satisfaction with the standard of living. Allardt (1976) found that material level of living and reported satisfaction were independent. Hankiss et al. (1978) reported similar levels of perceived quality of life for people living in countries with dissimilar scores on a developmental index. Michalos (1980b) reported that although Americans were over five times as vulnerable to violent crimes as Canadians, national surveys in 1973 and 1974 revealed that roughly 40% of respondents in both countries expressed some fear of walking alone at night in their own areas. It was anomalies such as these that prompted Campbell et al. (1976, p. 115) to speak of the 'dilemma' of social indicators research, namely, that

> We become most suspicious of bias or measurement inadequacy when subjective assessment come into conflict with objective situations, although such discrepancies taken substantively are almost the principal reason for the conduct of the study [of subjective indicators].

Most of the research on subjective social indicators has centred around problems involved in the measurement of satisfaction or happiness with particular domains (e.g., housing, family relations and health) and with life as a whole. Measures of life as a whole are referred to as *global* measures, in contrast to more limited *domain* measures. In the next two sections I will briefly review some of the most salient literature in this field from the twentieth century. For a thorough and extremely thought-provoking historical review of the literature on satisfaction and happiness beginning in about the seventh century B.C., one should read Tatarkiewicz (1976). The next section is on the theories, models or hypotheses that have been proposed in order to explain perceived anomalies, e.g., hypotheses about the role of expectations, aspirations and so on in the determination of feelings of satisfaction. In the section following this review I present some ideas on plausible next steps to take in order to increase our understanding at key points in the current stage of the discussion.

Overview of Previous Research

One of the first things that occurs to researchers interested in explaining anomalies in this field is that expectations have a lot to do with the way people feel about their objective circumstances. The hypothesis that reported satisfaction is a function of the perceived difference between achievement and expectations has been tested in a variety of experimental situations with mixed results. Confirming evidence has been reported by Spector (1956), Foa (1957), Hulin and Smith (1965), Ilgen (1969, 1971), Locke et al. (1970), Ilgen and Hamstra (1972), Greenstein (1972), Lewis (1973), Space (1974), Gelwick (1975), Al-Hoory (1976), and Campbell et al. (1976). Unsuccessful attempts to confirm the hypothesis have been reported by Kawakami (1967), Buckley (1969), Berkey (1971), Carey (1974), Hibbs (1975), Newton (1976), Wantz (1976), and Morgan (1976).

Although some people (e.g., Pelz and Andrews 1976) use the terms 'expectations' and 'aspirations' as synonyms, there are good logical and experimental reasons for avoiding such usage. This was recognized clearly in the early studies of Lewin et al. (1944). Logically or conceptually there is a difference between what one aspires, hopes, wants or would like to achieve and what one expects to achieve. For example, underdog candidates for all sorts of positions may have high aspirations but very moderate expectations. They need not, of course, but it is logically possible and it often happens. Aspiration implies a conative element that is lacking in expectation. One has an emotional or affective stake in aspirations that may be entirely missing from expectations. (Edwards and Tversky 1967 is a good place to begin exploring studies of the impact of desirability on probability assessments.)

The fundamental logical distinction between expectations and aspirations is supported by the experimental literature. While we have just seen that the hypothesis regarding satisfaction as a function of the gap between *expectation* and achievement has had at best equivocal success, the hypothesis regarding satisfaction as a function of the gap between *aspiration* and achievement has been almost uniformly successful. Using the same computerized bibliographic search procedures that uncovered the mixed reports about expectation and achievement, I found only a single unsuccessful attempt to link satisfaction to an aspiration-achievement gap, namely, Carpenter (1973). Successful attempts to find an association were reported by Thibaut and Kelly (1959), Patchen (1961a, b), Cook (1968), Bharadwaj and Wilkening (1974), Thompson (1975), Warr and Wall (1975), Campbell et al. (1976), Danielson (1977), Dorsett (1977) and Mason and Faulkenberry (1978).

Hamner and Harnett (1974) found that satisfaction in a competitive situation was a function of two comparisons which interacted, namely, the perceived achievement-aspiration difference mentioned above and the difference between one's own perceived achievement and that of one's selected reference person. The idea that satisfaction might be a function of the perceived difference between one's own status and that of a reference person or group has received indirect support from Davies (1962), Feierabend et al. (1969), Gurr (1970), Easterlin (1973, 1974), and Scott (1979). Duncan (1975a, p. 273) claimed that "the relevant source of satisfaction with one's standard of living is having more income than someone else, not just having more income". Gurr (1970, p. 52) cited a passage from Aristotle's *Politics* suggesting the antiquity of the hypothesis.

Cambell et al. (1976) tested the hypothesis directly using three reference groups (typical Americans, most close relatives and most close friends) and satisfaction with two particular domains (housing and neighbourhoods). In each case they found a positive association between reported satisfaction with the domain, and the gap between respondents' present status and the status of the reference groups as perceived by the respondents. In their most sophisticated model of satisfaction with particular domains of life, these authors have such social comparisons feeding directly into aspirations (as in Lewin et al. 1944, pp. 340–341), with the aspiration-achievement comparison directly related to satisfaction. Figure 2.1 illustrates their model. The most influential comparisons respondents made were not with other people, but with the most liked previous experiences they had had (see Fig. 2.1).

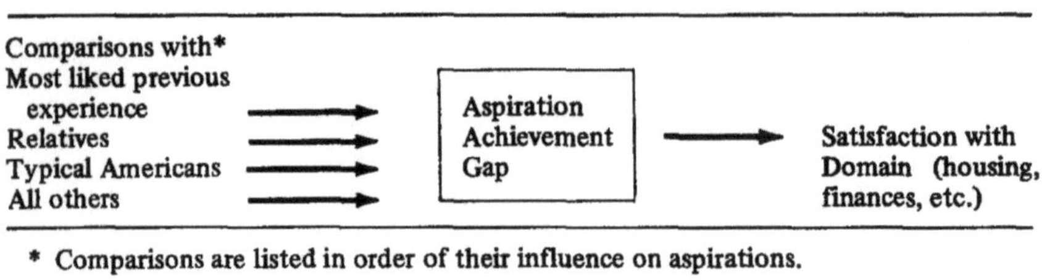

Fig. 2.1 Campbell et al. (1976) model of satisfaction with particular domains as a function of comparisons and an aspiration-achievement gap

Andrews and Withey (1976) also tested the social comparison hypothesis directly for one reference group (most people) and three domains (self-accomplishments, housing and national government). In each case they found the anticipated positive association.

Equity theory might be regarded as a particular species of Aristotle's old hypothesis insofar as it is based on a perceived difference between what one gets and what one thinks one is entitled to get, *given* what some reference person or group gets. As the theory has been developed since Adams (1963, 1965), it has led to mixed results. That, at any rate, is the conclusion reached by three reviewers of the literature, namely, Lawler (1968), Pritchard (1969), and Burgess and Nielsen (1974). Abrams (1972) and Strumpel (1972) both claimed that the reported satisfaction of their respondents was partly a function of the perceived equity of their situations. Andrews and Withey (1976) used an item that required respondents to make a judgment about the appropriateness or fairness of their housing, self-accomplishments and national government without necessarily making a comparison to any reference group. That seems to be another species of equity theory, and it at least yielded results consistent with the hypothesis that such judgments do influence reports of satisfaction concerning the three relevant domains.

Some researchers have found a positive association between goal setting and job satisfaction, even if the goals were not achieved, e.g., Latham and Kinne (1974), Kim and Hamner (1976), and Umstot et al. (1976). Others have found that it is not merely the presence of goals that contributes to job satisfaction (whether the goals are achieved or not), but it is participation in the goal setting process that is satisfying (Arvey et al. 1976). According to Umstot et al. (1976, p. 381), "A conservative weighing of the evidence suggests that goal setting has a strong, positive effect on productivity but an unknown effect on job satisfaction".

Some other theories that have a fairly direct relation to the ideas already discussed include cognitive dissonance theory (Festinger 1957; Brehm and Cohen 1962), adaptation-level theory (Helson 1964; Appley 1971), expected utility theory (Edwards and Tversky 1967) and attribution theory (Jones et al. 1971).

Next Steps

As the preceding brief overview suggests, there is no shortage of plausible models and more or less developed theories available to account for anomalies of reported satisfaction with various domains and with life as a whole. There are many more models and theories, and there is more experimental evidence than anyone could review in anything less than a long book. Campbell et al. (1976, p. 287) remarked that by 1972 there were over 3000 articles, books and dissertations written on job satisfaction alone! Nevertheless, these authors concluded (correctly, I think) that "However worthy generic explanatory constructs like tastes or aspirations may be, they fall far short of providing any very elaborated theory." (Campbell et al. 1976, p. 483).

Apart from constructing a 'very elaborated theory', there are still some important developmental steps that can be taken. In the first place there is a question of the effects of intercorrelations among measures of satisfaction in particular domains and for life as a whole. Weaver (1974) reported several significant intercorrelations among domain satisfaction scores. He concluded that

> The considerable interdependence among domain variables suggests that happiness is based on satisfaction in a number of different parts of life, that the employee whose happiness is significantly related to job satisfaction is also likely to experience satisfaction in other parts of life as well (Weaver 1974, pp. 838–839).

Although Weaver worked with a global measure of happiness with life as a whole rather than of satisfaction with life as a whole, the scores from the two measures generally correlate with Pearson *r*'s around 0.6–0.7 (McKennell 1978). Atkinson (1979, p. 14) reported that age and income were so highly intercorrelated that "any analysis of one of these factors must proceed with the effects of the other held constant". A systematic search for intercorrelation effects among domain satisfaction scores and life as a whole satisfaction and happiness scores would improve our understanding of such scores, and their change over time.

A second important question concerns the role of an aspiration-achievement gap in the explanation of satisfaction with particular domains and life as a whole. I have already noted that such a gap was found to be influential in reported satisfaction measures for housing, neighbourhoods, self-accomplishments and national government. Mason and Faulkenberry (1978) also found it influential in assessments of satisfaction with income and public safety. As Campbell et al. (1976) pointed out, so far no one has been able to design a questionnaire item that lends itself to repeated use across a variety of domains and that captures respondents' feelings about aspiration-achievement gaps. Consequently, different researchers focus on certain domains and invest the additional resources required to explore the relevant gaps in the limited areas. Thus, Campbell et al. (1976, p. 484) concluded that

> it remains quite conceivable that the general structuring of standards of comparison and aspiration levels might take quite a different form in other more disparate domains such as financial situation or marriage.

A similar suggestion was made by Duncan (1975a, p. 273). In other words, the model illustrated in Exhibit I may be appropriate for some domains and inappropriate for others. Clearly, what is required is the design and testing of a new efficient questionnaire item for a variety of domains and for life as a whole. Such an item is introduced and used in the following sections of this paper.

All previous tests of the hypothesis concerning the influence of an aspiration-achievement gap on reported satisfaction have involved the calculation of the gap from separate measures of aspiration and achievement. These procedures presume that the calculations researchers make are roughly identical to the calculations respondents make. The fact that relatively strong connections have been found between gap measures thus calculated and reported satisfaction measures suggests that the presumption is not entirely unfounded. Nevertheless, from the point of view of the basic assumption behind the study of perceptual or subjective indicators, the *perceived* gap between one's aspirations and achievements should be more closely related to reported satisfaction than the calculated gap. The gap we calculate for respondents may be significantly different from the gap they perceive on the basis of their own calculations and intuitions. The new efficient questionnaire item mentioned in the previous paragraph should allow us to capture the perceived gap between aspirations and achievements.

Method and Sample

In April 1979 I set out to try to pave the way for the important next steps described in the previous section. A campus mail questionnaire was distributed to the 867 members of the University of Guelph's Staff Association. This is the local union representing our office, clerical and technical staff. After three follow-up requests, a total of 357 or 41% of the questionnaires were received. Table 2.1 summarizes the sample.

According to our personnel department, the office, clerical and technical staff is 70% female and 30% male. Sixty-six percent are married and 34% are not. As you can see, then, the sample has more women and married folks than the population from which it was drawn. Moreover, the sample is nowhere near demographically representative of Guelph, Ontario or Canada. My guess would be that it is roughly representative of office, clerical and technical staffs in most universities in Canada and probably the United States. Whether one looks at the demographic characteristics (sex, age, marital status, education and family income) of university faculties, staffs or students, I suspect one would find considerable homogeneity. I imagine, for example, that our staff is more like the staff at York University or the University of Waterloo than it is like the staff at Canadian General Electric (which is also located in Guelph). Nevertheless, it is not necessary to speculate about what bigger group our 357 people might plausibly represent. It is a partially self-selected group with the composition specified in Table 2.1, and I'm not making any inferences about any other group. I should add, however, that there are some remarkable similarities in the results reported here and elsewhere in North America.

The questionnaires had 64 items in five pages and took about 20 min to fill out. Besides the opening demographic page, there were four pages with 13 items covering 12 domains and life as a whole. The four pages covered perceived satisfaction, the goal-achievement gap, life compared to average folks the same age and life compared to the best previous experience (To save space and shorten sentences I don't always put 'perceived' or 'reported' in front of 'satisfaction', 'goal-achievement gap' and so on. Similarly, I usually shorten phrases like 'satisfaction with free time activity' to 'free time activity'. In context these abbreviations should not be misleading).

Table 2.1 Sample composition

	N	Percent
Sex		
Male	80	22
Female	277	78
	357	100
Age		
18–34	249	69
35–44	42	12
45–64	64	18
65–up	2	1
	357	100
Marital status		
Single	112	31
Married	206	58
Separated	16	5
Divorced	15	4
Widowed	8	2
	357	100
Education		
Completed grade 8 or less	4	1
Completed 13 or less to 9	123	35
Completed some college, university, trade school	108	30
Degree, college or university	122	34
	357	100
Total family income		
0–$4 999	5	1
$5 000–$9 999	70	20
$10 000–$14 999	94	27
$15 000–$19 999	55	16
$20 000–$24 999	50	14
$25 000 and over	76	22
	330	100

All of the 53 substantive items called for a single checkmark on a seven point rating scale, with one off scale option called 'No opinion'. The instructions and format of my satisfaction items were adapted from Andrews and Withey (1976) with small changes. In particular, their scale has 'pleasant' and 'unhappy' where mine has 'very satisfying' and 'very dissatisfying.' My instructions were as followes.

> Below are some words and phrases that people use to identify various features of their lives. Each feature title has a scale beside it that runs from 'Terrible' to 'Delightful' in seven steps. In general we think of the numbers correlated with words such as the following:

1	2	3	4	5	6	7
Terrible	**Very Dissatisfying**	**Dissatisfying**	**Mixed**	**Satisfying**	**Very Satisfying**	**Delightful**

Please check the number on the scale beside each feature that comes closest to describing how you feel about that particular aspect *of your life these days.*

Twelve domain titles followed these instructions, namely, health, financial security, family life, friendship, housing, job, free time activity, education, self-esteem, area you live in, ability to get around and secure from crime. These were followed by the global question "How do you feel about your life as a whole?" Because my questionnaire was designed with one eye on using it in rural settings, I used 'area you live in' instead of the more common 'neighbourhood'. I considered 'transportation' and 'mobility', but finally settled for 'ability to get around'. In future studies other domains may be added or substituted.

The instructions and format of my goal-achievement gap items run thus:

Some people have certain goals or aspirations for various aspects of their lives. They aim for a particular sort of home, income, family life style and so on. Compared to your own aims or goals, for each of the features below, would you say that your life measures up perfectly now, fairly well, about half as well, fairly poorly or just not at all. Please check the percentage that best describes how closely your life now seems to approach *your own goals.*

Not at at	**Fairly poorly**		**Half as well as your goal**	**Fairly well**		**Matches your goal**	**No opinion**
0%	**20%**	**30%**	**50%**	**70%**	**80%**	**100%**	
1	**2**	**3**	**4**	**5**	**6**	**7**	**8**

The same twelve domain titles followed these instructions and were in turn followed by the global question "Now, considering your life as a whole, how does it measure up to your general aspirations or goals?"

The instructions and format of my average folks comparison items ran thus:

So far we have asked you to appraise several features of your life itself and in relation to your goals. Now we would like you to compare your life with that of other folks of your own age. Compared to average people of your age, for each of the features listed below, would you say that your life is a perfect fit (average), a bit better or worse, or far better or worse. Please check the number on the scale that comes closest to comparing your life to *the average.*

Far below average	**Worse than average**		**Average**	**Better than average**		**Far above average**	**No opinion**
1	**2**	**3**	**4**	**5**	**6**	**7**	**8**

Following the twelve domain titles, there was the global question "Now, considering your life as a whole, how does it measure up to the average for people your age?"

The instructions and format of my previous best comparison items ran thus:

Our final request is to have you compare your life now to your all time high. Compared to your own previous best experience, for each of the features listed below, would you say that your life now is far below the best it has been, worse than the best, matches the best, is better than your previous best, or far above the best it has ever been before. Please check the number on the scale that comes closest to comparing your life to *your previous best.*

Far below the best	**Worse than best**		**Matches the best**	**Better than best**		**Far above the best**	**No opinion**
1	**2**	**3**	**4**	**5**	**6**	**7**	**8**

Following the twelve domain titles, there was the global question "Now, considering your life as a whole, how does it measure up to the best in your previous experience?"

After this question, there was the following:

Finally, considering your life as a whole, would you describe it as very unhappy, an even mixture of unhappiness and happiness, happy, or very happy?

Very unhappy	**Unhappy**		**Mixed**	**Happy**		**Very happy**	**No opinion**
1	**2**	**3**	**4**	**5**	**6**	**7**	**8**

Notice that, with the exception of the satisfaction scale, two scale numbers but only one verbal description is provided for the areas between the midpoints and the extremes, e.g., '$_2$unhappy$_3$'. The aim was to eliminate 'noise' from disparate verbal cues (e.g., Andrews and Withey's insertion of 'unhappy' in a satisfaction scale), and to stay to a single scale-length.

Means, Standard Deviations and Skews

Table 2.2 summarizes some of the basic statistics of our diverse measures. The entries in the first four rows are arithmetic means of the means, standard deviations and skewness measures of the 12 domain scores taken collectively.

The skewness measures are those of the SPSS manual (Nie et al. 1975). Symmetric distributions have a zero value, while positive and negative values indicate clustering of values to the left and right of the mean, respectively. Thus, the top row of Table 2.2 tells us that the mean of the means of the 12 domain satisfaction scores was 5.18, the average standard deviation for these 12 scores was 1.20 and the average skew was −0.67 (i.e., the values were clustered to the right of the mean). The entries in the last five rows are for each of the five global items

Table 2.2 Means, standard deviations and skews

	Mean	Standard deviation	Skew
Average for 12 domains			
Satisfaction	5.18	1.20	−0.67
Goal-achievement	5.21	1.23	−0.81
Average folks	4.86	1.52	0.06
Previous best	4.51	1.37	−0.14
Global items			
Satisfaction	5.45	1.06	−1.02
Goal-achievement	5.19	1.06	−0.90
Average folks	5.06	1.12	−0.55
Previous best	4.81	1.28	−0.29
Happiness	5.36	1.28	−0.60

described earlier (i.e., life as a whole satisfaction, goal-achievement gap, average folks comparisons, previous best comparisons and happiness).

From Table 2.2 it's easy to see that, taken collectively, goal-achievement gap scores had the highest mean and the most skew, with rightside clustering. The average standard deviation for these scores was just barely bigger than that of the domain satisfaction scores, which was the smallest of the lot. The most variable set of scores of the four was that of average folks comparisons, which practically had a symmetric distribution. Insofar as Andrews and Withey (1976, pp. 206–210) are right about the virtues of symmetric distributions from the point of view of statistical operations, the average folks comparisons measures have some advantage over domain satisfaction measures.

Turning to the global measures, satisfaction with life as a whole had the highest mean, the lowest standard deviation and the greatest skew. As indicated earlier, this item was adapted from Andrews and Withey (1976). Although our samples were not comparable, they reported a mean of 5.30, a standard deviation of 1.05 and a skew of 1.05 for their comparable item (Their skewness measure is positive for rightside clustering). In terms of standard deviation and skew, my global goal-achievement gap measure was most similar to that of life satisfaction. However, the mean of the global happiness scores was most similar to the mean of life satisfaction scores.

Table 2.3 summarizes some of the basic statistics for the 12 domains and the four different kinds of indicators. In terms of satisfaction, highest mean ratings went to the ability to get around, security from crime, family life and health. These same four domains obtained highest mean rating for goal-achievement and comparisons with average folks, although the order of the four changed. For comparisons with the best of previous experience, the domains of health and security from crime were replaced in the top four by financial security and housing.

In terms of satisfaction, financial security had the lowest mean rating, followed by education and job. Since all of the respondents were employees of the university and probably realised that the results of my study would find their way to the

Table 2.3 Domain means, standard deviations and skews

	Means				Standard deviations				Skews			
	SAT	GOAL	AVE	BEST	SAT	GOAL	AVE	BEST	SAT	GOAL	AVE	BEST
Health	5.50	5.61	5.05	4.12	0.97	1.06	1.23	1.37	−0.51	−1.20	−0.23	0.26
Financial security	4.56	4.73	4.64	4.63	1.30	1.19	1.25	1.51	−0.58	−0.63	0.03	−0.39
Family life	5.51	5.47	5.24	4.76	1.34	1.40	1.37	1.43	−1.07	−1.18	−0.48	−0.08
Friendships	5.34	5.27	4.83	4.36	1.22	1.23	1.27	1.36	−0.61	−0.68	0.06	0.16
Housing	5.25	5.01	4.87	4.58	1.21	1.29	1.19	1.50	−0.72	−0.53	0.17	−0.08
Job	4.74	4.62	4.61	4.40	1.36	1.39	1.20	1.53	−0.48	−0.61	−0.15	0.00
Free time activity	5.09	5.02	4.75	4.40	1.32	1.25	1.18	1.30	−0.54	−0.76	0.15	0.18
Education	4.70	4.96	4.71	4.56	1.04	1.15	1.00	1.20	−0.49	−0.55	0.55	0.73
Self-esteem	5.02	5.24	4.74	4.57	1.07	1.09	1.15	1.15	−0.72	−0.81	−0.10	0.21
Area you live in	5.37	5.33	4.89	4.47	1.22	1.23	1.12	1.40	−0.63	−0.77	0.37	0.23
Ability to get around	5.58	5.57	4.98	4.74	1.21	1.28	1.19	1.37	−1.05	−1.18	−0.06	0.04
Secure from crime	5.53	5.69	5.01	4.57	1.14	1.14	1.21	1.27	−0.68	−0.84	0.36	0.47

SAT short for satisfaction, *GOAL* goal-achievement, *AVE* average folks comparison and *BEST* previous best comparison

powers that be, they may have been sending the powers a message. The rest of that message shows tip nicely in two other measures. Job had the lowest mean rating for goal-achievement and for comparisons with average folks of the same age as these respondents. Clearly, although these respondents are satisfied with their jobs, they are just barely satisfied. A score of 5 is labeled 'satisfying' and the mean score was 4.74. Moreover, their current jobs seem to take them half to two-thirds of the way toward their occupational goals, and to leave them slightly better off than they perceive average folks their age to be. In terms of their best previous experience with the 12 domains, the lowest mean rating went to health.

Intercorrelation

As indicated earlier, some researchers have found significant intercorrelation or covariation among domain and global indicators. Tables 2.4 and 2.5 summarize a series of partial correlations undertaken in order to find out how much of particular zero-order relationships might remain if conceptually distinct but relevant variables are controlled. For example, given that satisfaction with one's job and family life are each associated with one's satisfaction with life as a whole, how much of the associations remain if one of the domain variables is partialled out? In other words, how much of the associations are package deals in which several aspects of the quality of one's life are tied together?

Generally speaking, such analyses run the risk of being either unnecessary or misleading. Suppose, for example, that *A, B* and *C* represent any three variables. If *A* and *B* are completely unrelated, then partial correlations of either variable with *C* while controlling the other will yield results identical to zero-order correlations. Nothing in *A* is related to anything in *B*; so partialling is unnecessary. At the other extreme, if $A = B$ then partial correlations of either with *C* while controlling for the other will yield results of zero, because one is merely partialling a 'relationship out of itself' (Gordon 1968). In such cases, whatever *A* and *B* designate may be strongly associated with whatever *C* designates, and the partial correlation coefficient of zero may be misleading.

In Table 2.4 the dependent variable is my global measure of satisfaction with life as a whole, which hereafter will be abbreviated *S*. Column (1) gives the Pearson product moment coefficient *r* of each domain variable with *S*. Except for secure from crime, each domain variable is positively correlated with *S* above 0.27 with $P = 0.0001$ or better. Secure from crime correlates with *S* at 0.14 with $P = 0.005$.

Since Pearson's *r* measures only the linear association between variables and there was a possibility of curvilinear association, the same correlations were measured using the correlation ratio *eta* (Guilford and Fruchter 1978, pp. 296–300). The *eta* coefficients are listed in Column (2). The difference between *r* and *eta* values is a measure of the curvilinearity of the association between two variables (Guilford and Fruchter 1973). As Column (3) shows, with the exception of secure

Table 2.4 Correlations of domain, demographic and happiness scores with satisfaction scores

	(1)	(2)	(3)	(4)	(5)	(6)	(7)	(8)	(9)	(10)	(11)
Health	0.359	0.373	0.014	0.137	0.007	0.070	NS	0.132	0.011	0.062	NS
Financial security	0.400	0.409	0.009	0.212	0.001	0.196	0.001	0.226	0.001	0.220	0.001
Family life	0.602	0.661	0.059	0.393	0.001	0.257	0.001	0.380	0.001	0.245	0.001
Friendships	0.538	0.543	0.005	0.208	0.001	0.131	0.010	0.237	0.001	0.152	0.004
Housing	0.267	0.297	0.030	−0.089	0.05	−0.097	0.042	−0.056	NS	−0.062	NS
Job	0.343	0.355	0.012	0.133	0.008	0.133	0.009	0.156	0.003	0.161	0.003
Free time activity	0.413	0.448	0.035	0.131	0.009	0.122	0.015	0.093	0.052	0.074	NS
Education	0.359	0.376	0.017	−0.071	NS	−0.045	NS	−0.074	NS	0.050	NS
Self-esteem	0.454	0.477	0.023	0.172	0.001	0.139	0.007	0.152	0.004	0.132	0.011
Area you live in	0.283	0.347	0.064	0.049	NS	0.064	NS	0.058	NS	0.079	NS
Ability to get around	0.330	0.387	0.057	0.119	0.017	0.112	0.023	0.098	0.044	0.093	0.053
Secure from crime	0.135[a]	0.220	0.085	0.028	NS	0.053	NS	0.026	NS	0.052	NS

Explanations column code:
(1) Pierson r, P = 0.0001
(2) Eta
(3) Col. 2 minus Col. 1
(4) Correlation of domain listed at left with S, partialling out all other domain effects
(5) Significance levels of partial correlations in Col. 4, 319 degrees of freedom
(6) Correlation of domain with S, partialling out all other domain effects plus global happiness effects
(7) Significance levels of partial correlations in Col. 6, 316 degrees of freedom
(8) Correlation of domain with S, partialling out other domain effects plus five demographic variables (sex, age, marital status, education, family income)
(9) Significance levels of partial correlations in Col. 8, 303 degrees of freedom
(10) Correlation of domain with S, partialling out all other domain, happiness and demographic effects
(11) Significant levels of partial correlations in Col. 10, 300 degrees of freedom.
Significant levels less than 0.05 were uniformly labeled 'NS' for 'not statistically significant'
[a]P = 0.005

Table 2.5 Correlations of domain, demographic and satisfaction scores with happiness scores

	(1)	(2)	(3)	(4)	(5)	(6)	(7)	(8)	(9)	(10)	(11)
Health	0.330	0.349	0.019	0.175	0.001	0.139	0.007	0.184	0.001	0.151	0.004
Financial security	0.310	0.329	0.019	0.084	NS	−0.003	NS	0.060	NS	−0.033	NS
Family life	0.585	0.607	0.022	0.376	0.001	0.234	0.001	0.373	0.001	0.239	0.001
Friendships	0.509	0.528	0.019	0.228	0.001	0.153	0.003	0.257	0.001	0.172	0.001
Housing	0.246	0.306	0.060	0.015	NS						
Job	0.243	0.271	0.028	0.027	NS						
Free time activity	0.335	0.370	0.035	0.032	NS						
Education	0.292	0.325	0.033	−0.071	NS						
Self-esteem	0.364	0.378	0.014	0.111	0.023						
Area you live in	0.229	0.270	0.041	−0.018	NS						
Ability to get around	0.246	0.273	0.027	0.042	NS						
Secure from crime	0.078[a]	0.191	0.113	−0.067	NS						

Explanations column code
(1) Pearson r, P = 0.0001
(2) Eta
(3) Col. 2 minus Col. 1
(4) Correlation of domain listed at left with H, partialling out all other domain effects
(5) Significance levels of partial correlations in Col. 4, 319 degrees of freedom
(6) Correlation of domain with H, partialling out other domains plus S effects
(7) Significance levels of partial correlations in Col. 6, 316 degrees of freedom
(8) Correlation of domain with H, partialling out other domain effects plus five demographic variables
(9) Significance levels of partial correlations in Col. 8, 303 degrees of freedom
(10) Correlation of domain with H, partialling out all other domain, demographic and S effects
(11) Significance levels of partial correlations in Col. 10, 300 degrees of freedom
'NS' is short for 'not statistically significant'
The last 8 rows of columns (6) to (11) were omitted because there were no statistically significant associations
[a]NS

from crime, the difference between *r* and *eta* values never rose above 0.06, indicating practically no curvilinear association.

Column (4) shows the results of partialling out (statistically controlling) all other domain variables. In every case there was a fairly dramatic decrease in the correlation with *S*, indicating substantial covariation. Ignoring the three statistically insignificant correlations, the covariation ran from a maximum of 68% for free time activity to a minimum of 35% for family life. That is, 68% of the correlation coefficient measuring the linear association between satisfaction with free time activity and satisfaction with life as a whole represents shared covariation with the eleven other domain variables. Controlling the other eleven variables, the correlation between free time activity and *S* drops from 0.413 to 0.131. In the case of job satisfaction, when the covariation with all other domains is eliminated, the correlation with *S* drops from 0.343 to 0.133, a 61% decrease. The domain of family life has the highest correlation with *S*, $r = 0.602$, and also the least covariation with other domains, 35%. It would be a mistake, however, to infer uniqueness from strength of association. Friendship has a 0.538 correlation with *S*, 61% of which covaries with the eleven other domains. In general, the mean covariation of the eleven other domains with any particular domain-5 correlation was 59%. In other words, an average of nearly 60% of the association between satisfaction with any domain and satisfaction with life as a whole represents a package deal in which several aspects of the quality of one's life are tied together.

Column (6) of Table 2.4 shows the results of partialling out all other domains plus global happiness, which hereafter will be abbreviated *H*. I will have much more to say about relations between *S* and *H* later. Here it is sufficient to notice that the Pearson *r* association between *S* and *H* is 0.68 ($P = 0.0001$) and that following Andrews and Withey (1976) and McKennell (1978), I'm assuming *H* is a purer measure of affect than *S*. Thus, the point of partialling out *H* is to try to eliminate some of the affective component from *S*, leaving a purer cognitive component. Ignoring the four statistically insignificant correlations, in seven of the eight remaining partial correlations, the removal of *H* decreased the domain-*S* association still farther. Only the job-*S* association remained unchanged. The family life-*S* association, for example, dropped from 0.393 to 0.257.

Column (8) shows the results of partialling out all other domains plus five demographic variables (sex, age, marital status, education and family income). Ignoring the four insignificant correlations, comparison with Column (4) reveals that in five cases there was a further decrease in the domain-*S* association and in three cases there was an increase. The average change brought about by the partialling out of demographic variables was 0.02, hardly worth the bother. I suppose the demographic variables are relatively unimportant because of the homogeneity of the sample.

Column (10) represents the bottom line of this sort of statistical striptease. Here we have domain-*S* associations with all other domains, five demographic variables and happiness partialled out. So we're looking at domain-*S* associations in about as pure a form as anyone has ever looked at them. Comparison of Columns (10) and (1) are startling. First, only half of the associations are statistically significant in

Column (10). Second, the remaining significant associations are all severely diminished from Column (1). The average decrease in the domain-*S* associations from (1) to (10) is 62%.

As interesting as the preceding exercise may have been, it is worthwhile to remember the caveats introduced in the second paragraph of this section, and to recall Campbell et al. (1976, p. 122) warning of the danger of 'overcontrol'. "To overcontrol" they said, "is to adjust from view some contour of the data which is actually relevant in a substantive way to the more precise question being asked about reality." A case in point, for example, is the removal of *H* effects from domain-5 associations. Technically, as we saw, the amputation is possible. But is the resulting satisfaction measure somehow purer or more valid, or just more artifact? Is it more frank or more Frankenstein? At this point, I suspect it is the latter.

Table 2.5 summarizes a series of analyses that were patterned after those reviewed in Table 2.4. The basic difference is that the dependent variable in these analyses is *H,* the global measure of happiness. Inspection of the first columns of Tables 2.4 and 2.5 reveals immediately that *S* is more closely related than *H* to domain satisfaction. In every case the domain-*S* association is stronger than the domain-*H* association. There is one statistically insignificant domain-*H* association, for secure from crime (which was an oddball earlier too). The *eta* minus *r* values in Column (3) again indicate the absence of any significant curvilinearity. The average *eta-r* difference is only 0.03. When we move to Column (4), in which all other domains are partialled out, we are left with only four statistically significant correlations (health, family life, friendships and self-esteem). In fact, with the exception of the self esteem-*H* association, we could just as well have omitted the last eight rows of every column from (4) to (11). To make a potentially long story short, it seems to me that the associations in Table 2.5 suggest that *H* is not going to be as analytically useful as *S* as a basic dependent variable for quality of life studies.

Path Models of Satisfaction

Campbell's et al. (1976) model of satisfaction was introduced earlier and illustrated in Fig. 2.1. Because other researchers at the University of Michigan have worked with this model (Andrews and Withey 1976 for example), and in order to save space, I will hereafter refer to it as the 'Michigan model'. Given the brief literature review presented earlier and the historical antecedents documented in Tatarkiewicz (1976), there is no doubt that the *Michigan* model has very deep roots in Western civilization. To test the model directly for satisfaction and happiness with life as a whole, and for satisfaction with a dozen domains, I undertook a series of path analyses. Formal models similar to those employed here are discussed in detail in Kerlinger and Pedhazur (1973, pp. 307–314, 322–327), and Duncan ((1975b, pp. 42–44). So interested readers can consult those texts for detailed analyses of the formal features of path analysis generally and the Michigan model in particular.

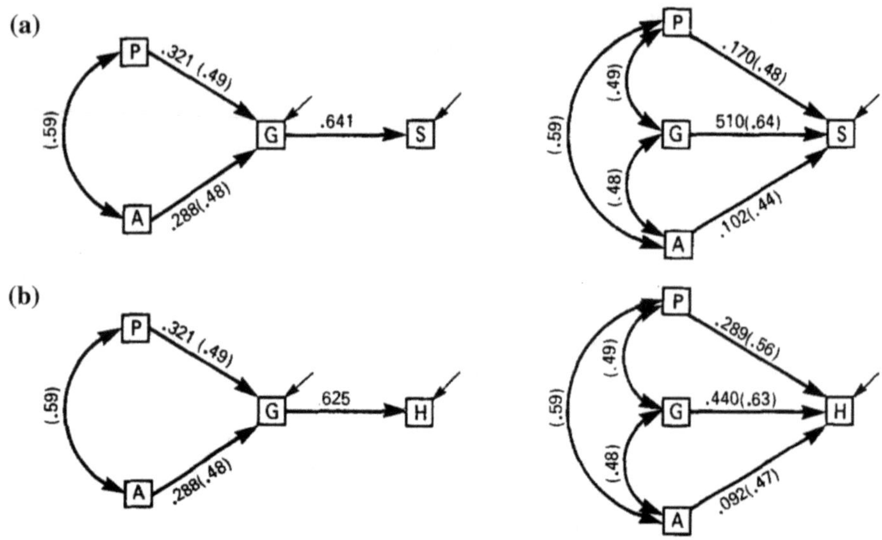

Fig. 2.2 **a** Satisfaction with life as a whole, **b** happiness with life as a whole

All of the path models considered here have the form of those in Fig. 2.2a. In all of the diagrams *S* and *H* are interpreted as usual, while *G* is short for the goal-achievement gap, *P* for comparisons with the best previous experience and *A* for comparisons with average folks of the same age. The arrows in the diagrams indicate proposed (hypothesized, theorized, imagined, etc.) causal relations, with effects named at the arrowheads and causes named at the end of the shafts. The small arrows without names at the end of their shafts represent error terms on the endogenous variables. The model on the left is the Michigan model and the model on the right is its most plausible competitor. Thus, in the Michigan model, *S* is supposed to be caused directly by G which is in turn directly caused by *P* and *A*. In its competitor, *S* is directly caused by *P, G* and *A*. The numbers in parentheses along the shafts are the zero-order correlation coefficients between the variables named at either end of the shafts, while the other numbers are standardized regression coefficients (betas) or path coefficients. In the Michigan model, the path coefficient connecting G to *S* is obtained by regressing *S* on *G,* and a multiple regression of *G* on *P* and *A* gives the path coefficients connecting these variables. The betas of the competitor are obtained from a multiple regression of *S on P, G* and *A*. For example, then, in the Michigan model of Fig. 2.2a, the numbers above the arrow from *P* to *G* indicate that the Pearson *r* between these variables is 0.49, and that there will be an average change of 0.32 in *G* for every unit change in *P* (when both *P* and *G* are standardized to have means of zero and standard deviations of one). The path coefficient is analogous to a partial correlation coefficient in that it indicates a relation between two variables with the effects of all others in the system held constant.

Testing the Michigan model means, in the present context, comparing its features to those of its competitor and answering the following question: Are all of the path coefficients in the Michigan model bigger than their alternatives in its competitor? In other words, does the Michigan model represent a system or structure of relationships that is stronger or tighter than the system represented by its competitor? A second question of interest concerns the relative strength of the connections from *P* to *G*, and *A* to *G*. Campbell et al. (1976) and Andrews and Withey (1976) found that the former (*P* to G) was uniformly stronger than the latter (*A* to *G*). So, the question is: Will the relative strength of these connections be duplicated here?

For a number of reasons that need not detain us, it is obviously possible to have data consistent or inconsistent with a hypothesis without the hypothesis being true or false, respectively. Since, if all other things are equal, beta values are liable to be lowered as the number of covarying predictor variables increases in a multiple regression, one must be especially cautious about assessing apparently supporting evidence for our models (Gordon 1968). Nevertheless, hypotheses should at least be regarded as live options as long as the results of tests are consistent with them. Thus, affirmative answers to the fundamental question raised above represent some support for the Michigan model as a relatively good explanatory account of reported satisfaction and happiness.

Inspection of Fig. 2.2a, b reveals that our basic question has an affirmative answer. In Fig. 2.2a, for example, *P* and *A* are stronger predictors of *G* than of *S*, as hypothesized in the Michigan model. *G* to *S* connections (betas) are the strongest in the systems whether one adopts the Michigan model or not. Similar remarks apply to Fig. 2.2b, with *H* substituted for *S*. Moreover, in both exhibits, the *P* to *G* connection is stronger than the *A* to *G* connection, as reported by Campbell et al. (1976).

Figure 2.3a–l summarize the results of testing the Michigan model in twelve domains. In these cases, *S*, *P*, *G* and *A* have to be interpreted as *domain specific*. For example, in Fig. 2.3a, *S* is short for satisfaction with one's own health, *P* for comparisons with the best previous experience of one's own health, *A* for comparisons of one's own health with that of average folks of one's age, and *G* for the gap between one's health goals and one's achievement of those goals. In all twelve domains the Michigan model looks superior to its competitor. In every domain *P* and *A* are better predictors of *G* than of *S*, and *G* is always the strongest predictor of *S*. With the single exception of free time activity, in every domain the path coefficient connecting *A* to *G* is bigger than that connecting *P* to *G*, *contrary* to hypothesis and to results obtained by Campbell et al. (1976) and Andrews and Withey (1976) for their domains of housing, neighborhood and self-accomplishment. (My 'area you live in' is analogous to the 'neighborhood' of Campbell et al. and 'self-esteem' is very roughly related (I guess) to Andrews and Withey's 'self accomplishments'.)

I don't know how to account for the discrepancy with respect to the relative relations between comparisons with the best previous experience and average folks. Maybe it's peculiar to this sample; maybe it's peculiar to Canadians. As indicated

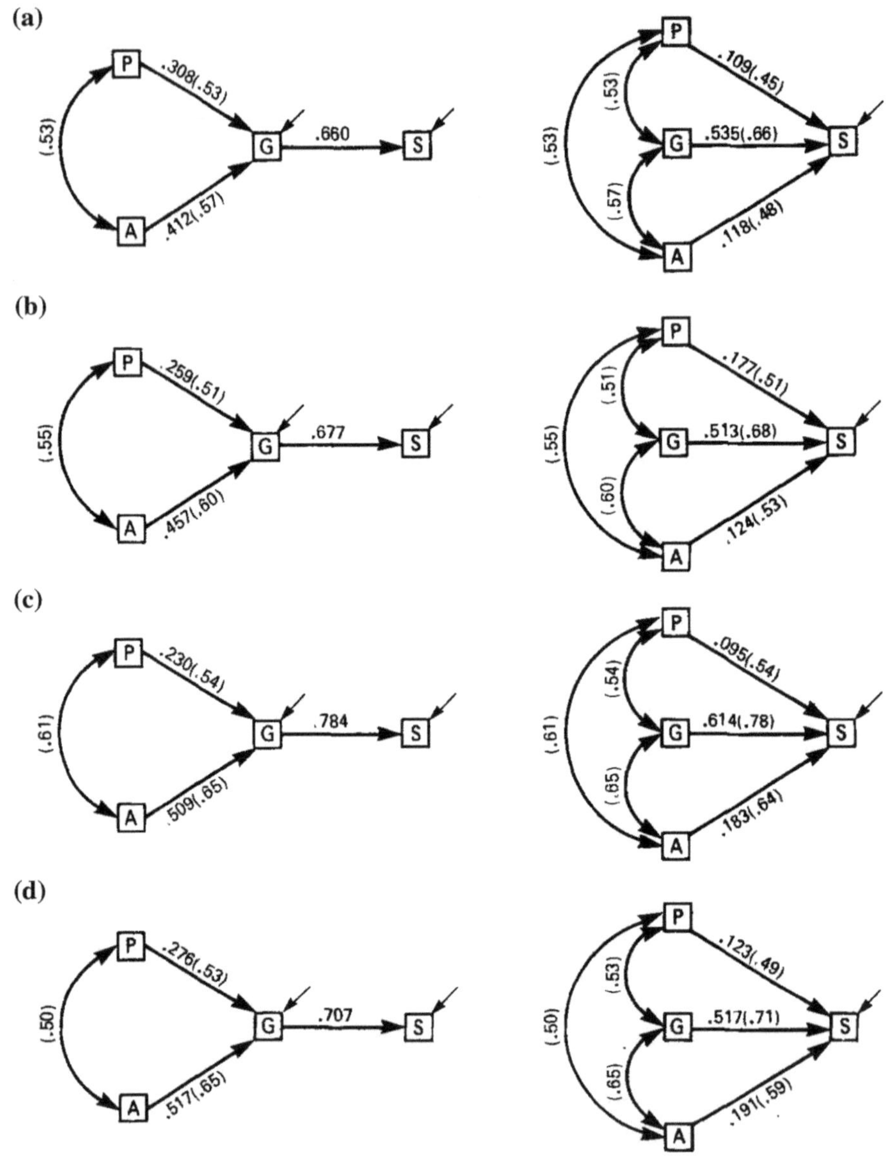

Fig. 2.3 **a** Satisfaction with health, **b** satisfaction with financial security, **c** satisfaction with family life, **d** satisfaction with friendships, **e** satisfaction with housing, **f** satisfaction with job, **g** satisfaction with free time activity, **h** satisfaction with education, **i** satisfaction with self-esteem, **j** satisfaction with area you live in, **k** satisfaction with ability to get around, **l** satisfaction with security from crime

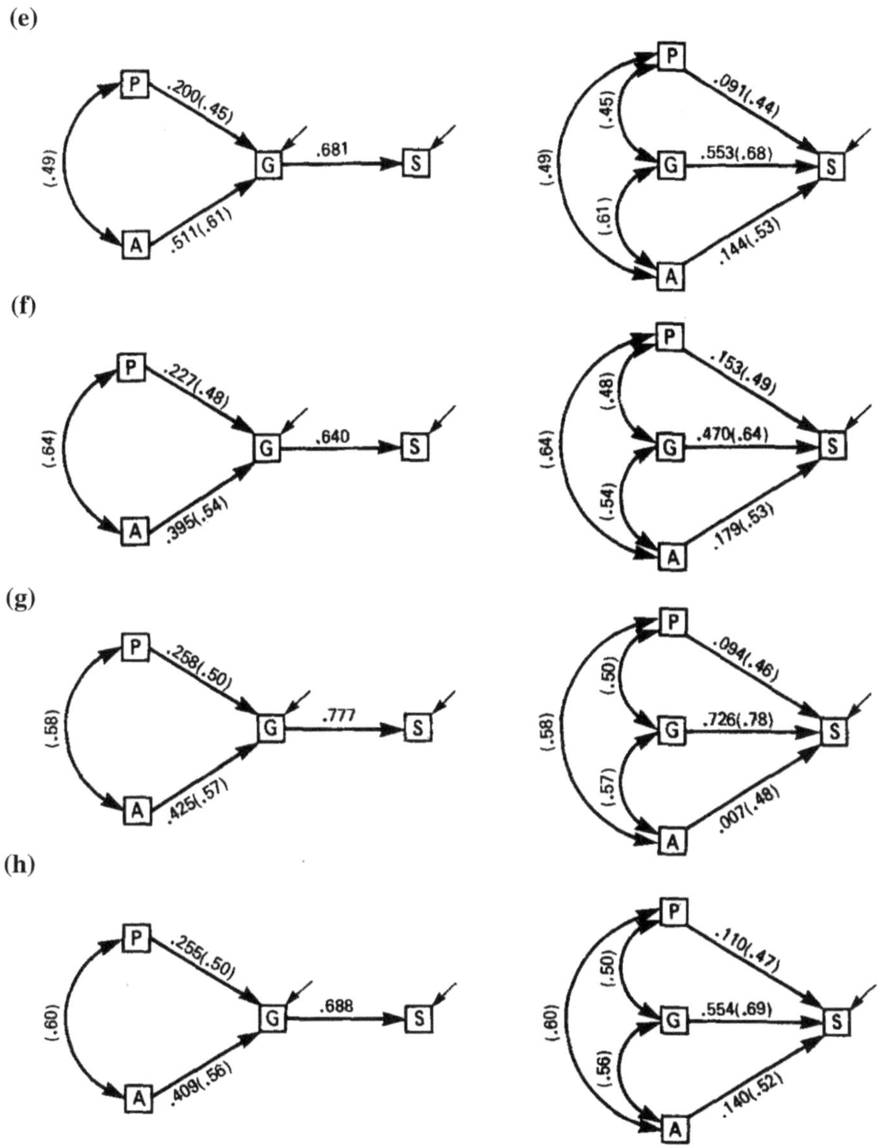

Fig. 2.3 (continued)

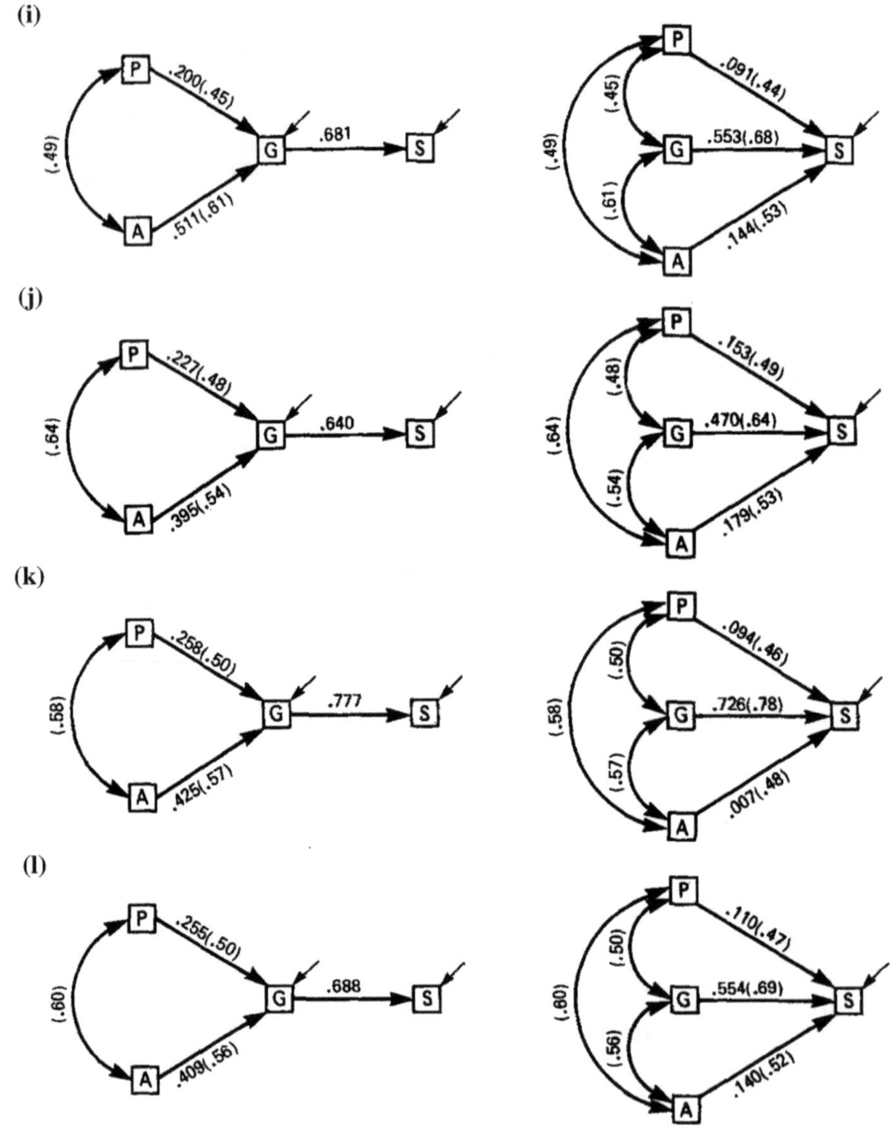

Fig. 2.3 (continued)

earlier, one of the motives behind this investigation was the suspicion that other domains may involve psychological processes different from those proposed in the Michigan model. Maybe they do.

The implications of confirmation of most of the postulated relations in the Michigan model are profound. Insofar as this type of model can be substantiated, human satisfaction is not just a brute fact to be accommodated like the wind and rain. It is to some extent manageable in the best sense and manipulable in the worst sense. By providing relevant experiences and information, people's goal-achievement gaps may be altered, with their satisfaction levels not far behind. Campbell et al. (1976, pp. 149–150) note that a tyrant might try to inflate the satisfaction levels of his or her subjects by restricting their experiences or giving them false reports about the status of their peers. Packard (1957), Key (1973), Michalos (1978a) and many others have argued that advertisers have attempted with more or less success to manipulate satisfaction and demand by providing unrealistic norms, e.g., strange guests who inspect glasses for soap marks, sniff carpets, squeeze toilet tissue, stroke the dust from the Exhibit tops, and so on. Confirmation of the Michigan model provides a picture of the psychology of satisfaction that is a necessary condition of carrying out such manipulation.

Insofar as satisfaction is generated as the Michigan model indicates, education and individual initiative have a fundamental role to play in the development of the good life for individuals and societies. Accurate perceptions of the real world have a vital role to play in the determination of satisfaction with that world. The proverbial Fool's Paradise may be regarded as the result of experiencing uninformed or

Table 2.6 Percent of variance explained in path models of Figs. 2.2a, b and 2.3a–l

Dependent variables	R^2 from 3 predictors*	Dependent variables	R^2 from 2 predictors**
Satisfaction with	($P = 0.001$)	Goal-achievement gap	($P = 0.001$)
Health	0.459	Health	0.398
Financial security	0.503	Financial security	0.406
Family life	0.650	Family life	0.455
Friendships	0.539	Friendships	0.484
Housing	0.499	Housing	0.377
Job	0.667	Job	0.397
Free time activity	0.556	Free time activity	0.423
Education	0.440	Education	0.137
Self-esteem	0.489	Self-esteem	0.402
Area you live in	0.471	Area you live in	0.322
Ability to get around	0.612	Ability to get around	0.374
Secure from crime	0.506	Secure from crime	0.359
Life as a whole	0.453	Life as a whole	0.295
Happiness with life as a whole	0.479		

*Goal-achievement gap, comparisons with previous best and average folks
**Comparisons with previous best and average folks

misinformed satisfaction. Thus, if knowledge is a reasonable thing (i.e. something to which principles of sound reasoning are applicable), then so is satisfaction, taste, etc. Here the dreams of all naturalistic value theorists loom large. Values may be psychologically connected to facts roughly as theoreticians have held they ought to be logically connected. Again, unfortunately, this is not the place to examine these implications, though one ought to be aware of them. (Michalos 1976, 1980a, Chap. 1 address some of the issues.)

Table 2.6 records the various percents of variance explained in the multiple regressions used to construct the paths in Fig. 2.3a–l. Some of these coefficients of determination (R^2) are fairly substantial, e.g. job (0.667), family life (0.650) and ability to get around (0.612). The percent of variance explained in *S* by *P, A* and *G* is, relative to the preceding figures, unimpressive (0.453). I did a bit better

Table 2.7 Multiple regression of satisfaction with life as a whole on domain satisfaction and demographic variables

	Predictors used		
	Six demographic variables	Ten domains[b]	Demographic and eleven domains[c]
Percent of variance explained	0.068	0.548	0.566 ($P = 0.001$)
Predictors			
Demographic variables	*Beta*	*Beta*	*Beta*
Marital status	−0.135	[a]	0.014
Family income	0.109	[a]	−0.028
Age	−0.153	[a]	−0.128
Sex	−0.115	[a]	−0.096
Education	−0.030	[a]	−0.013
Work status	−0.026	[a]	0.044
Satisfaction variables			
Family life	[a]	0.348	0.351
Friendships	[a]	0.195	0.202
Financial security	[a]	0.152	0.184
Self-esteem	[a]	0.131	0.105
Job	[a]	0.100	0.109
Health	[a]	0.107	0.101
Ability to get around	[a]	0.088	0.082
Free time activity	[a]	0.083	0.062
Housing	[a]	−0.049	−0.019
Education	[a]	−0.026	−0.041
Secure from crime	[a]	–	−0.005

[a]Predictor omitted

[b]‘Area you live in’ and ‘secure from crime’ had F-levels too low to enter equation

[c]‘Area you live in’ F-level was too low for admission

accounting for the variance in H (0.479). Allowing for some attenuation due to measurement error, it is safe to say that I am able to account for well over 50% of the explainable variance in all of my dependent variables. (See Andrews and Withey 1976, pp. 142–144, and Cochran 1970.)

As Table 2.7 shows, best predictive results were obtained from eleven domains and six demographic variables to S, namely, $R^2 = 0.566$. Attempting to predict H in the same way (Table 2.8), I was only able to reach an R^2 of 0.462, and even so a couple domains failed to be included in the equation due to unacceptably low F-levels.

Table 2.8 Multiple regression of happiness with life as a whole on domain satisfaction and demographic variables

	Predictors used		
	Five demographic variables	Eleven domains[b]	Demographic and ten domains[c]
Percent of variance explained	0.050	0.451	0.462 ($P = 0.001$)
Predictors			
Demographic variables	*Beta*	*Beta*	*Beta*
Family income	0.167	[a]	0.065
Marital status	−0.126	[a]	−0.033
Age	−0.078	[a]	−0.016
Sex	−0.060	[a]	−0.055
Education	−0.039	[a]	−0.023
Satisfaction variables			
Family life	[a]	0.384	0.391
Friendships	[a]	0.225	0.238
Health	[a]	0.121	0.124
Financial security	[a]	0.092	0.073
Self-esteem	[a]	0.070	0.066
Ability to get around	[a]	0.050	0.039
Secure from crime	[a]	−0.048	−0.048
Job	[a]	0.033	0.034
Education	[a]	−0.033	−0.039
Free time activity	[a]	0.027	0.023
Housing	[a]	0.005	–

[a]Predictor omitted
[b]'Area you live in' F-level was too low to enter equation
[c]'Housing' and 'area you live in' F-levels were too low for admission

Types of Satisfaction

Campbell et al. (1976, p. 10) wrote that

> It may be necessary to distinguish between a satisfaction which is associated with an experience of rising expectations and one which is associated with declining expectations. An individual who has achieved an aspiration toward which he has been moving may be said to experience the satisfaction of success. Another person may have lowered his aspiration level to the point which he can achieve, and he might be said to experience the satisfaction of resignation. The two individuals might be equally satisfied in the sense of fulfilled needs, but the affective content associated with success and resignation may well differ. In experiences of dissatisfaction, we might expect the affective content of disappointment and frustration to accompany any failure to achieve one's expectations.

This passage is instructive in a number of ways. In the first place, it may be noticed that the authors seem to use the terms 'aspiration' and 'expectation' as synonyms, a practice that ought to be discouraged. Second, the passage contains a hint of another assumption that is probably unwarranted. The basic view of these authors seems to be that satisfaction may be thought of as essentially a matter of need fulfillment, insofar as aspirations are somehow generated by needs. I suppose they would recognize some difference logically and psychologically between wanting something and needing something, but if they do, they never seem to allow the difference to emerge in their remarks about fulfillment. I have discussed these issues at length in Michalos (1978b), but here I only want to say that from the point of view of theorizing about and occasionally even managing satisfactions, it may be worthwhile to be scrupulously attentive to the difference between want and need fulfillment.

The third lesson to be learned from the quotation above is central to my purposes. That is the suggestion that one might begin to distinguish types of satisfaction on the basis of the significance of its affective component. McKennell (1978), Andrews and McKennell (1980), and McKennell and Andrews (1980), have explored this possibility with some success. McKennell (1978) suggested the following Boolean classification of people.

Subgroup	*Interpretation*	*Short name*
1. Satisfied – Happy	**Satisfaction of achievement**	**Achievers**
2. Satisfied – Unhappy	**Satisfaction of resignation**	**Resigned**
3. Dissatisfied – Happy	**Satisfaction of aspiration**	**Aspirers**
4. Dissatisfied – Unhappy	**Satisfaction of frustration**	**Frustrated**

Using this scheme, my sample was divided into the four groups illustrated in Table 2.9. Achievers had scores of 5–7 on *S* and *H*; Resigned had 5–7 *S* and 1–4 on *H*; Aspirers had 1–4 on *S* and 5–7 on *H*; Frustrated had 1–4 on *S* and *H*. Curiously and unfortunately only two people out of 348 classifiable respondents (0.6%) fell into the Aspirers group. Campbell et al. (1976, pp. 36, 165–168) and McKennell (1978, pp. 401–403) found the dissatisfied-happy combination (Aspirers) to be especially characteristic of youth, and the Guelph sample is relatively youthful.

Table 2.9 Achievers, resigned, aspirers and frustrated

Happiness	Satisfaction	
	Terrible-mixed (1–4)	Satisfied-delighted (5–7)
Very unhappy	Frustrated	Resigned
Mixed (1–4)	N = 46, 13.2% Group 4	N = 52, 14.9% Group 2
Happy	Aspirers	Achievers
Very happy (5–7)	N = 2, 0.6% Group 3	N = 248, 71.3% Group 1

Seventy percent of the respondents are 18–34 years old. Besides, you recall that in section "Means, Standard Deviations and Skews" it was pointed out that, so far as their jobs are concerned, these respondents are only half to two-thirds along the way to their goals. So, I expected to find more Aspirers in the group. It's worth mentioning, however, that the global goal-achievement gap mean (5.19) is higher than the job goal-achievement gap mean (4.62) for the total sample (Tables 2.2 and 2.3), which indicates that there is globally a smaller goal-achievement gap than one would suspect from considering only the job domain. At any rate, it would have been pointless to try to perform a statistical analysis with a two-membered Aspirers group. So I confined the discriminant analysis to the three remaining groups.

Discriminant analysis has not been especially popular with social indicators researchers, although it is available in *SPSS* and there are some nice discussions of it in Kleinbaum and Kupper (1978) and Thorndike (1978). Without such a procedure we might discriminate our three groups (Achievers, Resigned and Frustrated) by selecting, say, some demographic variables and inspecting the means and variances of these variables for each of the three groups. With the procedure we simply form composite scores based on some selected set of variables and discriminate the groups on the basis of these scores. Technically speaking, a linear combination or function of variables is constructed such that the variation of its values *between* any two groups will be greater than the variation of its values *within* the groups.

Tables 2.10, 2.11 and 2.12 summarize the results of a discriminant analysis of the three groups (Achievers, Resigned and Frustrated) on the basis of 12 domain satisfaction and 6 demographic scores. Table 2.10 lists the standardized discriminant function coefficients for the discriminating variables that had F levels sufficient to keep them in the equation. A single function accounted for 98% of all the variance in these variables, and the canonical correlation between this set of variables and the two variables (S and H) used to define the three groups was 0.712 ($P = 0.0001$). The second function was relatively worthless given the amount of variance left to be accounted for in the 12 variables and the statistically insignificant canonical correlation between it and H and S.

Inspection of the column under 'Function 1' reveals that family life is three times as important as its nearest rival, friendships, in determining the values of the function. Insofar as any single name would accurately describe what is captured by

Table 2.10 Standardized discriminant function coefficients

	Function 1	Function 2
Relative percent of variance explained in 12 variables	97.84	2.16
Canonical correlation	0.712 ($P = 0.0001$)	0.149 (NS)
Discriminators		
Satisfaction with		
Health	−0.117	0.198
Financial security	−0.108	−0.416
Family life	−0.610	0.276
Friendships	−0.219	0.093
Free time activity	−0.099	−0.451
Education	0.154	0.042
Self-esteem	−0.196	0.444
Ability to get around	−0.103	−0.417
Demography		
Sex	0.115	0.126
Marital status	0.147	−0.216
Work status	−0.175	0.363
Education	−0.103	−0.607

Function 1, one would have to say it is satisfaction with family life. Thus, given the question "Which domain satisfaction and demographic scores provide the maximum discrimination among Achievers, Resigned and Frustrated?", the answer is "Satisfaction with one's family life".

Table 2.11 lists the mean scores of each of the 12 variables of the discriminant functions for each of the 3 groups. The domain satisfaction means provide a splendid summary of the difference among the groups. Indeed, given the predominance of satisfaction with family life as a discriminating variable, one can practically imagine the three groups distinguished along that single axis. Visually speaking, the plots of the means of this variable for the three groups are very similar to the plots of the group centroids, i.e. similar to roughly the means of the means of the scores of each individual on each variable for each group.

In an earlier study of the quality of life in a rural township in Ontario, Michalos (1978c) reported that satisfaction with family life was the strongest predictor of personal life satisfaction. A pilot survey in Guelph in the fall of 1977 revealed the same thing. (No report was written on that study.) Accordingly, I'm beginning to suspect that satisfaction with family life really is the primary determinant of satisfaction with life as a whole for Canadians. Campbell et al. (1976, p. 85) reported that family life satisfaction was the strongest predictor of global well-being in their sample, and Andrews and Withey (1976, p. 169) had it in second place behind 'amount of fun'.

Table 2.11 Mean scores on variables in the discriminant function for three groups

	Dissatisfied + unhappy = frustrated (N = 42)	Satisfied + unhappy = resigned (N = 49)	Satisfied + happy = achievers (N = 224) Total = 315
Satisfaction with			
Health	4.83	5.31	5.69
Financial security	3.50	4.47	4.79
Family life	3.71	5.14	5.99
Friendships	3.93	5.00	5.68
Free time activity	3.91	5.00	5.39
Education (Sat.)	3.98	4.61	4.92
Self-esteem	4.02	4.74	5.32
Ability to get around	4.67	5.55	5.80
Sex[a]	1.91	1.78	1.76
Marital status[a]	2.26	1.98	1.79
Work status[a]	1.12	1.02	1.06
Education[a]	2.79	3.12	3.02

[a]Demographic variables

Table 2.12 summarizes the results of using the discriminant functions to predict group membership. Eighty-three percent of the cases were correctly classified. Perfect accuracy of classification would have given 100% figures along the left to right diagonal in Table 2.12. So it's apparent that the discriminant functions were strongest for predicting Achievers (98%) weakest for Resigned (18%), and pretty good for Frustrated (76%).

Several other discriminant analyses were undertaken with results similar to those just reported. When the three global predictors were used (goal-achievement gap, comparisons with previous best and average folks), two significant functions were obtained. The first function captured 95% of the variance in the three predictors and was dominated by the goal-achievement gap. The second function was led by comparisons with best previous experience.

Table 2.12 Results of predicting group membership from discriminant functions

Actual groups	Predicted groups		
	Frustrated	Resigned	Achievers
Frustrated (N = 42, 13%)	32 (76%)	4 (10%)	6 (14%)
Resigned (N = 49, 16%)	4 (8%)	9 (18%)	36 (74%)
Achievers (N = 224, 71%)	2 (1%)	3 (1%)	219 (98%)
Total N = 315			
83% of grouped cases correctly classified			

Conclusion

I set out to review the recent literature on satisfaction and happiness, to identify some plausible next steps to take along the frontiers of this area of research and to offer some suggestions to facilitate those steps. Using partial correlation techniques, substantial levels of covariation were found among all the variables that were used in predictions of satisfaction and happiness with life as a whole from satisfaction with specific domains (e.g. family life, health). Using path analysis, confirmation was found in a dozen domains for a model which has satisfaction as a function of a perceived goal-achievement gap, and the latter as a function of comparisons with previous best experience and the status of average folks. Using discriminant analysis, satisfaction with family life was found to be a powerful and predominant discriminator among three groups, identified as Frustrated (dissatisfied and unhappy), Resigned (satisfied and unhappy) and Achievers (satisfied and happy).

Acknowledgements I am grateful for the help of A.M. Blanchet, L. Ferraro, R.A. Logan, S. McNeill, J. Tofflemire and the generous members of our university Staff Association who gave up their time to fill out yet another questionnaire. F.M. Andrews. O.D. Duncan, J.J. Hubert, K.C. Land, S. Swaminathan and F.W. Young gave me plenty of good advice, for which I am also grateful. Of course, I alone am responsible for this final version of the paper.

References

Abrams, M. (1972). Social indicators and social equity. *New Society, 22,* 454–455.

Adams, J. S. (1963). Toward an understanding of inequity. *Journal of Abnormal and Social Psychology, 67,* 422–436.

Adams, J. S. (1965). Inequity in social exchange. In L. Berkowitz (Ed.), *Advances in experimental social psychology* (pp. 267–299). New York: Academic Press.

Al-Hoory, M. T. (1976). *Campsite selection as a decision-making process: A behavioral approach.* Doctoral dissertation, Utah State University, Logan, UT.

Allardt, E. (1976). Dimensions of welfare in the comparative Scandinavian study. *Acta Sociologica, 19,* 227–239.

Andrews, F. M., & McKennell, A. C. (1980). Measures of self-reported well-being: Their affective, cognitive, and other components. *Social Indicators Research, 8,* 127–155.

Andrews, F. M., & Withey, S. B. (1976). *Social indicators of well-being.* New York: Plenum Press.

Appley, M. H. (Ed.). (1971). *Adaptation-level theory.* New York: Academic Press.

Arvey, R. D., Dewhirst, H. D., & Boling, J. C. (1976). Relationships between goal clarity, participation in goal setting, and personality-characteristics on job satisfaction in a scientific organization. *Journal of Applied Psychology, 61,* 103–105.

Atkinson, T. H. (1979). *Trends in life satisfaction among Canadians 1968–1977.* Montreal, Quebec: Institute for Research on Public Policy.

Bharadwaj, L. K., & Wilkening, E. A. (1974). Occupational satisfaction of farm husbands and wives. *Human Relations, 27,* 739–753.

Bradburn, N. M., & Caplovitz, D. (1965). *Reports on happiness.* Chicago, IL: Aldine Pub. Co.

Brehm, J. W., & Cohen, A. R. (1962). *Explorations in cognitive dissonance.* New York: Wiley.

Buckley, H. D. (1969). *The relationship of achievement and satisfaction to anticipated environmental stress of transfer students in the State University of New York.* Doctoral dissertation, Syracuse University, Syracuse, NY.
Burgess, R. L., & Nielson, J. M. (1974). Distributive justice and the balance of power. *American Sociological Review, 39,* 427–443.
Campbell, A. (1972). Aspiration, satisfaction and fulfillment. In A. Campbell & P. E. Converse (Eds.), *The human meaning of social change* (pp. 441–466). New York: Russell Sage Foundation.
Campbell, A., Converse, P. E., & Rodgers, W. L. (1976). *The quality of American life.* New York: Russell Sage Foundation.
Cantril, H. (1965). *The pattern of human concerns.* New Brunswick, NJ: Rutgers University Press.
Carey, J. F. (1974). *A study of dissonance in the classroom setting: Its relationship to teacher job satisfaction, student achievement and school satisfaction.* Doctoral dissertation, University of Maryland, College Park, MD.
Carpenter, S. S. (1973). *User satisfaction with a planned physical environment.* Doctoral dissertation, United States International University, San Diego, CA.
Cochran, W. G. (1970). Some effects of errors of measurement on multiple correlation. *Journal of the American Statistical Association, 65,* 22–34.
Cook, D. M. (1968). *The psychological impact on management of selected procedures in managerial accounting.* Doctoral dissertation, University of Texas, Austin, TX.
Danielson, L. C. (1977). *Effects of success and failure on aspiration level, problem solving performance, and satisfaction with performance.* Doctoral dissertation, Pennsylvania State University, University Park, PA.
Davies, J. C. (1962). Toward a theory of revolution. *American Sociological Review, 27,* 5–18.
Dorsett, K. G. (1977). *A study of levels of job satisfaction and job aspiration among black clerical employees in city and county Governments of Greensboro, Guilford County, North Carolina.* Doctoral dissertation, University of North Carolina, Greensboro, NC.
Duncan, O. D. (1975a). Does money buy satisfaction? *Social Indicators Research, 2,* 267–274.
Duncan, O. D. (1975b). *Introduction to structural equation models.* New York: Academic Press.
Easterlin, R. A. (1973). Does money buy happiness? *The Public Interest, 30,* 3–10.
Easterlin, R. A. (1974). Does Economic Growth Improve the Human Lot? Some Empirical Evidence. In P.A. David & M.W. Reder (Eds.), *Nations and households in economic growth* (pp. 89–125). New York: Academic Press.
Edwards, W., & Tversky, A. (Eds.). (1967). *Decision making.* Middlesex, England: Penguin Books Ltd..
Feierabend, I, K., Feierabend, R. L., & Nesvold, B. A. (1969). Social change and political violence: Cross-national patterns. In H. D. Graham & T. R. Gun (Eds.), *Violence in America* (Vol. 2, pp. 498–509). Washington, DC, USA: Government Printed Office.
Festinger, L. (1957). *A theory of cognitive dissonance.* Stanford, CA: Stanford University Press.
Foa, V. G. (1957). Relation of worker's expectation to satisfaction with the supervisor. *Personnel Psychology, 10,* 161–168.
Gelwick, B. P. (1975). *The adult woman student and her perceptions and expectations of the university environment.* Doctoral dissertation, University of Missouri, Columbia, MO.
Gordon, R. A. (1968). Issues in multiple regression. *The American Journal of Sociology, 73,* 592–616.
Greenstein, G. (1972). *A study of the relationships between teachers' feelings of general satisfaction and the needs and expectations fulfillment qualities of their organizational press.* Doctoral dissertation, Syracuse University, Syracuse, NY.
Guilford, J. P., & Fruchter, B. (1973). *Fundamental Statistics in Psychology and Education.* McGraw Hill Education: New York.
Gurr, T. R. (1970). *Why men rebel.* Princeton, NJ: Princeton University Press.
Hamner, W. C., & Harnett, D. L. (1974). Goal setting, performance and satisfaction in an interdependent task. *Organizational Behavior and Human Performance, 12,* 217–230.

Hankiss, E., Manchin, R., & Fiistes (1978). *Cross-cultural quality of life research: An outline for a conceptual framework and some methodological issues*. Budapest: Center for Quality of Life Research, Hungarian Academy of Sciences.
Helson, H. (1964). *Adaption-level theory: An experimental and systematic approach to behavior*. New York: Harper and Row, Inc.
Hibbs, C. W. (1975). *Selected factors affecting client satisfaction in a university counselling center*. Doctoral dissertation, University of Iowa, Iowa City.
Hulin, C. L., & Smith, P. C. (1965). A linear model of job satisfaction. *Journal of Applied Psychology, 49,* 206–216.
Ilgen, D. R. (1969). *Satisfaction with performance as a function of the initial level of expected performance and the deviation from expectation*. Doctoral dissertation, University of Illinois, Urbana, IL.
Ilgen, D. R. (1971). Satisfaction with performance as a function of the initial level of expected performance and the deviations from expectations. *Organizational Behavior and Human Performance, 6,* 345–361.
Ilgen, D. R., & Hamstra, B. W. (1972). Performance satisfaction as a function of the difference between expected and reported performance at five levels of reported performance. *Organizational Behavior and Human Performance, 7,* 359–370.
Jones, E. E., et al. (1971). *Attribution: Perceiving the causes of behavior*. Morristown, NJ: General Learning Press.
Kawakami, D. T. (1967). *Changes in self-evaluation and expression of satisfaction with vocational decision*. Doctoral dissertation, Columbia University, New York.
Kerlinger, F. N., & Pedhazur, E. J. (1973). *Multiple regression in behavioral research*. New York: Holt, Rinehart and Winston, Inc.
Key, B. W. (1973). *Subliminal seduction*. New York: The New American Library.
Kim, J. S., & Hamner, W. C. (1976). Effect of performance feedback and goal setting on productivity and satisfaction in an organizational setting. *Journal of Applied Psychology, 61,* 48–57.
Kleinbaum, D. G., & Kupper, L. L. (1978). *Applied regression analysis and other multivariable methods*. North Scituate, MA: Duxbury Press.
Kuhn, T. S. (1962). *The structure of scientific revolutions*. Chicago: University of Chicago Press.
Kuhn, T. S. (1977). *The essential tension*. Chicago: University of Chicago Press.
Latham, G. P., & Kinne, S. B. (1974). Improving job performance through training in goal setting. *Journal of Applied Psychology, 59,* 187–191.
Lawler, E. E. (1968). Equity theory as a predictor of productivity and work quality. *Psychological Bulletin, 70,* 596–610.
Lewin, K., et al. (1944). Level of aspiration. In J. McV. Hunt (Ed.), *Personality and the behavior disorders* (pp. 333–378). New York: Ronald Press Co.
Lewis, S. A. (1973). *Perceived competence, success-failure, and performance feedback in outcome satisfaction and expectancy behavior*. Doctoral dissertation, State University of New York, Buffalo, NY.
Locke, E. A., Cartledge, N., & Knerr, C. S. (1970). Studies of the relationships between satisfaction, goal setting and performance. *Organizational Behavior and Human Performance, 5,* 135–158.
Mason, R., & Faulkenberry, G. D. (1978). Aspirations, achievements and life satisfactions. *Social Indicators Research, 5,* 133–150.
McKennell, A. C. (1978). Cognition and affect in perception of well-being. *Social Indicators Research, 5,* 389–426.
McKennell, A. C., & Andrews, F. M. (1980). Models of cognition and affect in perceptions of well-being. *Social Indicators Research, 8,* 257–298.
Michalos, A. C. (1976). The morality of cognitive decision-making. In M. Brand & D. Walton (Eds.), *The Winnipeg conference on action theory* (pp. 325–340). Dordrecht: D. Reidel Pub. Co.

Michalos, A. C. (1978a). Advertising: Its logic, ethics and economics. A paper read at the Informal Logic Conference at the University of Windsor, ON, June 26–28, 1978.
Michalos, A. C. (1978b). *Foundations of decision-making*. Ottawa: Canadian Library of Philosophy.
Michalos, A. C. (1978c). Satisfaction with life and housing in rural Ontario. A paper presented at the Rural Sociological Society meeting in San Francisco, August 31, 1978.
Michalos, A. C. (1980a). *Foundations, population and health; North American Social Report, Volume One*. Dordrecht: D. Reidel Pub. Co.
Michalos, A. C. (1980b). *Crime, justice and politics; North American Social Report, Volume Two*. Dordrecht: D. Reidel Pub. Co.
Morgan, S. M. (1976). *The relationship between congruent student and supervisor expectations, student performance, and student satisfaction in counselling practica*. Doctoral dissertation, University of Tennessee, Knoxville, TN.
Nie, N. H., et al. (1975). *Statistical package for the social sciences*. New York: McGraw-Hill Book Co.
Newton, R. M. (1976). *Supervisor expectations and behavior: Effects of consistent-inconsistent supervisory pairings on supervisee satisfaction with supervision, perceptions of supervisory relationships and rated counsellor competency*. Doctoral dissertation, University of Missouri, Columbia, MO.
Packard, V. (1957). *The hidden persuaders* New York: David McKay Co.
Patchen, M. (1961a). *The choice of wage comparisons*. Englewood Cliffs, NJ: Prentice-Hall, Inc.
Patchen, M. (1961b). A conceptual framework and some empirical data regarding comparisons of social rewards. *Sociometry, 24,* 136–156.
Pelz, D. C., & Andrews, F. M. (1976). *Scientists in Organizations*. Ann Arbor, MI: Institute for Social Research.
Pritchard, R. D. (1969). Equity theory: A review and critique. *Organizational Behavior and Human Performance, 4,* 176–211.
Schneider, M. (1975). The quality of life in large American cities: Objective and subjective social indicators. *Social Indicators Research, 1,* 495–509.
Scott, J. P. (1979). Single rural elders. *Alternative Lifestyles, 2,* 359–378.
Space, M. A. (1974). *Vocational role image, perceptions of employers' expectations, and job satisfaction in novice nurses*. Doctoral dissertation, Columbia University, New York.
Spector, A. J. (1956). Expectations fulfillment and morale. *Journal of Abnormal and Social Psychology, 52,* 51–56.
Strumpet, B. (1972). Economic well-being as an object of social measurement. In B. Strumpel (Ed.), *Subjective elements of well-being* (pp. 75–122). Paris: OECD.
Tatarkiewicz, W. (1976). *Analysis of happiness*. The Hague: Martinus Nijhoff.
Thibaut, J. W., & KeUey, H. H. (1959). *The social psychology of groups*. New York: Wiley.
Thompson, A. P. (1975). *Subjective expectations and job facet predictability in job satisfaction*. Doctoral dissertation, University of Western Ontario, London, ON.
Thorndike, R. M. (1978). *Correlational procedures for research*. Gardner Press, Inc., New York.
Umstot, D. D., Bell, C. H., & Mitchell, T. R. (1976). Effects of job enrichment and task goals on satisfaction and productivity: Implications for job design. *Journal of Applied Psychology, 61,* 379–394.
Wantz, R. A. (1976). *A Multivariate Analysis of Client Expectation, Client Satisfaction, and Client Personality Characteristics at the Ball State University Counselling Practicum Clinic*. Doctoral dissertation, Ball State University, Muncie, IN.
Warr, P., & Wall, T. (1975). *Work at well-being*. Middlesex, England: Penguin Books, Ltd.
Weaver, P. J. (1974). *A person-environment analysis of performance, satisfaction, and expectancies of job trainees*. Doctoral dissertation, University of Michigan, Ann Arbor, MI.

Chapter 3
Multiple Discrepancies Theory (MDT)

Alex C. Michalos

Introduction

The aim of this paper is to present a fairly thorough and rigorous account of multiple discrepancies theory (MDT), review its historical antecedents and submit it to some empirical tests. The basic hypotheses of the theory are given in the next section, which is followed by a section reviewing the supporting evidence for its several hypotheses taken individually or in groups. The hypotheses are illustrated graphically and algebraically in the next section. Following the illustrative section, there is a section describing the sample of 700 University of Guelph undergraduates on whom the theory was tested, and the methods used. Then there is a section reviewing general results and comparing these to some results of earlier studies, followed by a review of results for MDT and a discussion.

Basic Hypotheses

The basic hypotheses of MDT are as follows:

H1 Reported net satisfaction is a function of perceived discrepancies between what one has and wants, relevant others have, the best one has had in the past, expected to have 3 years ago, expects to have after 5 years, deserves and needs.

Michalos, A.C.: 1985. Multiple Discrepancies Theory (MDT) Social Indicators Research, 16, pp. 347–413. 0303-8300/85.10 © 1985 by D. Reidel Publishing Company.

A.C. Michalos (✉)
University of Northern British Columbia, Prince George, BC, Canada
e-mail: michalos@brandonu.ca

A.C. Michalos, *Development of Quality of Life Theory and Its Instruments*,
DOI 10.1007/978-3-319-51149-8_3

H2 All perceived discrepancies, except that between what one has and wants, are functions of objectively measurable discrepancies, which also have direct effects on satisfaction and actions.
H3 The perceived discrepancy between what one has and wants is a mediating variable between all other perceived discrepancies and reported net satisfaction.
H4 The pursuit and maintenance of net satisfaction motivates human action in direct proportion to the perceived expected levels of net satisfaction.
H5 All discrepancies, satisfaction and actions are directly and indirectly affected by age, sex, education, ethnicity, income, selfesteem and social support.
H6 Objectively measurable discrepancies are functions of human action and conditioners.

Supporting Evidence

Since I have already written an extensive review of the literature related to MDT in Michalos (1985), I will not undertake that task again here. However, it will be worthwhile to briefly indicate the variety of insights from several well-known theories that are incorporated into MDT.

Although nobody has bound together as many hypotheses or articulated a theory of multiple discrepancies as systematically as I have here, a number of people have worked with two or more discrepancy hypotheses in conjunction. As I have mentioned in all my earlier publications, I originally followed Campbell, Converse and Rodgers (1976) and Andrews and Withey (1976) fairly directly. Crosby (1982) used several gap hypotheses in conjunction, and cited seven other people who had also used multiple discrepancies, namely, Davis (1959), Runciman (1966), Gurr (1970), Williams (1975), Berkowitz (1968), Adams (1965) and Patchen (1961). Goodman (1974) and Oldham et al. (1982) should also be listed as labourers in the same vineyard.

H1 refers to seven different perceived discrepancies. The idea that net satisfaction is a function of the perceived discrepancy or gap between what one has and wants is at least as old as the stoic philosophy of Zeno of Citium around 300 B.C. In the form of aspiration theory, Lewin et al. (1944) gave the idea a new start. More recent confirmations of the basic hypothesis have been reported by Bledsoe et al. (1980), Canter and Rees (1982), Cherrington and England (1980), Campbellet al. (1976), Andrews and Withey (1976), Michalos (1980a, 1982a, 1983a) and Crosby (1976, 1982).

The idea that net satisfaction is a function of the perceived discrepancy between what one has and relevant others have can also be found before the birth of Jesus Christ, namely, in Aristotle's *Politics* in the fourth century B.C. In the form of reference group theory, Merton and Kitt (1950) gave the hypothesis a provocative new start. Recent confirmations have come from Oldham and Miller (1979), Appelgryn and Plug (1981), Hatfield and Huseman (1982), Duncan (1975), Campbell et al. (1976), Andrews and Withey (1976), Crosby (1976, 1982), Oldham et al. (1982), Goodman (1974), Michalos (1980a, 1982a, 1983a). Wills (1981, 1983) considers this sort of theory (by its other popular name, "social comparison theory") from the point of view of its usefulness in explaining people's behaviour and attitudes regarding help-seeking decisions, self-evaluation and self-enhancement.

Confirmations of the hypothesis that net satisfaction is a function of the perceived gap between what one has now and the best one has ever had in the past have been reported by Campbell et al. (1976) and Michalos (1980a, 1982a, 1983a). Suls and Sanders (1982) present evidence supporting a developmental model in which evaluations based on this sort of perceived discrepancy occur in children around the ages of 4–5, while "social comparisons with similar others" occur a bit later around the age of 9.

Equity theorists have found considerable support for the hypothesis that net satisfaction is a function of the perceived gap between what one has and what one deserves. For examples, see Hatfield et al. (1982), Walster et al. (1976), Adams and Freedman (1976) and Goodman and Friedman (1971). In ordinary English one may distinguish an equitable distribution in which each person gets whatever is due to him or her from an equal distribution in which each person gets the same as every other person. (See Michalos (1982b) for more on this). However, equity theorists usually ignore this distinction and define equitable relationships as those in which "all participants are receiving equal relative outcomes" (Walster et al. 1976, pp. 2, 7). Cook (1975, p. 376) took a third and more relativistic view, asserting that "a state of equity is said to exist if the actual allocation of outcomes coincides with *p*'s beliefs about how they should be distributed…."

The hypothesis that net satisfaction is a function of the perceived discrepancy between what one has and expected to have was given a fairly systematic treatment by Festinger (1957). As indicated by several authors in Abelson et al. (1968), Festinger's theory of cognitive dissonance mixed several kinds of discrepancies together, although there was a tendency to emphasize the gap between expected and actual states of affairs. Support for this hypothesis has been reported by Campbell et al. (1976), Weintraub (1981), Oliver (1980), Ross et al. (1982); and many others cited in Abelson et al. (1968).

Person-environment fit theorists have hypothesized that, among other things, net satisfaction is a function of the perceived fit between what a person has (resources, abilities) and what a person needs. Considerable support for this hypothesis has been reported in excellent review articles by Harrison (1978, 1983) and Caplan (1979, 1983). Kurella (1979) and Booth et al. (1979) have also reported support for a similar sort of hypothesis.

The seventh gap hypothesis incorporated into H1 involves the perceived discrepancy between what one has now and expects to have in the future (after five years). One would expect that optimism about the future would bring satisfaction, and there is some experimental evidence supporting this idea, e.g., Goodman (1966).

H1 refers to reported satisfaction because the survey research procedures used to test MDT rely on personal reports. Although I usually omit the word "reported", strictly speaking it is essential. Usually, I think, things are regarded and reported as satisfying if and only if on balance they are satisfying. So, typically, "satisfaction" has the force of "net satisfaction", and "dissatisfaction" has the force of "net dissatisfaction", Scales running from "very satisfied" to "very dissatisfied" presuppose that respondents are reporting net assessments.

H2 affirms ontological realist or objectivist assumptions, namely, that there is a world relatively independent of this or that person, containing things with more or less objectively measurable properties, which are more or less objectively comparable. (Festinger 1957; Crosby 1982 emphasize a similar point.) For example, according to H2, the perceived discrepancy between what one earns and some relevant other person earns is to some extent a function of a real or objectively measurable discrepancy; the perceived discrepancies between needs for nourishment or warmth and their attainment are to some extent functions of real or objectively measurable discrepancies; and so on. While I strongly suspect and there is some evidence that the mixture of objectively measurable and perceived discrepancies is a bit like a horse and rabbit stew, with perceived discrepancies represented by the horse, I will have little more to say on the matter here. The only exception to this realist assumption is in the case of perceived gaps between what one has and wants. In Michalos (1978) I gave a dispositional analysis of wanting which might allow one to distinguish objectively measurable from perceived wants. After performing many thought experiments on this view, I am still not persuaded that one could operationalize the two kinds of wanting in distinct ways. Moreover, I suspect that one could always regard dispositional wants as particularistic or adventitious needs as defined in Michalos (1978). If the latter is true, then it would be redundant to introduce objectively measurable wants as a partial determinant of perceived wants. These considerations led me to treat perceived wants as an exception in H2. H2 also affirms that objectively measurable discrepancies have a direct impact on net satisfaction and human action, as will become clearer shortly.

H3 is relatively straightforward, saying that the perceived gap between what one has and wants serves as a mediator between all other perceived gaps and net satisfaction. This hypothesis was confirmed by Campbell et al. (1976) and Michalos (1980a, 1982a, 1983a). H1 and H3 taken together imply that perceived discrepancies have both direct and indirect (mediated) effects on reported net satisfaction. In Michalos (1980a, 1982a, 1983a), I compared two models, one with and one without a mediating variable, and I recommended the former. I was unable to see the obvious, namely, that a combination of the two models would provide a more accurate account of the dynamics of satisfaction than either model could provide separately. Here I have tried to articulate this insight.

H4 connects net satisfaction to human action in a fairly traditional utilitarian way. (For examples, see Kauder 1965, Luce and Raiffa 1957, Festinger 1957, Edwards and Tversky 1967, Kuhn 1974 and Harsanyi 1982.) The main difference between what is going on here and what has traditionally gone on in utilitarian discussions is that here we do not begin with utility, happiness, satisfaction or even preferences. From the crude utilitarianism of Shaftesbury (1711) to the most recent sophisticated utilitarianism of Harsanyi (1982), this view always begins with some sort of a given affect-laden attitude or interest, e.g., preferences. It is precisely this foundation, this given element in all utilitarian theories, that MDT is designed to break through and explain. By the time H4 arrives on the scene, the most important innovative and explanatory work of MDT is virtually complete. At this point, one might go the way of a variety of utilitarians or naturalistic value theorists.

According to H5, discrepancies are directly and indirectly affected by certain demographic elements and/or conditioners. Although such elements have not been found to be relatively powerful predictors of satisfaction, they do have some impact. On average, perhaps as much as 10% of the variance in reported net satisfaction can be explained by demographic variables. Generally speaking, the best and most recent literature reviews regarding the impact of demographic elements on satisfaction and happiness are in Diener (1984) and Veenhoven (1984). Examples of studies showing that age, sex, education, ethnicity and income have an impact on satisfaction and/or happiness include Campbell et al. (1976) and Andrews and Withey (1976). A variety of researchers have found one or more of these variables related to satisfaction with life as a whole or to satisfaction with some domain of life. For example, Weaver (1980) found job satisfaction and age positively associated; Rhyne (1981) and Glenn (1981) found that sex had a differential affect on marital satisfaction. Barnett and Nietzel (1979) reported that personal self-esteem had an impact on marital satisfaction, and Diener (1984, p. 558) cited eleven studies indicating that "high self-esteem is one of the strongest predictors of [subjective well-being]". The importance of a variety of species of social support, measured in a variety of ways, is thoroughly documented in excellent articles by Caplan (1979), Turner et al. (1983), Abbey and Andrews (1985) and Gottlieb (1984). LaRocco et al. (1980) review several studies and provide a careful analysis of data on the moderating effects of social support on job strain (dissatisfaction). Their conclusion is that social support has greater direct than indirect effects.

The point of H6 is primarily to indicate that human action, including especially one's own, has a direct effect on the objectively measurable discrepancies of one's life, as do the previously mentioned demographic and/or conditioning elements. It is assumed, of course, that there is some time lag and directionality involved, and that events and actions are not their own causes or motives.

The basic hypotheses of MDT refer to functions without specifying them as linear or nonlinear. Equity theorists (e.g., Walster et al. 1976) and person-environment fit theorists (e.g., Harrison 1978, 1983) have tended to predict and find U-shaped relationships between reported net satisfaction and their independent variables. There is evidence that people who get more or less than they think they deserve are dissatisfied, with those who get more being less dissatisfied than those who get less. There is also some evidence that people in a work environment that is too complex or too simple for their particular needs or wants are relatively less satisfied than people whose work environment fits their needs or wants fairly closely. At this point, we don't know if U-shaped relationships obtain between perceived discrepancies between what one has and deserves, and has and needs on the one hand, and what one has and wants on the other. It strikes me as likely that human agents alter their wants (wittingly or not) so as to maintain a minimum level of net satisfaction, which is essentially what aspiration theorists have always said. So, rather than expecting a nonlinear relationship between the perceived gap between what one has and wants and the other gaps, I would expect internal adjustments to be made that would tend to keep the relationship linear.

Hypotheses Illustrated

Figure 3.1 illustrates the relationships postulated in the basic hypotheses. In this figure, capital letters stand for items in boxes (e.g., A stands for objectively measurable discrepancies) and numbers following letters stand for paths connecting items in boxes (e.g., A1 stands for the path connecting objectively measurable discrepancies to perceived discrepancies). Thus, our basic hypotheses H1-H6 yield the following derived hypotheses expressed in terms of Fig. 3.1.

DH1 Objectively measurable discrepancies (A) are a function of anagent's own action along the path El and conditioners along the path F1. Briefly, this may be expressed

$A = f(E1, F1)$ (From H6)

DH2 Perceived discrepancies (B) are a function of objectively measurable discrepancies along the path A1 and the conditioners along the path F2. Briefly, this is

$B = f(A1, F2)$ (From H2, 5)

DH3 The perceived discrepancy between what one has and wants (C) is a function of all other perceived discrepancies along the path Bl, objectively measurable discrepancies along the path A2, and the conditioners along the path F3. Briefly,

$C = f(B1, A2, F3)$ (From HI, 3, 5)

DH4 Reported net satisfaction (D) is a function of the perceived discrepancy between what one has and wants along the path C1, objectively measurable discrepancies along the path A3, all other perceived discrepancies directly along the path B2, and the conditioners along the path F4. Briefly,

$D = f(C1, A3, B2, F4)$ (From Hl, 3, 5)

DH5 An agent's action (E) is a function of reported net satisfaction along the path Dl, objectively measurable discrepancies along the path A4, all other perceived discrepancies directly along the path B3, and the conditioners along the path F5. Briefly,

$E = f(D1, A4, B3, F5)$ (From H2, 4, 5)

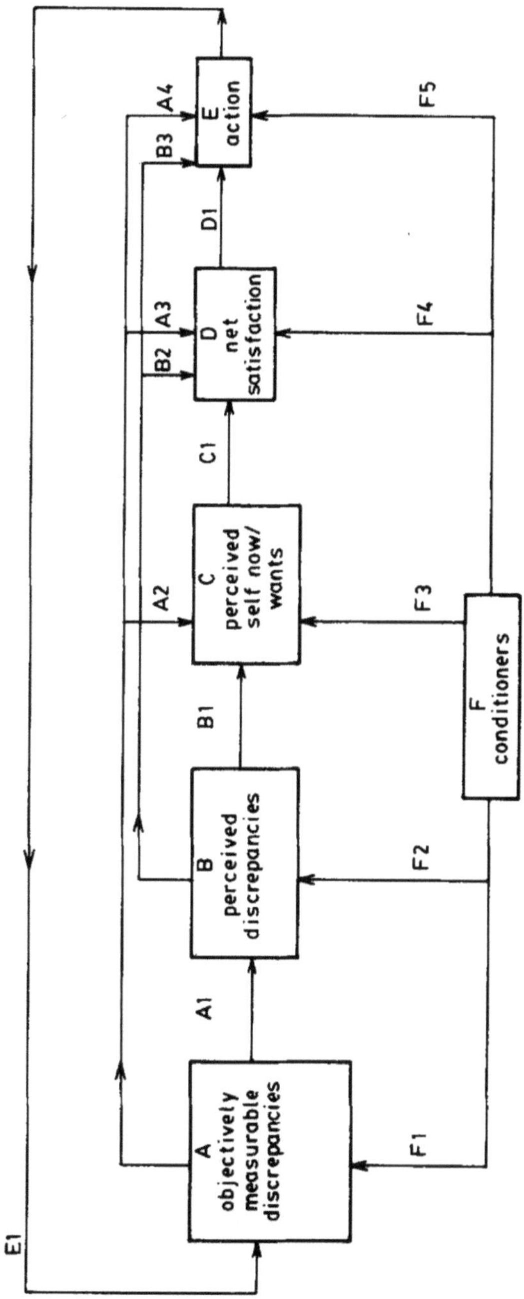

Fig. 3.1 Multiple discrepancies theory

The general idea expressed in H4 is that people tend to try to maximize net satisfaction. DH5 provides a bit more information about the sources of resources and restrictions that help and hinder people from achieving their aims. Exactly which aspect of an agent's situation will become the focus of attention depends on the perceived relative expected net satisfaction attached to action directed to that aspect. For example, if one perceives greater expected net satisfaction connected to action designed to alter objectively measurable conditions of one's life rather than to action designed to alter one's own desires, one would tend to perform the former rather than the latter. Thus, if it is likely to be more satisfying to earn more money relative to one's peers than to try to want fewer material goods, one would tend to pursue a course of action designed to earn more money. If the prospects for closing the income gap between relevant others and oneself are practically hopeless, one would tend to focus on a more profitable course of action, such as trying to limit one's own desires. (Compare Corollaries IV. 1 and 1.2 in Walster et al. 1976; Festinger 1957, pp. 6, 31 and 182.)

DH5 provides a number of potential avenues of intervention for those interested in altering people's net satisfaction. By noticing the relative impact (statistically, the beta value) of each relevant variable on net satisfaction, one can identify the place to intervene to get the biggest bang for one's buck. For example, if it turns out that, say, perceived social comparisons have relatively less impact on net satisfaction than perceived inequities, then one might be wise to focus one's interventions on altering the latter rather than the former.

Figure 3.2 illustrates in greater detail the central core of relationships expressed in Fig. 3.1, ignoring all references to objectively measurable discrepancies. In Fig. 3.2, each perceived discrepancy in box B has an abbreviation, namely Ba for "the perceived discrepancy between what one has now and relevant others have", Bb for "the perceived discrepancy between what one has now and the best one has had in the past", and so on to Bf. Similarly, each conditioner in box F has an abbreviation, namely, Fa for "age", Fb for "sex", and so on to Fg. The path labeled B1 in Fig. 3.1 is unpacked into its six constituents Bla–Blf in Fig. 3.2. To keep the Exhibit relatively simple, the seven items in box F are not unpacked. Strictly speaking, as will be shown below, every path labeled with an F should be unpacked into seven constituents labeled, for example, F4a, F4b and so on. Thus, the derived hypotheses DH3 and DH4 yield the following expanded derived hypotheses expressed in terms of Fig. 3.2.

$$\text{EDH3.C} = \text{f}(\mathbf{B}1\text{a}\ldots\mathbf{B}1\text{f}, \text{F3a}\ldots\text{F3g})$$

EDH3 says that the perceived discrepancy between what one has and wants is a function of 6 other perceived discrepancies and 7 conditioners. Exactly how many and which of the elements of EDH3 will survive empirical testing is at present unknown. Much of what is known about these elements was briefly reviewed above and in Michalos (1980a, 1982a, 1983a, 1985).

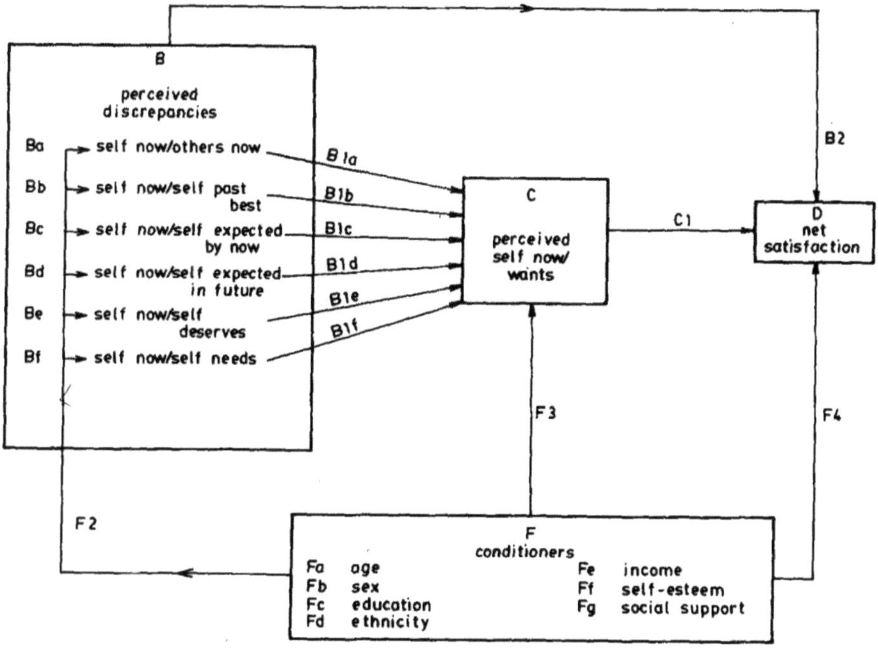

Fig. 3.2 Perceptual core of MDT

From DH4, one may derive the following expanded derived hypothesis in terms of Fig. 3.2.

$$\text{EDH4.} \quad \mathrm{D} = \mathrm{f}(\mathrm{C1}, \mathbf{B}2\mathrm{a}\ldots\mathbf{B}2\mathrm{f}, \mathrm{F3a}\ldots\mathrm{F3g}, \mathrm{F4a}\ldots\mathrm{F4g})$$

EDH4 says that reported net satisfaction is a function directly of 7 perceived discrepancies, indirectly of 6 of these mediated by the discrepancy between what one has and wants, and directly and indirectly of age, sex, education, ethnicity, income, self-esteem and social support. Fig. 3.2 and EDH4 are alternative representations of the perceptual core of MDT that will be our primary focus of attention in following sections.

Sample and Methods

In order to test the current version of MDT articulated in the previous sections, a convenience sample of 700 University of Guelph undergraduates was drawn from the 3130 students enrolled in the 1984 summer term (May and June). The composition of the sample is described in Table 3.1. Briefly, of the 683 usable questionnaires obtained, 54% came from females, 70% from students aged 20–25, 84%

Table 3.1 Sample composition

Sex	N	%	Work status	N	%
Males	314	46	Unemployed	471	69
Females	368	54	Employed 10 h	68	10
Total	682	100	Employed 20 h	55	8
			Employed 30 h	34	5
Age	*N*	%	Employed 40 h	54	8
17–19	60	9	Total	682	100
20–22	345	50			
23–25	135	20	*Formal education*	*N*	%
26–30	75	11	1 year or less	150	22
31–35	34	5	2 years	177	26
36 and up	33	5	3 years	191	28
Total	682	100	4 years	89	13
			5 years	14	2
Marital status	*N*	%	Diploma/degree	61	9
Single	571	84.0	Total	682	100
Married	83	12.0			
Widowed	1	0.1	*Major studies*	*N*	%
Separated	15	2.0	General	57	8
Divorced	12	1.9	Natural sciences	30	4
Total	682	100.0	Biological sciences	161	24
			Social sciences	182	27
			Humanities	24	3
			Engineering	21	3
			Commerce	35	5
			Other	172	26
			Total	682	100

from single people, 76% had 3 years or less of university, and 51% were majoring in biological or social sciences. Official registration statistics indicated that in the total enrollment there were 57% females, 71% aged 20–25, 85% single, and 78% had 3 years or less of university. So the sample was in fact fairly representative of the student body that term.

The questionnaire was an extended version of those described in Michalos (1980a, 1982a, 1983a). It had a demographic page with 7 questions yielding the information in Table 3.1, an instruction page, a page defining the terms designating the 12 domains (Appendix B), and 8 pages containing items involving the assessment of domain and global satisfaction from 8 different perspectives. A 7-point Likert-type scale was provided on each of these pages to obtain data relevant to the 7 discrepancies mentioned in H1 of MDT and to the basic satisfaction ratings. An off-scale category was available in every case to allow people to opt out by checking ‘No opinion’.

Basic satisfaction ratings were taken on my revised delightful—terrible scale. For example, the global item asked “How do you feel about your life as a whole right now?” and the response categories ran from “terrible” (=1 point), through “mixed dissatisfying and satisfying” (=4) to “delightful” (=7).

Assessments of the discrepancies between what one has and wants were obtained in the next battery of questions. For example, the global item asked “Consider your life as a whole. How does it measure up to your general aspirations or what you want?” and the response categories ran from “not at all” (=1), through “half as well as what you want” (=4) to “matches or is better than what you want” (=7).

Assessments of the discrepancies between what one has and relevant others have were obtained next. The global item asked “Consider your life as a whole. How does it measure up to the average for most people your own age in this area?” and the response categories ran from “far below average” (=1), through “average” (=4) to “far above average” (=7).

Assessments of the discrepancies between what one has and deserves were next. The global item asked “Consider your life as a whole. How does it measure up to the life you think you deserve?” and the responses ran from “far below what is deserved” (=1), through “matches exactly what is deserved” (=4) to “far above what is deserved” (=7).

Assessments of the discrepancies between what one has and needs were next. The global item asked “Consider your life as a whole. How does it measure up to what you think you need?” and the responses ran from “far below what is needed” (=1), through “matches exactly what is needed” (=4) to “far above what is needed” (=7).

Assessments of the discrepancies between what one has and expected to have 3 years ago at this point in life were next. The basic question was briefly “Compared to what you expected to have, does your life offer extremely less (=1), about what you expected (=4) or extremely more (=7)?”

Assessments of the discrepancies between what one has and expects to have 5 years in the future were next. Unfortunately, the question was worded ambiguously.[1] Preceding the list of 12 domains, it was asked “… consider how you would rate your own life, as it is at present, in comparison to what you expect it will be five years from now. Do you expect it [later] to offer extremely less, much more, etc.?” The reference point of this question is life 5 years from now. However, the global item asked “Now, using the same scale, consider your life as a whole. How does it [now] measure up to what you expect five years from now?” The reference point of this question is life as it is now. If respondents noticed the difference, then their responses to the global item should have been roughly opposite to their domain item responses. In fact, the mean of the mean responses to the 12 domain items was 4.5 and the mean response to the global item was 4.4 (Table 3.2), indicating that respondents apparently answered the thirteenth item on the page from the same point of view that they answered the other 12. Thus, although these

Table 3.2 Mean scores

	A	B	C	D	E	F	G	H	Mean
	Self now	Self wants	Self others	Self de served	Self needs	Self pro gress	Self future	Self best	B-H
Health	5.3	5.3	4.7	4.1	3.8	3.9	4.3	3.5	4.2
Financial security	4.2	3.8	4.1	3.7	3.2	3.7	4.6	3.4	3.8
Family relations	5.2	5.3	4.9	4.2	3.9	4.2	4.3	4.1	4.4
Paid employment	3.7	2.9	3.3	3.1	2.7	3.2	4.7	2.8	3.2
Friendships	5.2	5.2	4.7	4.1	3.8	4.2	4.4	4.0	4.3
Housing	5.1	4.7	4.5	4.0	3.9	4.1	4.5	3.7	4.2
Area lived in	5.1	4.9	4.6	4.1	4.0	4.1	4.5	3.7	4.3
Recreation	4.9	4.8	4.4	3.8	3.6	3.9	4.4	3.6	4.1
Religion	4.8	4.9	4.5	4.1	3.7	4.1	4.3	3.8	4.2
Self-esteem	5.1	5.1	4.7	3.9	3.7	4.2	4.6	4.2	4.3
Transportation	4.7	4.5	4.2	3.8	3.6	3.9	4.5	3.6	4.0
Education	5.1	5.1	5.0	4.1	3.8	4.5	4.8	4.8	4.6
Mean	4.9	4.7	4.7	3.9	3.6	4.0	4.5	3.8	4.2/4.1
Whole life	5.0	4.9	4.8	4.0	3.7	4.2	4.4	4.1	4.3
Happiness	5.0								

13 questions were consistently answered from the same reference point, this distant point differed from the current reference point used in all the other discrepancy items.

Assessments of the discrepancies between what one has and the best one has ever had in the past were next. The global item asked "Consider your life as a whole. How does it measure up to the best in your previous experience?" and the responses ran from "far below the previous best" (=1), through "matches the previous best" (=4) to "far above the previous best" (=7).

Assessments of happiness with life as a whole were based on the question "Considering your life as a whole, would you describe it as very unhappy (=1), unhappy (=2 or 3), mixed (=4), happy (=5 or 6), or very happy (=7)?"

The conditioners measured directly included age, sex and education. Selfesteem was measured indirectly using the domain satisfaction score, and social support was also measured indirectly using the mean of the satisfaction scores for family relations and friendships. I assumed that perceived selfesteem and perceived satisfaction with self-esteem would be highly correlated, and that if one had relatively satisfying relations with friends and family, then one had relatively good social support. Both of these assumptions are being tested with field studies now in progress, although they already have some support in the literature; e.g., see Turner et al. (1983) and Wills (1983). Instead of collecting data on incomes, which I suspected would be similar for most students or misleading as a result of scholarships, grants or bursaries, average length of weekly employment time was measured. In Canada, if not everywhere else, it is not likely that full-time students take on part-time paid employment unless they have financial problems. So the time invested in such employment might be a reasonable indirect measure of economic status. Ethnicity was not measured in this survey.

General Results

Table 3.2 summarizes the results from the 8 batteries of substantive questions. The third row from the bottom gives the means of the domain mean scores for the 8 sets of scores. The ratings on the delightful-terrible scale had the highest mean, 4.9. Life as a whole had a mean score of 5 on this scale,

which was exactly the same as the score for happiness with life as a whole. The Pearson correlation of these two global items was $r = 0.67$ ($P \leqslant 0.001$). The gap between what one has and needs was generally perceived as the greatest of the 7. It had a mean of 3.6 for the 12 domains and 3.7 for life as a whole. The discrepancies between what one has and wants, and what one has and relevant others have yielded the same means, 4.7. These were the highest means for the 7. On average, there was a difference of 0.15 between the mean of the mean domain scores and its corresponding global mean.

For the 12 domains, satisfaction with health had the highest mean, 5.3, and satisfaction with paid employment had the lowest mean, 3.7. For university undergraduates, these are quite reasonable results. Considering the means of mean domain discrepancy scores (in the extreme righthand column), it is clear that on average respondents' current university education tended to provide the smallest discrepancies. The mean of means for the 7 scales was 4.6. Again, on average it was paid employment that yielded the greatest discrepancy, 3.2.

Tables 3.3, 3.4 and 3.5 show the relative impact of domain scores on global scores for the 7 sorts of discrepancies. Table 3.3 shows that for 3 types of discrepancies (self-others, self-deserved and self-best), the domain of selfesteem has the greatest impact on its corresponding global discrepancy score, and for 3 others (self-needs, self-progress and self-future) the domain of education has the greatest impact. For the self-wants discrepancy, the domain of financial security has the greatest impact on the global score. Only 3 of 12 domains have a significant impact on all of the 7 global discrepancy

Tables 3.4 and 3.5 show that males and females had slightly different profiles of domain impacts on global discrepancies. For both groups, only the domain of self-esteem had an impact on all of the 7 global discrepancy scores. However, males had on average 5.3 domains with significant impacts on their global discrepancy scores, while females averaged 7.1. That seems to indicate that female global discrepancy scores have a broader base than their male counterparts. In total figures, 37 (44%) of 84 possible domain gaps had significant impacts on corresponding global gaps for makes while 50 (60%) had significant impacts for females.

Table 3.3 Multiple regression of global scores on domain scores

	Self wants	Self others	Self deserved	Self needs	Self progress	Self future	Self best
Percent of variance explained[a]	53	53	58	58	50	55	54
	$N = 315$	$N = 326$	$N = 294$	$N = 315$	$N = 327$	$N = 380$	$N = 329$
Predictors	*Beta*	*Beta*	*Beta*	*Beta*	*Beta*	*Beta*	*Beta*
Health	0.105[d]	0.130[b]	e	e	0.099[d]	e	0.150[a]
Financial security	0.212[a]	0.186[a]	0.170[a]	0.233[a]	0.196[a]	0.173[b]	0.097[d]
Family relations	e	e	0.128[b]	e	e	0.111[c]	0.083[d]
Paid employment	e	e	0.100[d]	e	e	e	e
Friendships	0.189[a]	0.144[a]	0.112[c]	0.156[a]	0.176[a]	e	0.189[a]
Housing	0.195[a]	0.143[a]	e	e	e	e	e
Area lived in	e	e	0.205[a]	0.208[a]	0.094[d]	e	0.154[a]
Recreation	0.108[d]	e	0.142[a]	0.130[b]	0.138[b]	0.123[c]	e
Religion	e	0.082[d]	0.09[d]	e	e	0.095[d]	e
Self-Esteem	0.191[a]	0.266[a]	0.209[a]	0.243[a]	0.193[a]	0.167[a]	0.323[a]
Transportation	e	0.123[b]	e	e	e	0.126[d]	0.085[d]
Education	0.208[a]	0.260[a]	0.159[a]	0.249[a]	0.261[a]	0.186[a]	0.241[a]

[a] $P \leqslant 0.001$
[b] $P \leqslant 0.005$
[c] $P \leqslant 0.01$
[d] $P \leqslant 0.05$
[e] Significance level too low to enter equation

Table 3.6 gives the results of regressing global satisfaction on 12 domains and 6 demographic variables. The most striking feature of the three regressions (for the whole group, males and females) is the relative insignificance of the demographic variables. As indicated earlier, most studies have found such variables to have relatively little impact on global satisfaction. Our program *(SPSS)* would not allow variables to enter regression equations unless they yielded values with a statistical significance level of 0.05, and that criterion was rigorous enough to keep out all the demographic variables. Presumably, the relatively homogeneous demographics of this sample of university under graduates was largely responsible for these variables having no distinctive explanatory power. Satisfaction in 2 domains had no impact on global satisfaction, namely, the area lived in and transportation. Satisfaction with selfesteem had the greatest relative impact on global satisfaction for all three groups, and satisfaction with friendships was second. Satisfaction with religion and family relations had no impact on global satisfaction for males, but some impact for females. Fifty-three percent of the variance in global satisfaction was explained by satisfaction in 9 domains for the whole group. For males, 46% was explained by satisfaction in 5 domains and for females, 54% was explained by satisfaction in 7

Table 3.4 Multiple regression of global scores on domain scores: Males

	Self wants	Self others	Self deserved	Self needs	Self progress	Self future	Self best
Percent of variance explained[a]	52	54	59	53	58	48	57
	N = 140	N = 146	N = 133	N = 140	N = 146	N = 165	N = 145
Predictors	*Beta*	*Beta*	*Beta*	*Beta*	*Beta*	*Beta*	*Beta*
Health	0.211[b]	0.122[d]	0.131[d]	e	0.164[c]	e	0.228[a]
Financial security	0.210[b]	0.246[a]	0.289[a]	0.243[a]	0.239[a]	e	0.188[a]
Family relations	e	e	e	e	e	e	e
Paid employment	e	e	e	e	e	e	e
Friendships	0.188[c]	0.132[d]	0.142[d]	0.175[c]	0.211[a]	e	e
Housing	0.218[a]	0.183[c]	e	e	e	0.261[a]	e
Area lived in	e	e	0.262[a]	0.242[a]	e	e	0.150°
Recreation	e	e	0.131[d]	e	e	e	e
Religion	e	e	e	e	e	0.128[d]	e
Self-Esteem	0.158[d]	0.246[a]	0.239[a]	0.255[a]	0.258[a]	0.273[a]	0.468[a]
Transportation	e	e	e	e	e	e	e
Education	0.228[a]	0.296[a]	e	0.268[a]	0.306[a]	0.216[b]	0.265[a]

[a]$P \leqslant 0.001$
[b]$P \leqslant 0.005$
[c]$P \leqslant 0.01$
[d]$P \leqslant 0.05$
[e]Significance level too low to enter equation

domains. Again, therefore, the global satisfaction of females was influenced by more domains than that of males.

Table 3.7 gives the results of regressing global happiness on 12 domains and 6 demographic variables. Again, the latter had no significant impact on happiness. Satisfaction in 6 domains had no impact on happiness, namely, the area lived in, transportation, religion, recreation, housing and financial security. Again, satisfaction with self-esteem had the greatest relative impact on happiness, and satisfaction with friendships was second. Satisfaction with family relations and education had no impact on happiness for males, but some impact for females. Thirty-nine percent of the variance in happiness was explained by satisfaction in 6 domains for the whole group. For males, 33% was explained by satisfaction in 4 domains and for females, 43% was explained by satisfaction in 6 domains. Again, therefore, female happiness was influenced by more domains than that of males.

Tables 3.8 and 3.9 provide comparisons between this sample of university students and three previous samples described in Michalos (1980a, 1982a, 1983a). The first involved members of the University of Guelph's office and clerical staff, the second involved rural senior citizens in Huron County, Ontario, and the third

Table 3.5 Multiple regression of global scores on domain scores: Females

	Self wants	Self others	Self deserved	Self needs	Self progress	Self future	Self best
Percent of variance explained[a]	55 $N = 170$	49 $N = 175$	56 $N = 152$	62 $N = 170$	Al $N = 176$	60 $N = 176$	54 $N = 179$
Predictors	*Beta*	*Beta*	*Beta*	*Beta*	*Beta*	*Beta*	*Beta*
Health	e	e	e	0.119[d]	e	e	e
Financial security	0.221[a]	0.205[a]	e	0.146[b]	0.154[c]	0.192[c]	e
Family relations	e	e	0.206[a]	e	0.124[d]	0.139[c]	0.113[d]
Paid employment	e	e	0.159[b]	0.136[d]	e	e	e
Friendships	0.177[b]	0.156[c]	0.140	0.165[b]	0.130[d]	e	0.237[a]
Housing	0.161[c]	e	e	e	e	e	e
Area lived in	e	0.156[c]	0.187[b]	0.172[a]	0.126[d]	e	0.182[a]
Recreation	0.149[d]	0.169[c]	0.124[d]	0.121[d]	0.165[c]	0.196[a]	e
Religion	0.128[d]	e	0.163[b]	e	0.186[b]	e	0.180[b]
Self-Esteem	0.197[b]	0.277[a]	0.178[b]	0.208[a]	0.125[d]	0.163[c]	0.256[a]
Transportation	e	e	e	e	e	0.155[d]	0.123[d]
Education	0.188[b]	0.237[a]	0.266[a]	0.228[a]	0.234[a]	0.145[b]	0.205[a]

[a]$P \leqslant 0.001$
[b]$P \leqslant 0.005$
[c]$P \leqslant 0.01$
[d]$P \leqslant 0.05$
[e]Significance level too low to enter equation scores, financial security, self-esteem and education

involved all residents 18 years and older in the Northern Ontario community of Cochrane. Both exhibits show that the predictive power of domain satisfaction scores for global satisfaction and happiness is fairly stable across the 4 samples. Typically domain satisfaction scores can account for a bit over half the variance in global satisfaction scores, and a bit over a third of the variance in happiness scores. Table 3.8 shows that satisfaction with self-esteem is the only variable to appear in the top 3 predictors of global satisfaction for 3 of the 4 samples. Table 3.9 shows that satisfaction with friendships and health appear in the top 3 for 3 of the 4 samples.

Results for MDT

Tables 3.10 and 3.11 provide overviews of the success of MDT in its application to the undergraduate data-set. In these exhibits a successful prediction is understood as a predicted path coefficient with a (beta) value *and* a significance level of at least 0.05. This dual standard is a conservative combination of fairly common practice

Table 3.6 Multiple regression of satisfaction with life as a whole on satisfaction with 12 domains and 6 demographic variables

	Whole group	Males	Females
Percent of variance explained[a]	53 (N = 296)	46 (N = 140)	54 (N = 149)
Predictors Satisfaction with:	*Beta*	*Beta*	*Beta*
Health	0.117[c]	[e]	[e]
Financial security	0.112[c]	0.179[b]	0.154[c]
Family relations	0.133[b]	[e]	0.142[d]
Paid employment	0.092[d]	[e]	[e]
Friendships	0.172[a]	0.235[a]	0.204[b]
Housing	0.121[b]	[e]	[e]
Area lived in	[e]	[e]	[e]
Recreation	0.122[c]	0.163[d]	0.143[d]
Religion	[e]	[e]	0.160[c]
Self-Esteem	0.308[a]	0.344[a]	0.290[a]
Transportation	[e]	[e]	[e]
Education	0.160[a]	0.208[b]	0.173[b]
Demographic variables			
Sex	[e]	–	–
Age	[e]	[e]	[e]
Marital status	[e]	[e]	[e]
Work status	[e]	[e]	[e]
Education level	[e]	[e]	[e]
Course of study	[e]	[e]	[e]

[a]$P \leqslant 0.001$
[b]$P \leqslant 0.005$
[c]$P \leqslant 0.01$
[d]$P \leqslant 0.05$
[e]Significance level too low to enter equation

(Reis 1982) and a proposal by Land (1969). A successful prediction ratio (ratio of successful to total predictions) may be used as one measure of a theory's adequacy, although it is certainly not the only or, perhaps, even the most important measure.

There were 771 successful out of a total of 2184 predictions, for a success rate of 35% (Table 3.10). Only 528 of all these predictions involved the direct or indirect effects of perceived discrepancies, and these yielded 289 successes for a 55% rate of success. By "direct effects of perceived discrepancies" I mean predictions of satisfaction or happiness from perceived discrepancies, and by "indirect effects" I mean predictions of the gap between what one has and wants from the other six discrepancies. Sixty-two percent of the predicted indirect effects were successful, compared to 49% of the direct effects. The highest success rates were obtained for the two global variables, happiness (54%) and satisfaction with life as a whole (49%). The average domain satisfaction success rate was 34%, including a maximum of 37% for self-esteem and a minimum of 29% for education.

Table 3.7 Multiple regression of happiness with life as a whole on satisfaction with 12 domains and 6 demographic variables

	Whole group	Males	Females
Percent of variance explained[a]	39 (N = 296)	33 (N = 140)	43 (N = 149)
Predictors Satisfaction with:	*Beta*	*Beta*	*Beta*
Health	0.168[a]	0.173[d]	0.189[b]
Financial security	e	e	e
Family relations	0.141[b]	e	0.174[c]
Paid employment	0.180[a]	0.231[a]	0.137[d]
Friendships	0.212[a]	0.242[a]	0.230[a]
Housing	e	e	e
Area lived in	e	e	e
Recreation	e	e	e
Religion	e	e	e
Self-Esteem	0.255[a]	0.290[a]	0.249[a]
Transportation	e	e	e
Education	0.123[c]	e	0.142[d]
Demographic variables			
Sex	e	–	–
Age	e	e	e
Marital status	e	e	e
Work status	e	e	e
Education level	e	e	e
Course of study	e	e	e

[a]$P \leqslant 0.001$
[b]$P \leqslant 0.005$
[c]$P \leqslant 0.01$
[d]$P \leqslant 0.05$
[e]Significance level too low to enter equation

Successful prediction ratios provide a minimum measure of a theory's adequacy. A more substantial measure is provided by a theory's explanatory power. The percent of variance explained in one's dependent (criterion) variables by one's independent (explanatory, predictor) variables provides a good measure of a theory's explanatory power. Table 3.10 lists the percent of variance explained in each of our basic 14 dependent variables beginning with happiness (49%) and global satisfaction (53%). On average 57% of the variance in domain satisfaction scores is explained by MDT, with a high of 79% for family relations and a low of 35% for education. To some extent the high percent of variance explained in satisfaction with family relations and friendships is the result of social support being defined by the mean of the mean scores for the former two variables. As it happened, the mean of each of the former two variables was 5.2, while the variance of the family relations variable was 1.51 and that of friendships was 1.44. Ignoring these possible anomalies, MDT was still able to explain 50% or more of the variance in 7 of the

Table 3.8 Comparison of satisfaction regressions for University Clerical Staff, Rural Seniors, Northern Community and Guelph Students

	1979 Clerical staff	1981 Rural seniors	1982 Northern community	1984 Guelph university undergraduates
Percent of variance explained in satisfaction with life as a whole[a]	57 (N = 312)	49 (*N* = 273)	53 (*N* = 328)	53 (*N* = 296)
Predictors Satisfaction with:	*Beta*	*Beta*	*Beta*	*Beta*
Health	0.107	0.180(2)	0.169(3)	0.117
Financial security	0.152(3)[d]	−0.011	0.242(1)	0.112
Family relations	0.348(1)	0.102	0.101	0.133
Paid employment	0.100	c	b	0.092
Friendships	0.195(2)	0.080	0.068	0.172(2)
Housing	−0.049	0.207(1)	0.095	0.121
Area lived in	b	0.010	0.133	b
Recreation	0.083	0.077	0.052	0.122
Religion	c	0.134	0.065	b
Self-Esteem	0.131	0.174(3)	0.192(2)	0.308(1)
Transportation	0.088	0.046	0.059	b
Government services	c	0.134	0.042	c
Spouse	c	0.057	c	c
Education	−0.026	c	c	0.160(3)

[a]$P \leqslant 0.001$
[b]Significance level too low to enter equation
[c]Not in equation
[d]Numbers in parentheses indicate the variable's rank of influence

remaining 10 domain satisfaction scores. It was most successful in accounting for satisfaction with financial security (58%), paid employment (59%), recreation activity (56%), religion (62%) and self-esteem (58%).

Table 3.11 summarizes the success rates of each of our predictor variables. The 7 discrepancy variables had an average success rate of 58%, ranging from 100% for the self-want discrepancy to 15% for the self-future discrepancy. That is, every time we predicted that the self-want discrepancy variable would have a significant effect, it did; but only 15% of the predicted effects of the self-future variable were confirmed. In fact, the self-others discrepancy variable was also practically infallible, with a success rate of 99%. The third most successful discrepancy predictor was self-needs (62%). Since I had never used this variable before, it was very encouraging to find it so successful. It surpassed the self-best (53%) predictor, which was the third basic variable in my earlier studies and the self-deserved (47%) predictor, which was another new one. The self-progress (32%) variable was also new and fairly successful.

The last two columns of Table 3.11 list the numbers and percents of direct and indirect effects of our predictors. Since the self-wants discrepancy variable was only

Table 3.9 Comparison of happiness regressions for University Clerical Staff, Rural Seniors, Northern Community and Guelph students

	1979 Clerical staff	1981 Rural seniors	1982 Northern community	1984 Guelph university under graduates
Percent of variance explained in happiness with life as a whole[a]	45 ($N = 312$)	32 ($N = 273$)	36 ($N = 328$)	39 ($N = 296$)
Predictors Satisfaction with:	*Beta*	*Beta*	*Beta*	*Beta*
Health	0.121(3)	0.116(3)	0.181(2)	0.168
Financial security	0.092	0.057	0.211(1)	b
Family relations	0.384(1)	−0.028	0.090	0.141
Paid employment	0.033	c	0.092	0.180(3)
Friendships	0.225(2)	0.228(2)	0.011	0.212(2)
Housing	0.005	−0.010	0.095	b
Area lived in	b	0.014	0.048	b
Recreation	0.027	0.035	0.049	b
Religion	c	0.012	0.026	b
Self-Esteem	0.070	0.086	0.144(3)	0.255(1)
Transportation	0.050	0.046	b	b
Government services	c	0.080	0.033	c
Spouse	c	0.298(1)	c	c
Education	−0.033	c	c	c
Secure from crime	−0.048	c	c	0.123

[a]$P \leqslant 0.001$
[b]Significance level too low to enter equation
[c]Not in equation
[d]Numbers in parentheses indicate the variable's rank order of influence

used in direct predictions of satisfaction and happiness, its 42 successes yielded a 100% prediction success rate. All other discrepancy variables were used to make direct and indirect predictions as indicated earlier. Thus, for example, the self-others discrepancy variable had 80 successful predictions, of which 41 were direct and 39 were indirect. Since 42 of the predictions made from this variable were direct, its success rate for direct predictions was 41/42 = 98%. Its success rate for indirect predictions was 100%. Hence, both the *total* and the *distribution* of predicted effects of this variable were almost exactly as MDT predicted. The self-needs discrepancy variable had the third best total (62%), indirect (95%) and average (63%) prediction success rates. In fact, the indirect prediction success rates were higher than the direct rates for each of the 6 variables that had both kinds of predictions, indicating a clear need for H3 in MDT.

The two satisfaction variables, self-esteem and social support, had total success rates of 33% and 58%, respectively (Table 3.11). Unlike the discrepancy variables, the direct prediction success rates were higher than the indirect rates for these

Table 3.10 Summary of prediction success rates, by dependent variables

	Whole group	Males	Females	Total
All effects				
N successes	305	225	241	771
N predictions	798	693	693	2184
Success rate (%)	38	33	35	35
All gap effects				
N successes	105	91	93	289
N predictions	176	176	176	528
Success rate (%)	60	52	53	55
Direct gap effects				
N successes	49	47	47	143
N predictions	98	98	98	294
Success rate (%)	50	48	48	49
Indirect gap effects				
N successes	56	44	46	146
N predictions	78	78	78	234
Success rate (%)	72	56	59	62
All effects by domains				
Happiness				
N successes	7	6	7	20
N predictions	13	12	12	37
Success rate (%)	54	50	58	54
% Vai. exp.	49	45	53	
Global satisfaction				
N successes	32	25	24	81
N predictions	61	53	53	167
Success rate (%)	53	47	45	49
% Var. exp.	53	50	56	
Health satisfaction				
N successes	22	18	17	57
N predictions	61	53	53	167
Success late (%)	36	34	32	34
% Var. exp.	50	46	53	
Financial security sat.				
N successes	21	19	20	60
N predictions	61	53	53	167
Success rate (%)	34	36	38	36
% Var. exp.	58	59	59	
Family relations sat.				
N successes	24	17	18	59
N predictions	61	53	53	167
Success rate (%)	39	32	34	35

(continued)

Table 3.10 (continued)

	Whole group	Males	Females	Total
% Var. exp.	79	77	81	
	Whole group	Males	Females	Total
Paid employment sat.				
N successes	25	12	23	60
N piedictions	61	53	53	167
Success rate (%)	41	23	43	36
% Var. exp.	59	55	68	
Friendships sat.				
N successes	21	17	19	57
N predictions	61	53	53	167
Success rate (%)	34	32	36	34
% Var. exp.	75	76	74	
Housing sat.				
N successes	24	18	16	58
N predictions	61	53	53	167
Success rate (%)	39	34	30	35
% Var. exp.	44	46	44	
Area sat.				
N successes	23	17	14	54
N predictions	61	53	53	167
Success rate (%)	38	32	26	32
% Var. exp.	48	49	46	
Recreation sat.				
N successes	21	14	19	54
N predictions	61	53	53	167
Success rate (%)	34	26	36	32
% Var. exp.	56	53	58	
Religion sat.				
N successes	21	13	17	51
N predictions	61	53	53	167
Success rate (%)	34	25	32	31
% Var. exp.	62	70	58	
Self-esteem sat.				
N successes	20	15	18	53
N predictions	53	45	45	143
Success rate (%)	38	33	40	37
% Var. exp.	58	54	61	
Transportation sat.				
N successes	24	20	15	59
N predictions	61	53	53	167
Success rate (%)	39	38	28	35

(continued)

Table 3.10 (continued)

	Whole group	Males	Females	Total
% Var. exp.	55	52	57	
Education sat.				
N successes	20	14	14	48
N predictions	61	53	53	167
Success rate (%)	33	26	26	29
% Var. exp.	35	34	37	

variables. For social support the direct rate was a very solid 83%, compared to a 55% indirect rate.

As indicated earlier, these variables were used as surrogate measures pending further tests with alternatives. Presumably the surrogate satisfaction measures would have some method effects resulting from the similarity of items (Diener 1984). Still, whatever method effects there are, they seem to be at best erratic. For example, Tables 3.6 and 3.7 show that often there is no significant relation between global satisfaction, happiness and one or another domain satisfaction score in spite of the similarities in the format of the items. Furthermore, as I have just mentioned, the two surrogate variables in particular are not uniformly successful as predictors.

The four demographic predictors had an average total prediction success rate of 19% with a high of 29% for age and a low of 7% for educational level (Table 3.11). In every case there were higher indirect than direct rates. Given the results presented earlier, one would have expected these variables to have low individual success rates, but there was no reason to expect that their indirect rates would be higher than their direct rates. This seems to demand some rethinking of H5 of MDT.

Figure 3.3, Tables 3.12, 3.13, 3.14, 3.15, 3.16, 3.17, 3.18, 3.19, 3.20, 3.21, 3.22, 3.23 and 3.24 show the detailed results of applying MDT to happiness, global and twelve domains of satisfaction. Fig. 3.3 graphically illustrates the application of MDT to satisfaction with life as a whole for 635 respondents. Fifty-three percent of the variance was explained. The solid lines leading to net satisfaction represent the results of regressing this variable on the other thirteen in the diagram. The dashed lines leading to self-wants represent the results of regressing this variable on the six discrepancy and six conditioning variables. Thirty-nine percent of the variance in self-wants was explained by those twelve predictors. The dotted lines leading to the column of six discrepancy variables from the six conditioners represent the results of regressing each of the former on the latter set. The number in each of the six discrepancy boxes indicates the percent of variance explained by the 6 conditioning variables. For example, the latter variables explained 19% of the variance in self-others scores, 10% in self-deserved scores, etc.

The three columns of numbers attached to the solid, dashed and dotted lines are standardized regression coefficients (Betas) or path coefficients. For example, the number 0.246[a] above the arrow from self-wants to net satisfaction is a path coefficient indicating that for every unit of change in self-wants there will be a change of 25% of a unit in net satisfaction (when both variables are standardized to have

Table 3.11 Prediction success rates, by predictors

Predictors	Whole group	Males	Females	Total	Direct	Indirect
Self-Wants						
N successes	14	14	14	42	42	0
N predictions	14	14	14	42	42	0
Rate (%)	100	100	100	100	100	0
Self-Others						
N successes	27	27	26	80	41	39
N predictions	27	27	27	81	42	39
Rate (%)	100	100	96	99	98	100
Self-Deserved						
N successes	16	9	13	38	17	21
N predictions	27	27	27	81	42	39
Rate (%)	59	33	48	47	40	54
Self-Needs						
N successes	17	15	18	50	13	37
N predictions	27	27	27	81	42	39
Rate (%)	63	56	67	62	31	95
Self-Progress						
N successes	9	8	9	26	10	16
N predictions	27	27	27	81	42	39
Rate (%)	33	30	33	32	24	41
Self-Future						
N successes	3	6	3	12	5	7
N predictions	27	27	27	81	42	39
Rate (%)	11	22	11	15	12	18
Self-Best						
N successes	19	12	12	43	16	27
N predictions	27	27	27	81	42	39
Rate (%)	70	44	44	53	38	69
Sex						
N successes	20	–	–	20	1	19
N predictions	105	–	–	105	14	91
Rate (%)	19			19	7	21
Age						
N successes	36	26	29	91	5	86
N predictions	105	105	105	315	42	273
Rate (%)	34	25	28	29	12	32
Work status						
N successes	27	25	17	69	6	63
N predictions	105	105	105	315	42	273
Rate (%)	26	24	16	22	14	23

(continued)

Table 3.11 (continued)

Predictors	Whole group	Males	Females	Total	Direct	Indirect
	Whole group	Males	Females	Total	Direct	Indirect
Education level						
N successes	6	3	11	21	2	19
N predictions	105	105	105	315	42	273
Rate (%)	6	3	11	7	5	7
Self-esteem						
N successes	40	28	29	97	20	77
N predictions	97	97	97	291	39	252
Rate (%)	41	29	30	33	51	31
Social support						
N successes	71	52	61	184	35	149
N predictions	105	105	105	315	42	273
Rate (%)	68	50	58	58	83	55

means of zero and standard deviations of one). Figuratively speaking, for every full step in self-wants, there will be a quarter of a step in net satisfaction. In order to interpret the dotted lines, follow each line first as far to the left and then as far down the page as it will go. For example, the number 0.303[a] at the head of the column on the left is on a line that goes all the way down to self-esteem. Following that, 0.174[a] goes all the way down to social support, and so on. The superscripts on these Betas indicate statistical significance levels. From Fig. 3.3 on into Appendix A, I adopt the convention that a means $p \leqslant 0.001$, b: $p \leqslant 0.005$, c: $p \leqslant 0.01$ and d: $p \leqslant 0.05$.

Because Fig. 3.3 is relatively difficult to read compared to the tables in Tables 3.12, 3.13, 3.14, 3.15, 3.16, 3.17, 3.18, 3.19, 3.20, 3.21, 3.22, 3.23 and 3.24, I have not drawn any more diagrams. All other summaries of results of applying MDT are presented as in Table 3.12, for happiness with life as a whole. In this exhibit, each set of figures represents a separate regression, with the word at the top of the set indicating the dependent variable. For example, the extreme right column indicates the results of regressing happiness on the thirteen predictors follows for all these exhibits.

SO: Self-Other	A: Age
SD: Self-Deserved	S: Sex
SN: Self-Needs	WS: Work Status
SP: Self-Progress	E: Education
SH: Self-Future	SE: Self-Esteem
SB: Self-Best	SS: Social Support
SW: Self-Wants	

Betas and their significance levels are listed, followed by the squared multiple correlation coefficient (R^2) and its significance level, and finally the number (N) of

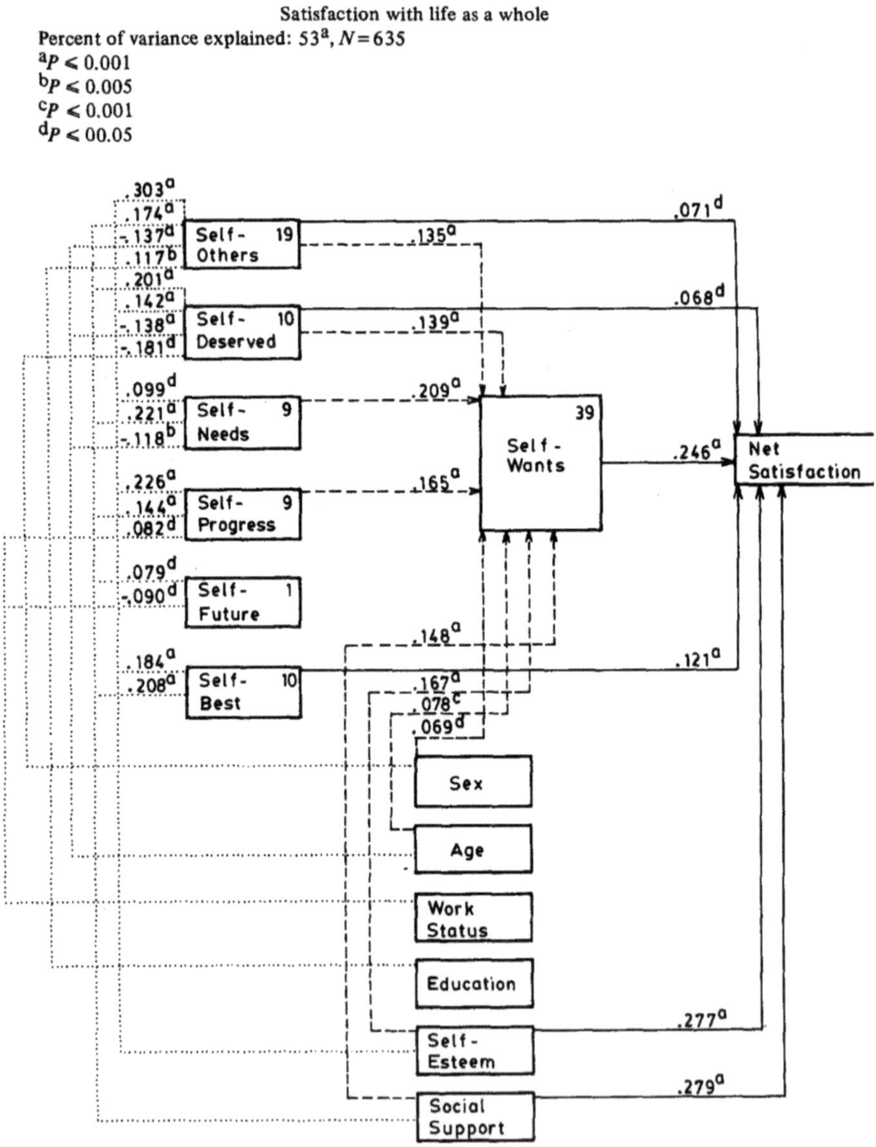

Fig. 3.3 Satisfactin with life as a whole, Percent of variance explained: 53^{a}, $N = 635$, **a** $P \leqslant 0.001$, b $P \leqslant 0.005$, C $P \leqslant 0.001$, d $P \leqslant 00.05$

cases involved. The latter number is only given for the primary regression. For example, then, this column of numbers indicates that 49% of the variance in happiness with life as a whole was explained by MDT (cf. 39% in Table 3.7), the most influential variable was social support (Beta = 0.235^{a}) and the most influential discrepancy variable was self-wants (0.172^{a}). The second column from the right

Table 3.12 Happiness with life as a whole

Self-Others	Self-Deserved	Self-Needs	Self-Wants	Happiness
$A = -0.137^{a}$	$A = -0.138^{a}$	$A = -0.118^{b}$	$SO = 0.135^{a}$	$SO = 0.129^{a}$
$S = 0$	$S = -0.081^{d}$	$S = 0$	$SD = 0.139^{a}$	$SD = 0.103^{b}$
$WS = 0$	$WS = 0$	$WS = 0$	$SN = 0.209^{a}$	$SN = 0$
$E = 0.117^{b}$	$E = 0$	$E = 0$	$SP = 0.165^{a}$	$SP = 0$
$SE = 0.303^{a}$	$SE = 0.142^{a}$	$SE = 0.099^{d}$	$SH = 0$	$SH = 0$
$SS = 0.174^{a}$	$SS = 0.201^{a}$	$SS = 0.221^{a}$	$SB = 0$	$SB = 0.214^{a}$
$R^2 = 0.19^{a}$	$R^2 = 0.10^{a}$	$R^2 = 0.09^{a}$	$A = 0.078^{c}$	$A = 0$
			$S = 0.069^{d}$	$S = 0$
Self-Progress	Self-Future	Self-Best	$WS = 0$	$WS = 0.086^{a}$
			$E = 0$	$E = 0$
$A = 0$	$A = 0$	$A = 0$	$SE = 0.167^{a}$	$SE = 0.183^{a}$
$S = 0$	$S = -0.090^{d}$	$S = 0$	$SS = 0.148^{a}$	$SS = 0.235^{a}$
$WS = -0.082^{d}$	$WS = 0$	$WS = 0$	$R^2 = 0.39^{a}$	$SW = 0.172^{a}$
$E = 0$	$E = 0$	$E = 0$		$R^2 = 0.49^{a}$
$SE = 0.226^{a}$	$SE = 0$	$SE = 0.184^{a}$		$N = 635$
$SS = 0.144^{a}$	$SS = 0.079^{d}$	$SS = 0.208^{a}$		
$R^2 = 0.09^{a}$	$R^2 = 0.01^{d}$	$R^2 = 0.10^{a}$		

$^{a}P \leqslant 0.001$
$^{b}P \leqslant 0.005$
$^{c}P \leqslant 0.01$
$^{d}P \leqslant 0.05$
0 Significance level too low to enter equation

Table 3.13 Satisfaction with health

Self-Others	Self-Deserved	Self-Needs	Self-Wants	Satisfaction
$A = 0$	$A = 0$	$A = 0$	$SO = 0.390^{a}$	$SO = 0.173^{a}$
$S = 0$	$S = -0.102^{b}$	$S = 0$	$SD = 0.079^{d}$	$SD = 0.069^{d}$
$WS = 0$	$WS = 0$	$WS = 0$	$SN = 0.134^{a}$	$SN = 0$
$E = 0$	$E = 0$	$E = 0$	$SP = 0.104^{b}$	$SP = 0$
$SE = 0.188^{a}$	$SE = 0.127^{a}$	$SE = 0.144^{a}$	$SH = -0.101^{a}$	$SH = 0$
$SS = 0$	$SS = 0$	$SS = 0$	$SB = 0.149^{a}$	$SB = 0$
$R^2 = 0.03^{a}$	$R^2 = 0.03^{a}$	$R^2 = 0.02^{a}$	$A = 0$	$A = -0.058^{a}$
			$S = 0.108^{a}$	$S = 0$
Self-Progress	Self-Future	Self-Best	$WS = 0$	$WS = 0$
			$E = 0$	$E = 0$
$A = 0$	$A = 0$	$A = 0$	$SE = 0.175^{a}$	$SE = 0.088^{b}$
$S = 0$	$S = 0$	$S = -0.106^{c}$	$SS = 0$	$SS = 0.098^{a}$
$WS = 0$	$WS = 0$	$WS = 0$	$R^2 = 0.49^{a}$	$SW = 0.498^{a}$
$E = 0$	$E = 0$	$E = 0$		$R^2 = 0.50^{a}$
$SE = 0.213^{a}$	$SE = 0$	$SE = 0.173^{a}$		$N = 647$
$SS = 0$	$SS = 0.127^{a}$	$SS = 0$		
$R^2 = 0.04^{a}$	$R^2 = 0.02^{a}$	$R^2 = 0.04^{a}$		

$^{a}P \leqslant 0.001$
$^{b}P \leqslant 0.005$
$^{c}P \leqslant 0.01$
$^{d}P \leqslant 0.05$
0 Significance level too low to enter equation

Table 3.14 Satisfaction with financial security

Self-Others	Self-Deserved	Self-Needs	Self-Wants	Satisfaction
A = –0.256[a]	A = –0.170[a]	A = –0.149[a]	SO = 0.211[a]	SO = 0.254[a]
S = 0	S = 0	S = 0	SD = 0.155[a]	SD = 0
WS = 0.156[a]	WS = 0	WS = 0	SN = 0.319[a]	SN = 0.178[a]
E = 0	E = 0	E = 0	SP = 0	SP = 0
SE = 0	SE = 0	SE = 0	SH = 0	SH = 0
SS = 0.096[c]	SS = 0.091[d]	SS = 0.084[c]	SB = 0.166[a]	SB = 0.118[a]
R^2 = 0.08[a]	R^2 = 0.04[a]	R^2 = 0.03[a]	A = 0.119[a]	A = 0
			S = 0	S = 0
Self-Progress	Self-Future	Self-Best	WS = 0	WS = 0
			E = 0	E = 0
A = –0.188[a]	A = 0	A = 0.046[a]	SE = 0	SE = 0
S = 0	S = 0	S = 0	SS = 0	SS = 0.076[b]
WS = 0	WS = 0	WS = 0	R^2 = 0.46[a]	SW = 0.356[a]
E = 0	E = 0	E = 0		R^2 = 0.58[a]
SE = 0	SE = 0	SE = 0		N = 646
SS = 0.127[a]	SS = 0.119[b]	SS = 0		
R^2 = 0.05[a]	R^2 = 0.01[b]	R^2 = 0.05[a]		

[a]$P \leqslant 0.01$
[b]$P \leqslant 0.05$
[c]$P \leqslant 0.01$
[d]$P \leqslant 0.05$
0 Significance level too low to enter equation

Table 3.15 Satisfaction with family relations

Self-Others	Self-Deserved	Self-Needs	Self-Wants	Satisfaction
A = –0.086[c]	A = 0	A = –0.114[a]	SO = 0.321[a]	SO = 0.189[a]
S = 0	S = 0	S = 0	SD = 0.114[a]	SD = 0
WS = 0	WS = –0.097	WS = 0	SN = 0.199[a]	SN = 0.113[a]
E = 0	E = 0	E = 0	SP = 0	SP = 0
SE = 0	SE = 0	SE = 0	SH = –0.061[d]	SH = 0
SS = 0.573[a]	SS = 0.448[a]	SS = 0.489[a]	SB = 0.099[a]	SB = 0
R^2 = 0.34[a]	R^2 = 0.20[a]	R^2 = 0.26[a]	A = 0	A = 0
			S = 0	S = –0.042[d]
Self-Progress	Self-Future	Self-Best	WS = 0	WS = 0
			E = 0	E = 0
A = 0	A = 0	A = –0.073[d]	SE = 0	SE = – 0.063[d]
S = 0	S = 0	S = 0	SS = 0.251[a]	SS = 0.5 37[a]
WS = –0.073[d]	WS = –0.144[a]	WS = 0	R^2 = 0.60[a]	SW = 0.222[a]
E = 0	E = 0	E = 0		R^2 = 0.79[a]
SE = 0	SE = 0	SE = 0		N = 641
SS = 0.404[a]	SS = 0.176[a]	SS = 0.411[a]		
R^2 = 0.16[a]	R^2 = 0.05[a]	R^2 = 0.18[a]		

[a]$P \leqslant 0.001$
[b]$P \leqslant 0.005$
[c]$P \leqslant 0.01$
[d]$P \leqslant 0.05$
0 Significance level too low to enter equation

Table 3.16 Satisfaction with paid employment

Self-Others	Self-Deserved	Self-Needs	Self-Wants	Satisfaction
A = –0.205[a]	A = 0	A = –0.126[c]	SO = 0.269[a]	SO = 0.244[a]
S = 0	S = 0	S = –0.112[d]	SD = 0.160[a]	SD = 0
WS = 0.5 20[a]	WS = 0.159[a]	WS = 0.290[a]	SN = 0.222[a]	SN = 0
E = 0	E = 0	E = 0	SP = 0	SP = 0.091[d]
SE = 0	SE = 0	SE = 0	SH = 0	SH = 0
SS = 0.088[d]	SS = 0.110[d]	SS = 0	SB = 0.094[d]	SB = 0
R^2 = 0.27[a]	R^2 = 0.03[a]	R^2 = 0.09[a]	A = 0	A = 0
			S = 0	S = 0
Self-Progress	Self-Future	Self-Best	WS = 0.182[a]	WS = 0.222[a]
			E = 0	E = 0
A = –0.152[a]	A = 0	A = –0.239[a]	SE = 0	SE = 0
S = 0	S = 0	S = 0	SS = 0	SS = .115[a]
WS = 0.202[a]	WS = –0.094[d]	WS = 0.493[a]	R^2 = 0.49[a]	SW = 0.390[a]
E = 0	E = 0	E = 0		R^2 = 0.59[a]
SE = 0	SE = 0.107[c]	SE = 0		N = 371
SS = 0.093[d]	SS = 0	SS = 0		
R^2 = 0.06[a]	R^2 = 0.02[c]	R^2 = 0.24[a]		

[a]$P \leqslant 0.001$
[b]$P \leqslant 0.005$
[c]$P \leqslant 0.01$
[d]$P \leqslant 0.05$
0 Significance level too low to enter equation

Table 3.17 Satisfaction with friendships

Self-Others	Self-Deserved	Self-Needs	Self-Wants	Satisfaction
A = 0	A = 0	A = 0	SO = 0.341[a]	SO = 0.142[a]
S = 0	S = 0	S = 0	SD = 0.081[c]	SD = 0
WS = 0	WS = 0	WS = 0	SN = 0.096[c]	SN = 0
E = 0	E = 0	E = 0	SP = 0	SP = 0
SE = 0.143[a]	SE = 0	SE = 0.093[b]	SH = 0	SH = 0
SS = 0.521[a]	SS = 0.387[a]	SS = 0.410[a]	SB = 0.094[b]	SB = 0.095[a]
R^2 = 0.34[a]	R^2 = 0.15[a]	R^2 = 0.20[a]	A = 0.082[b]	A = 0
			S = 0	S = 0
Self-Progress	Self-Future	Self-Best	WS = 0	WS = 0
			E = 0	E = 0
A = 0	A = –0.109[a]	A = 0	SE = 0.113[a]	SE = 0
S = 0	S = 0	S = 0	SS = 0.262[a]	SS = 0.540[a]
WS = 0	WS = 0	WS = 0	R^2 = 0.56[a]	SW = 0.243[a]
E = 0	E = 0	E = 0		R^2 = 0.75[a]
SE = 0.085[d]	SE = 0	SE = 0		N = 650
SS = 0.336[a]	SS = 0.089[d]	SS = 0.426[a]		
R^2 = 0.14[a]	R^2 = 0.02[a]	R^2 = 0.18[a]		

[a]$P \leqslant 0.001$
[b]$P \leqslant 0.005$
[c]P $\leqslant 0.01$
[d]$P \leqslant 0.05$
0 Significance level too low to enter equation

Table 3.18 Satisfaction with housing

Self-Others	Self-Deserved	Self-Needs	Self-Wants	Satisfaction
A = –0.166[a]	A = –0.098[d]	A = –0.118[b]	SO = 0.306[a]	SO = 0.248[a]
S = 0.080[d]	S = 0	S = 0	SD = 0.084[d]	SD = 0.114[b]
WS = 0.128[a]	WS = 0	WS = 0	SN = 0.113[c]	SN = 0
E = 0	E = 0	E = 0.097[d]	SP = 0.110[c]	SP = 0.080[d]
SE = 0	SE = 0	SE = 0	SH = 0	SH = 0
SS = 0.131[a]	SS = 0	SS = 0.108[c]	SB = 0.166[a]	SB = 0
R^2 = 0.06[a]	R^2 = 0.01[d]	R^2 = 0.03[c]	A = 0	A = 0
			S = 0	S = 0
Self-Progress	Self-Future	Self-Best	WS = 0	WS = 0
			E = 0	E = 0
A = –0.222[a]	A = 0	A = 0	SE = 0	SE = 0.66[d]
S = 0	S = 0	S = 0	SS = 0	SS = 0.147[a]
WS = 0.84[d]	ws = o	ws = o	R^2 = 0.37[a]	SW = 0.325[a]
E = 0.097[d]	E = 0	E = 0.79[d]		R^2 = 0.44[a]
SE = 0	SE = 0	SE = 0		N = 644
SS = 0	SS = 0	SS = 0.089[d]		
R^2 = 0.04[a]	R^2 = 0	R^2 = 0.01[d]		

[a]P $\leqslant$ 0.001
[b]P $\leqslant$ 0.005
[c]P $\leqslant$ 0.01
[d]P $\leqslant$ 0.05
0 Significance level too low to enter equation

Table 3.19 Satisfaction with area lived in

Self-Others	Self-Deserved	Self-Needs	Self-Wants	Satisfaction
A = 0	A = –0.088[d]	A = –0.083[d]	SO = 0.210[a]	SO = 0.234[a]
S = 0.086[d]	S = 0	S = 0	SD = 0	SD = 0.073[d]
WS = 0	WS = 0	WS = 0.104[c]	SN = 0.206[a]	SN = 0
E = 0	E = 0	E = 0	SP = 0.137[a]	SP = 0.076[d]
SE = 0	SE = 0	SE = 0	SH = -0.114[a]	SH = 0
SS = 0.097[c]	SS = 0.086[d]	SS = 0.082[d]	SB = 0.209[a]	SB = 0
R^2 = 0.02[d]	R^2 = 0.01[d]	R^2 = 0.02[d]	A = 0	A = 0
Self-Progress	Self-Future	Self-Best	S = 0	S = 0
			WS = 0.066[d]	WS = 0
			E = 0	E = 0
A = -0.186[a]	A = 0	A = 0	SE = 0	SE = 0
S = 0	S = 0	S = 0.0 77[d]	SS = 0	SS = 0.197[a]
WS = 0	WS = –0.116[b]	WS = 0	R^2 = 0.37[a]	SW = 0.408[a]
E = 0.089[d]	E = 0	E = 0		R^2 = 0.48[a]
SE = 0	SE = 0	SE = 0		N = 644
SS = 0	SS = 0	SS = 0.089[d]		
R^2 = 0.03[b]	R^2 = 0.01[b]	R^2 = 0.01[d]		

[a]P $\leqslant$ 0.001
[b]P $\leqslant$ 0.005
[c]P $\leqslant$ 0.01
[d]P $\leqslant$ 0.05
0 Significance level too low to enter equation

Table 3.20 Satisfaction with recreation activity

Self-Others	Self-Deserved	Self-Needs	Self-Wants	Satisfaction
A = 0	A = 0	A = 0	SO = 0.393[a]	SO = 0.282[a]
S = –0.094[c]	S = 0	S = 0	SD = 0	SD = 0
WS = 0	WS = 0	WS = 0	SN = 0.129[a]	SN = 0
E = 0	E = 0	E = 0	SP = 0.154[a]	SP = 0
SE = 0.175[a]	SE = 0.118[b]	SE = 0.120[b]	SH = 0	SH = 0
SS = 0.214[a]	SS = 0.139[a]	SS = 0.171[a]	SB = 0.143[a]	SB = 0.094[b]
R^2 = 0.11[a]	R^2 = 0.04[a]	R^2 = 0.05[a]	A = 0	A = 0
Self-Progress	Self-Future	Self-Best	S = 0	S = 0
			WS = 0	WS = 0
			E = 0	E = 0
A = 0	A = −0.078[d]	A = 0	SE = 0.091[b]	SE = 0.057[d]
S = 0	S = 0	S = 0	SS = 0	SS = 0.125[a]
WS = 0	WS = 0	WS = 0	R^2 = 0.48[a]	SW = 0.415[a]
E = 0	E = 0	E = 0		R^2 = 0.56[a]
SE = 0.157[a]	SE = 0	SE = 0		N = 646
SS = 0.112[c]	SS = 0	SS = 0.162[a]		
R^2 = 0.05[a]	R^2 = 0.01[d]	R^2 = 0.03[a]		

[a] $P \leqslant 0.001$
[b] $P \leqslant 0.005$
[c] $P \leqslant 0.01$
[d] $P \leqslant 0.05$
0 Significance level too low to enter equation

Table 3.21 Satisfaction with religion

Self-Others	Self-Deserved	Self-Needs	Self-Wants	Satisfaction
A = 0	A = 0	A = 0	SO = 0.340[a]	SO = 0.384[a]
S = 0	S = 0	S = 0	SD = 0	SD = 0
WS = 0	WS = 0	WS = 0	SN = 0.247[a]	SN = –0.091[d]
E = 0	E = 0	E = 0	SP = 0	SP = 0
SE = 0.182[a]	SE = 0.137[b]	SE = 0.157[b]	SH = 0	SH = 0
SS = 0.140[b]	SS = 0	SS = 0.136[c]	SB = 0.154[a]	SB = 0.142[a]
R^2 = 0.07[a]	R^2 = 0.02[b]	R^2 = 0.05[b]	A = 0	A = 0
Self-Progress	Self-Future	Self-Best	S = 0	S = 0
			WS = 0	WS = 0
			E = 0	E = 0
A = 0	A = 0	A = 0	SE = 0.098[d]	SE = 0.104[b]
S = 0	S = 0.107[d]	S = 0	SS = 0.113[c]	SS = 0.073[d]
WS = 0	WS = 0	WS = 0	R^2 = 0.45[a]	SW = 0.400[a]
E = 0	E = 0	E = 0		R^2 = 0.62[a]
SE = 0.115[d]	SE = 0	SE = 0.106[d]		N = 396
SS = 0.143[b]	SS = 0	SS = 0.155[b]		
R^2 = 0.04[b]	R^2 = 0.01[d]	R^2 = 0.04[b]		

[a] $P \leqslant 0.001$
[b] $P \leqslant 0.005$
[c] $P \leqslant 0.01$
[d] $P \leqslant 0.05$
0 Significance level too low to enter equation

Table 3.22 Satisfaction with self-esteem

Self-Others	Self-Deserved	Self-Needs	Self-Wants	Satisfaction
A = 0	A = 0	A = 0	SO = 0.458[a]	SO = 0.276[a]
S = –0.124[a]	S = –0.139[a]	S = –0.148[a]	SD = 0	SD = 0.068[d]
WS = 0	WS = 0	WS = 0	SN = 0.187[a]	SN = 0
E = 0	E = 0	E = 0	SP = 0	SP = 0
SS = 0.254[a]	SS = 0.160[a]	SS = 0.235[a]	SH = 0	SH = 0
R^2 = 0.08[a]	R^2 = 0.04[a]	R^2 = 0.07[a]	SB = 0.155[a]	SB = 0
Self-Progress	Self-Future	Self-Best	A = 0	A = 0
			S = 0	S = 0
			WS = 0	WS = 0
			E = 0	E = 0
A = 0	A = 0	A = 0.121[b]	SS = 0.080[c]	SS = 0.127[a]
S = –0.105[c]	S = 0	S = 0	R^2 = 0.50[a]	SW = 0.463[a]
WS = 0	WS = –0.108[b]	WS = 0		R^2 = 0.58[a]
E = 0	E = 0	E = 0		N = 644
SS = 0.222[a]	SS = 0.113[b]	SS = 0.236[a]		
R^2 = 0.06[a]	R^2 = 0.02[b]	R^2 = 0.06[a]		

[a] $P \leqslant 0.001$
[b] $P \leqslant 0.005$
[c] $P \leqslant 0.01$
[d] $P \leqslant 0.05$
0 Significance level too low to enter equation

Table 3.23 Satisfaction with transportation

Self-Others	Self-Deserved	Self-Needs	Self-Wants	Satisfaction
A = –0.112[c]	A = 0	A = 0.123[b]	SO = 0.244[a]	SO = 0.268[a]
S = 0	S = 0	S = –0.077[d]	SD = 0.109[d]	SD = 0
WS = 0.103[c]	WS = 0.103[c]	WS = 0	SN = 0.254[a]	SN = 0.151[a]
E = 0	E = 0	E = 0	SP = 0.079[d]	SP = 0
SE = 0	SE = 0	SE = 0	SH = 0	SH = 0
SS = 0	SS = 0	SS = 0.080[d]	SB = 0.179[a]	SB = 0
R^2 = 0.01[c]	R^2 = 0.01[c]	R^2 = 0.02[d]	A = 0.128[a]	A = 0.082[b]
Self-Progress	Self-Future	Self-Best	S = 0	S = 0
			WS = 0	WS = 0
			E = 0	E = 0
A = –0.140[a]	A = 0	A = –0.144[a]	SE = 0	SE = 0.146[a]
S = 0	S = 0	S = 0.081[d]	SS = 0	SS = 0
WS = 0.113[b]	WS = –0.083[d]	WS = 0.172[a]	R^2 = 0.51[a]	SW = 0.408[a]
E = 0	E = 0	E = 0		R^2 = 0.55[a]
SE = 0	SE = 0.091[d]	SE = 0		N = 631
SS = 0	SS = 0	SS = 0		
R^2 = 0.02[a]	R^2 = 0.01[d]	R^2 = 0.04[a]		

[a] $P \leqslant 0.001$
[b] $P \leqslant 0.005$
[c] $P \leqslant 0.01$
[d] $P \leqslant 0.05$
0 Significance level too low to enter equation

Table 3.24 Satisfaction with education

Self-Others	Self-Deserved	Self-Needs	Self-Wants	Satisfaction
A = 0	A = 0	A = 0	SO = 0.164^{a}	SO = 0.180^{a}
S = 0	S = –0.082^{d}	S = 0	SD = 0.133^{a}	SD = 0.087^{d}
WS = 0	WS = 0	WS = 0	SN = 0.283^{a}	SN = 0
E = 0.187^{a}	E = 0	E = 0	SP = 0	SP = 0
SE = 0.202^{a}	SE = 0	SE = 0	SH = 0	SH = 0
SS = 0	SS = 0.116^{b}	SS = 0.132^{a}	SB = 0.101^{c}	SB = 0.198^{a}
R^2 = 0.08^{a}	R^2 = 0.02^{b}	R^2 = 0.02^{a}	A = 0	A = 0
Self-Progress	Self-Future	Self-Best	S = 0	S = 0
			WS = 0	WS = 0
			E = 0	E = 0
A = 0	A = 0	A = 0.079^{d}	SE = 0.120^{a}	SE = 0
S = –0.088^{d}	S = 0	S = 0	SS = 0	SS = 0.179^{a}
WS = 0	WS = –0.134^{a}	WS = 0	R^2 = 0.28^{a}	SW = 0.285^{a}
E = 0	E = 0	E = 0		R^2 = 0.35^{a}
SE = 0	SE = 0	SE = 0.115^{b}		*N* = 645
SS = 0.126^{a}	SS = 0	SS = 0		
R^2 = 0.02^{b}	R^2 = 0.02^{a}	R^2 = 0.02^{d}		

indicates that 39% of the variance in self-wants scores was explained by the 12 predictors listed in that column, and the selfneeds discrepancy variable was the most influential predictor (0.209^{a}). The column headed "self-needs" indicates that 9% of the variance in this discrepancy variable was explained by the 6 variables listed below it, led by social support (0.221^{a}).

It would obviously take more space than one can allow in an article to review each of the detailed Exhibits. However, it is possible to call your attention to a few notable features. Hereafter, it will be convenient to distinguish two kinds of indirect effects, namely, effects on the self-wants discrepancy variable and effects on any of the other six discrepancy variables. I will refer to the former as "second-level" and to the latter as "third-level" effects.

Figure 3.3 and Table 3.12 show that social support has the greatest direct effect on happiness and global satisfaction, but not the greatest second-level effect. The perceived discrepancy between what one has and needs has the greatest second-level effect on these two global variables.

Given the enormous literature regarding the impact of social support on self-perceived health, one would have expected it to have had a similar significant impact on perceived satisfaction with health. Table 3.13 shows that this is not the case for this data-set. On the other hand, self-esteem has significant second and third-level Effects.

Satisfaction with financial security and paid employment tend to be dominated by the perceived self-wants discrepancy (Tables 3.14 and 3.16), while self-esteem has no effect at all on the former variable and almost no effect on the latter.

Curiously, self-esteem has relatively little impact on satisfaction with family relations and friendships (Tables 3.15 and 3.17). However, the social comparison variable (self-others) has strong second-level effects in both cases.

Satisfaction with housing in largely determined by the self-wants and self- others discrepancies, with the latter (self-others) mainly influenced positively by social support and work status, and negatively by age (Table 3.18).

Satisfaction with housing is largely determined by the self-wants and self- tion are all strongly dominated by the self-wants and self-others discrepancies (Tables 3.20, 3.21, 3.22 and 3.23). Social support has significant first and third-level effects, but no second-level effects on satisfaction with recreation activity (Table 3.20). Social comparison has a surprisingly high impact on satisfaction with religion, especially since the latter is defined simply as "your spiritual fulfilment" (Table 3.22).

Given the variety of discrepancy hypotheses available in the literature, the question has been raised about the relative importance of each type, e.g., by Goodman (1974) and Diener (1984). The investigations reported in Michalos (1980a, 1982a, 1983a) indicated a fairly clear and consistent rank ordering of impact of perceived discrepancies on net satisfaction. In a total of 68 regressions, using three gap variables as predictors and some (domain or global) satisfaction or happiness variable as criteria, 65 times the gap between what one has and wants had the greatest impact (highest Beta value). The gap between what one has and relevant others have came in second 46 times, and the gap between what one has and the best one has ever had in the past came in third 50 times. There were only 6 times in which a variable involving the gap between what one has now and expects to have in five years was used, and in every case this variable ranked fourth behind the others and accounted for a negligible percent of the explained variance in the dependent variables.

Table 3.25 summarizes the relative impacts of discrepancy types on satisfaction and happiness for this data-set. For example, the self-wants variable has the greatest impact 38 times, second-greatest 4 times and fourth-greatest once. Thus, the self-wants variable is typically the most influential of all seven discrepancy variables. The self-others variable is typically second. In order to aggregate all the rankings in Table 3.25 to obtain a general view, I assigned each variable a weight. Six points were given to a variable for each time it was first, five points for each second, and so on to one for sixth place. Then the products were summed to get a total weight for each variable. Using this scheme, it is clear that the three discrepancy variables that I have worked with most are the three most influential, namely, self-wants, self- others and self-best.

In terms of the familiar theories reviewed earlier, one might say that Table 3.25 shows that aspiration theory (self-wants) is superior to social comparison theory (self-others), that equity theory (self-deserved) is slightly superior to person-environment fit theory (self-needs), and that cognitive dissonance theory (insofar as it involves future expectations (self-future)) is the least powerful of the lot. Given the artificiality of the weighting scheme, the limitations of the data-set and the severe reduction of the familiar theories to the few representative items in

Table 3.25 Comparison of relative impacts of discrepancy types on satisfaction and happiness

	Firsts	Seconds	Thirds	Fourths	Fifths	Sixths	Sevenths	Total weight
Self wants	38	4	0	1	0	0	0	251
Self others	3	31	6	0	0	0	0	197
Self deserved	0	0	11	4	1	0	0	58
Self needs	0	1	9	3	0	0	0	50
Self progress	0	1	5	2	0	0	0	35
Self future	0	0	1	3	0	1	0	14
Self best	2	6	6	2	0	0	0	97

Table 3.26 Comparison of relative impacts of discrepancy types, self-esteem and social support on satisfaction and happiness

	Firsts	Seconds	Thirds	Fourths	Fifths	Sixths	Sevenths	Total weight
Self wants	31	4	5	1	0	1	0	230
Self others	1	29	3	4	3	1	0	182
Self deserved	0	0	3	5	6	2	0	41
Self needs	0	0	7	4	2	0	0	44
Self progress	0	0	3	4	3	0	0	30
Self future	0	0	0	1	2	2	0	14
Self best	1	2	4	9	0	0	0	59
Self esteem	1	2	5	6	5	1	0	65
Social support	9	4	12	5	2	2	0	143

my questionnaire, one should not press the significance of this rank ordering very far. Still, I believe it is the first time anyone has ever tried to systematically assess the relative superiority of these theories.

Table 3.26 is like the one before it, with the addition of self-esteem and social support. After self-wants and self-others, social support has the greatest relative impact out of the nine variables.

Appendix Tables 3.27, 3.28, 3.29, 3.30, 3.31, 3.32, 3.33, 3.34, 3.35, 3.36, 3.37, 3.38, 3.39, 3.40 give detailed results of applying MDT to the happiness, global and domain satisfaction of males and females. The overviews given in Tables 3.10, 3.11, 3.25 and 3.26 cover this material too. On average MDT explained 48% of the variance in the global variables for males and 55% for females. For males, on average 56% of the variance in domain satisfaction was explained, compared to 58% for females. For both groups, the highest R^2's went to satisfaction with family relations and the lowest to satisfaction with education.

Table 3.27 Satisfaction with life as a whole

		Males		
Self-Others	Self-Deserved	Self-Needs	Self-Wants	Satisfaction
A = 0	A = – 0.165[b]	A = –0.125[d]	SO = 0.173[b]	SO = 0.110[d]
WS = 0	WS= 0	WS= 0	SD = 0	SD= 0
E = 0	E = 0	E = 0	SN = 0.261[a]	SN = 0
SE = 0.260[a]	SE = 0.176[b]	SE = 0.149[c]	SP = 0.186[a]	SP = 0
SS = 0.237[a]	SS = 0.138[d]	SS = 0.187[b]	SH = 0	SH = – 0.093[d]
R^2 = 0.16[a]	R^2 = 0.09[a]	R^2= 0.09[2]	SB = 0	SB = 0.129[c]
Self-Progress	Self-Future	Self-Best	A = 0	A = 0
			WS = 0	WS= 0
			E = 0	E = 0
A = 0	A = 0	A = 0	SE = 0.176[a]	SE = 0.252[a]
WS = 0.132[d]	WS = –0.119[d]	WS = 0	SS = 0.122[d]	SS = 0.262[a]
E = 0	E = 0	E = 0	R^2 = 0.38[a]	SW= 0.266[a]
SE = 0.218[a]	SE = 0	SE = 0.209[a]		R^2 = 0.50[a]
SS = 0.145[c]	SS = 0	SS = 0.186[b]		N = 283
R^2 = 0.09[a]	R^2 = 0.01[d]	R^2 = 0.10[a]		
		Females		
Self-Others	Self-Deserved	Self-Needs	Self-Wants	Satisfaction
A = –0.137[c]	A = 0	A = –0.121[d]	SO = 0.111[d]	SO = 0
WS = 0	WS = 0	WS = 0	SD = 0.167[b]	SD = 0.104[c]
E = 0.158[b]	E = 0	E = 0	SN = 0.185[a]	SN = 0
SE = 0.337[a]	SE = 0	SE = 0	SP = 0.167[a]	SP = 0
SS = 0.142[c]	SS = 0.305[a]	SS = 0.268[a]	SH = 0	SH = 0
R^2 = 0.20[a]	R^2 = 0.09[a]	R^2 = 0.08[a]	SB = 0	SB = 0.130[b]
Self-Progress	Self-Future	Self-Best	A = 0	A = 0
			WS = 0	WS = 0
			E = 0	E = 0
A = 0	A = –0.141[c]	A = 0	SE = 0.166[a]	SE = 0.305[a]
WS = 0	WS = 0	WS = 0	SS = 0.165[a]	SS = 0.278[a]
E = 0	E = 0	E = 0	R^2 = 0.40[a]	SW = 0.256[a]
SE = 0.235[a]	SE = 0	SE = 0.160[b]		R^2 = 0.56[a]
SS = 0.140[c]	SS = 0.150[b]	SS = 0.228[a]		N =340

Again, only a few of the interesting results in these exhibits can be emphasized. Notice, for example, that age has six negative third-level effects on female satisfaction with paid employment, but only one such effect for males (Table 3.32). Social support has only two effects on male satisfaction with recreation activity, but seven effects on female satisfaction (Table 3.36). Educational level has a single direct effect on male and female satisfaction with religion, but it is positive for males and negative for females (Table 3.37). Self-esteem has only one direct effect

Table 3.28 Happiness with life as a whole

Males				
Self-Others	Self-Deserved	Self-Needs	Self-Wants	Happiness
A = 0	A = –0.165[b]	A = –0.125[d]	SO = 0.173[b]	SO = 0.152[b]
WS = 0	WS = 0	WS = 0	SD = 0	SD = 0.109[b]
E = 0	E = 0	E = 0	SN = 0.261[a]	SN = 0
SE = 0.260[a]	SE = 0.176[b]	SE = 0.149[c]	SP = 0.186[a]	SP = 0
SS = 0.237[a]	SS = 0.138[d]	SS = 0.187[b]	SH = 0	SH = 0
R^2 = 0.16[a]	R^2 = 0.09[a]	R^2 = 0.09[a]	SB = 0	SB = 0.270[a]
Self-Progress	Self-Future	Self-Best	A = 0	A = 0
			WS = 0	WS = 0
			E = 0	E = 0
A = 0	A = 0	A = 0	SE = 0.176[a]	SE = 0.175[a]
WS = –0.132[d]	WS = –0.119[d]	WS = 0	SS = 0.122[d]	SS = 0.205[a]
E = 0	E = 0	E = 0	R^2 = 0.38[a]	SW= 0.108[d]
SE = 0.218[a]	SE = 0	SE = 0.209[a]		R^2 = 0.45[a]
SS = 0.145[c]	SS = 0	SS = 0.186[b]		N = 283
R^2 = 0.09[a]	R^2 = 0.01[d]	R^2 = 0.10[a]		
Females				
Self-Others	Self-Deserved	Self-Needs	Self-Wants	Happiness
A = –0.137[c]	A = 0	A = –0.121[d]	SO = 0.111[d]	SO = 0.113[c]
WS = 0	WS = 0	WS = 0	SD = 0.167[b]	SD = 0
E = 0.158[b]	E = 0	E = 0	SN = 0.185[a]	SN = 0.125[b]
SE = 0.337[a]	SE = 0	SE = 0	SP = 0.167[a]	SP = 0
SS = 0.142[c]	SS = 0.305[a]	SS = 0.268[a]	SH = 0	SH = 0
R^2 = 0.20[a]	R^2 = 0.09[a]	R^2 = 0.08[a]	SB = 0	SB = 0.164[a]
Self-Progress	Self-Future	Self-Best	A = 0	A = 0
			WS = 0	WS = 0.095[c]
			E = 0	E = 0
A = 0	A = –0.141[c]	A = 0	SE = 0.166[a]	SE = 0.219[a]
WS = 0	WS = 0	WS = 0	SS = 0.165[a]	SS = 0.246[a]
E = 0	E = 0	E = 0	R^2 = 0.40[a]	SW = 0.207[a]
SE = 0.235[a]	SE = 0	SE = 0.160[b]		R^2 = 0.53[a]
SS = 0.140[c]	SS = 0.150[b]	SS = 0.228[a]		N = 340
R^2 = 0.09[a]	R^2 = 0.04[a]	R^2 = 0.10[a]		

on male satisfaction with transportation, but it has one direct and three indirect effects on female satisfaction (Table 3.39). Work status has all six third-level effects on male satisfaction with transportation, but only one such effect for females.

Table 3.29 Satisfaction with health

		Males		
Self-Others	Self-Deserved	Self-Needs	Self-Wants	Satisfaction
A = 0	A = 0	A = 0	SO = 0.427[a]	SO = 0.189[a]
WS = 0	WS = 0	WS = 0	SD = 0	SD = 0
E = 0	E = 0	E = 0	SN = 0.128[c]	SN = 0
SE = 0.180[b]	SE = 0.155[b]	SE = 0.117[d]	SP= 0.139[c]	SP= 0
SS = 0	SS = 0	SS = 0	SH = –0.129[b]	SH = -0.088[d]
R^2 = 0.03[b]	R^2 = 0.02[b]	R^2 = 0.01[d]	SB = 0.105[d]	SB = 0
Self-Progress	Self-Future	Self-Best	A = 0	A = 0
			WS= 0	WS= 0
			E = 0	E = 0
A = 0	A = 0	A = 0	SE = 0.160[a]	SE = 0
WS = 0	WS = 0	WS = -0.137[d]	SS = 0.106[d]	SS = 0.167[a]
E = 0	E = 0	E = 0	R^2 = 0.48[a]	SW= 0.491[a]
SE = 0.150[c]	SE = 0	SE = 0.115[d]		R^2 = 0.46[a]
SS = 0	SS = 0.115[d]	SS = 0		N = 296
R^2 = 0.02[c]	R^2 = 0.01[d]	R^2 = 0.02[c]		
		Females		
Self-Others	Self-Deserved	Self-Needs	Self-Wants	Satisfaction
A = 0	A = 0	A = 0	SO = 0.364[a]	SO = 0.168[a]
WS = 0	WS = 0	WS= –0.129[C]	SD = 0	SD = 0.129[b]
E = 0.178[a]	E = 0	E = 0.112[d]	SN = 0.178[a]	SN = 0
SE = 0	SE = 0	SE = 0	SP = 0.126[c]	SP = 0
SS = 0	SS = 0	SS = 0.163[b]	SH = –0.081[d]	SH = 0
R^2 = 0.03[a]	R^2 = 0	R^2 = 0.04[a]	SB = 0.190[a]	SB = 0
			A = 0	A = 0
Self-Progress	Self-Future	Self-Best	WS = 0	WS = 0
			E = 0	E = 0
A = 0	A = 0	A = 0	SE = 0.151[a]	SE = 0.160[a]
WS = 0	WS = 0	WS = 0	SS = 0	SS = 0
E = 0	E = 0	E = 0	R^2 = 0.49[a]	SW = 0.493[a]
SE = 0.257[a]	SE = 0	SE = 0.206[a]		R^2 = 0.53[a]
SS = 0	SS = 0.149[b]	SS = 0		N = 341
R^2 = 0.06[a]	R^2 = 0.02[b]	R^2 = 0.04[a]		

Discussion

Having completed our analysis of the Guelph undergraduate data-set with MDT, there are a few loose ends that should be nailed down. In the first place, it may have been noticed that all but one of the variables used here (viz, social support) are based on single item measures, in spite of the fact that generally speaking if all other

Table 3.30 Satisfaction with financial security

Males				
Self-Others	Self-Deserved	Self-Needs	Self-Wants	Satisfaction
A = –0.296[a]	A = –0.157[c]	A = –0.188[a]	SO = 0.245[a]	SO = 0.284[a]
WS = 0.179[b]	WS = 0	WS = 0	SD = 0.250[a]	SD = 0
E = 0	E = 0	E = 0	SN = 0.246[a]	SN = 0.172[a]
SE = 0	SE = 0	SE = 0	SP = 0	SP = –0.100[d]
SS = 0.122[d]	SS = 0	SS = 0	SH = 0	SH = –0.077[d]
R^2 = 0.11[a]	R^2 = 0.02[c]	R^2 = 0.03[a]	SB = 0.113[d]	SB = 0.153[b]
Self-Progress	Self-Future	Self-Best	A = 0.125[c]	A = 0
			WS = 0	WS = 0
			E = 0	E = 0
A = –0.234[a]	A = 0	A = –0.282[a]	SE = 0	SE = 0
WS = 0	WS = 0	WS = 0.171[b]	SS = 0	SS = 0
E = 0	E = 0	E = 0	R^2 = 0.42[a]	SW = 0.401[a]
SE = 0	SE = 0	SE = 0		R^2 = 0.59[a]
SS = 0	SS = 0	SS = 0		*N* = 293
R^2 = 0.05[a]	R^2 = 0	R^2 = 0.08[a]		
Females				
Self-Others	Self-Deserved	Self-Needs	Self-Wants	Satisfaction
A = –0.176[a]	A = –0.182[a]	A = –0.109[d]	SO = 0.180[a]	SO = 0.200[a]
WS = 0.132[d]	WS = 0	WS = 0	SD = 0	SD = 0.120[c]
E = 0	E = 0	E = 0	SN = 0.415[a]	SN = 0.155[b]
SE = 0	SE = 0	SE = 0	SP = 0	SP = 0.128[b]
SS = 0	SS = 0	SS = 0	SH = 0	SH = 0
R^2 = 0.03[b]	R^2 = 0.03[a]	R^2 = 0.01[d]	SB = 0.255[a]	SB = 0
Self-Progress	Self-Future	Self-Best	A = 0.091[d]	A = 0
			WS = 0	WS = 0
			E = 0	E = 0
A = –0.136[c]	A = 0	A = –0.116[d]	SE = 0	SE = 0
WS = 0	WS = 0	WS = 0.182[a]	SS = 0.079[d]	SS = 0.112[b]
E = 0	E = 0	E = 0	R^2 = 0.51[a]	SW = 0.324[a]
SE = 0	SE = 0	SE = 0		R^2 = 0.59[a]
SS = 0.211[a]	SS = 0.182[a]	SS = 0		*N* = 341
R^2 = 0.06[a]	R^2 = 0.03[a]	R^2 = 0.03[a]		

things are equal, multi-item measures (indexes, scales) tend to have higher levels of reliability (Zeller and Carmines 1980; Andersonet al. 1983). The main reason for using single item measures with some face validity here is that I am primarily interested in tracing the boundaries or scope of MDT in terms of its domains of applicability. I want to have a rough idea fairly early about where this sort of theory is likely to work. Besides this basic consideration, there is also the problem of

Table 3.31 Satisfaction with family relations

Males				
Self-Others	Self-Deserved	Self-Needs	Self-Wants	Satisfaction
A = –0.127[c]	A = 0	A = –0.123[c]	SO = 0.378[a]	SO = 0.160[a]
WS = 0	WS = 0	WS = 0	SD = 0	SD = 0
E = 0	E = 0	E = 0	SN = 0.281[a]	SN = 0.173[a]
SE = 0	SE = 0	SE = 0	SP = 0	SP = 0
SS = 0.532[a]	SS = 0.443[a]	SS = 0.535[a]	SH = 0	SH = 0
R^2 = 0.31[a]	R^2 = 0.19[a]	R^2 = 0.32[a]	SB = 0.104[d]	SB = 0
Self-Progress	Self-Future	Self-Best	A = 0	A = 0
			WS = 0	WS = 0
			E = 0	E = 0
A = 0	A = 0	A = 0	SE = 0	SE = 0
WS = 0	WS = 0	WS = 0	SS = 0.156[b]	SS = 0.485[a]
E = 0	E = 0	E = 0	R^2 = 0.57[a]	SW = 0.222[a]
SE = –0.122[d]	SE = 0	SE = 0		R^2 = 0.77[a]
SS = 0.413[a]	SS = 0.160[c]	SS = 0.358[a]		N =290
R^2 = 0.15[a]	R^2 = 0.02[c]	R^2 = 0.13[a]		
Females				
Self-Others	Self-Deserved	Self-Needs	Self-Wants	Satisfaction
A = 0	A = 0	A= –0.116[c]	SO = 0.300[a]	SO = 0.219[a]
WS = 0	WS = –0.148[b]	WS = 0	SD = 0.154[a]	SD = 0
E = 0	E = 0	E = 0	SN = 0.165[a]	SN = 0.085[c]
SE = 0	SE = 0	SE = 0	SP = 0	SP = 0
SS = 0.607[a]	SS = 0.468[a]	SS = 0.468[a]	SH = 0	SH = 0
R^2 = 0.37[a]	R^2 = 0.23[a]	R^2 = 0.23[a]	SB = 0	SB = 0
Self-Progress	Self-Future	Self-Best	A = 0	A = 0
			WS = 0	WS = 0
			E = 0	E = 0
A = 0	A = 0	A = 0	SE = 0	SE = –0.069[c]
WS = 0	WS = –0.198[a]	WS = 0	SS = 0.340[a]	SS = 0.544[a]
E = 0	E = 0	E = 0	R^2 = 0.62[a]	SW = 0.215[a]
SE = 0	SE = 0	SE = 0		R^2 = 0.81[a]
SS = 0.430[a]	SS = 0.189[a]	SS = 0.473[a]		N = 341
R^2 = 0.18[a]	R^2 = 0.07[a]	R^2 = 0.22[a]		

increasing the length of the questionnaire with the use of multiitem measures. Moreover, as Schuessler (1982) had admirably shown, there is no guarantee that the more items a measure has, the more reliable it will be. For all these reasons, then, it seems wise to stay with single item measures for now.

The construct validity of the D-T scale of Andrews and Withey (1976) was thoroughly examined by these authors, and my delightful-terrible scale is simply a

Table 3.32 Satisfaction with paid employment

		Males		
Self-Others	Self-Deserved	Self-Needs	Self-Wants	Satisfaction
A = 0	A = 0	A = 0	SO = 0.377[a]	SO = 0.324[a]
WS = 0.478[a]	WS = 0	WS = 0.228[a]	SD = 0.168[c]	SD = 0
E = 0	E = 0	E = 0	SN = 0.171[d]	SN = 0
SE = 0	SE = 0	SE = 0	SP = 0	SP = 0
SS = 0.172[b]	SS = 0	SS = 0	SH = 0	SH = 0
R^2 = 0.26[a]	R^2 = 0	R^2 = 0.05[a]	SB = 0	SB = 0
Self-Progress	Self-Future	Self-Best	A = 0	A = 0
			WS = 0.196[a]	WS = 0.240[a]
			E = 0	E = 0
A = 0	A = 0	A = –0.196[b]	SE = 0	SE = 0
WS = 0	WS = 0	WS = 0.387[a]	SS = 0	SS = 0
E = 0	E = 0	E = 0	R^2 = 0.49[a]	SW = 0.334[a]
SE = 0	SE = 0	SE = 0		R^2 = 0.55[a]
SS = 0	SS = 0	SS = 0		*N* = 173
R^2 = 0	R^2 = 0	R^2 = 0.14[a]		
		Females		
Self-Others	Self-Deserved	Self-Needs	Self-Wants	Satisfaction
A = –0.270[a]	A = –0.182[c]	A = –0.176[c]	SO = 0.228[a]	SO = 0.195[a]
WS = 0.529[a]	WS = 0.224[a]	WS = 0.319[a]	SD = 0.167[c]	SD = 0.188[a]
E = 0	E = 0	E = 0	SN = 0.326[a]	SN = 0
SE = 0	SE = 0	SE = 0	SP = 0	SP = 0
SS = 0	SS = 0	SS = 0	SH = 0	SH = 0.133[b]
R^2 = 0.27[a]	R^2 = 0.05[a]	R^2 = 0.10[a]	SB = 0	SB = 0
Self-Progress	Self-Future	Self-Best	A = 0	A = 0
			WS = 0.203[a]	WS = 0.231[a]
			E = 0	E = 0
A = –0.152[d]	A = –0.126[d]	A = –0.270[a]	SE = 0	SE = 0
WS = 0.266[a]	WS = 0	WS = 0.595[a]	SS = 0	SS = 0.169[a]
E = 0	E = 0	E = 0	R^2 = 0.49[a]	SW = 0.369[a]
SE = 0	SE = 0	SE = 0		R^2 = 0.68[a]
SS = 0.121[d]	SS = 0.163[b]	SS = 0		*N* =192
R^2 = 0.08[a]	R^2 = 0.04[a]	R^2 = 0.34[a]		

linguistically purer version of their scale. The original scale had "approximately 65% valid variance" and "roughly eight percent of the total variance can be attributed to method effects" (Andrews and Withey 1976, p. 189). I suppose that my delightful-terrible scale has fairly similar characteristics.

All of the perceived discrepancy measures are designed on the working assumption that people have distinct and identifiable levels of wants, needs,

Table 3.33 Satisfaction with friendships

		Males		
Self-Others	Self-Deserved	Self-Needs	Self-Wants	Satisfaction
A = 0	A = 0	A = 0	SO = 0.387[a]	SO = 0.201[a]
WS = 0	WS = 0	WS = 0	SD = 0	SD = 0
E = 0	E = 0	E = 0	SN = 0.087[d]	SN = 0
SE = 0.170[a]	SE = 0	SE = 0.190[a]	SP = 0.100[d]	SP = 0
SS = 0.547[a]	SS = 0.361[a]	SS = 0.413[a]	SH = 0	SH = 0
R^2 = 0.38[a]	R^2 = 0.13[a]	R^2 = 0.25[a]	SB = 0	SB = 0.101[b]
Self-Progress	Self-Future	Self-Best	A = 0.093[c]	A = 0
			WS = 0	WS = 0
			E = 0	E = 0
A = 0	A = 0	A = 0	SE = 0.122[b]	SE = 0
WS = 0	WS = 0	WS = 0	SS = 0.304[a]	SS = 0.528[a]
E = 0	E = 0	E = 0	R^2 = 0.60[a]	SW = 0.191[a]
SE = 0	SE = 0	SE = 0		R^2 = 0.76[a]
SS = 0.348[a]	SS = 0	SS = 0.433[a]		N = 294
R^2 = 0.12[a]	R^2 = 0	R^2 = 0.19[a]		
		Females		
Self-Others	Self-Deserved	Self-Needs	Self-Wants	Satisfaction
A = 0	A = 0	A = 0	SO = 0.331[a]	SO = 0.082[d]
WS = 0	WS = 0	WS = 0	SD = 0	SD = 0
E = 0	E = 0	E = 0	SN = 0.147[b]	SN = 0
SE = 0.117[c]	SE = 0	SE = 0	SP = 0	SP = 0.104[b]
SS = 0.502[a]	SS = 0.417[a]	SS = 0.407[a]	SH = 0	SH = 0
R^2 = 0.30[a]	R^2 = 0.17[a]	R^2 = 0.16[a]	SB = 0.132[b]	SB = 0
Self-Progress	Self-Future	Self-Best	A = 0.081[d]	A = 0
			WS = 0	WS = 0
			E = 0	E = 0
A = 0	A = −0.204[a]	A = 0	SE = 0.104[c]	SE = 0
WS = 0	WS = 0	WS = 0.138[b]	SS = 0.237[a]	SS = 0.556[a]
E = 0	E = 0	E = 0	R^2 = 0.52[a]	SW = 0.284[a]
SE = 0.129[c]	SE = 0	SE = 0		R^2 = 0.74[a]
SS = 0.329[a]	SS = 0	SS = 0.408[a]		N = 345
R^2 = 0.15[a]	R^1 = 0.04[a]	R^2 = 0.19[a]		

expectations and so on. But it is more likely that any levels of experienced wants, etc. are vaguely bounded by intervals which obscurely blend into perceivable chunks (Michalos 1967). Following a suggestion from Samuel Stouffer, Rodman (1963) used the idea of an interval, "wider range of values" or "value-stretch" to account for the apparently contradictory findings in delinquency studies showing that society is based upon both a "common value system" and a

Table 3.34 Satisfaction with housing

		Males		
Self-Others	Self-Deserved	Self-Needs	Self-Wants	Satisfaction
A = –0.231[a]	A = 0	A = 0	SO = 0.369[a]	SO = 0.244[a]
WS = 0.186[a]	WS = 0	WS = 0	SD = 0.219[a]	SD = 0.175[a]
E = 0	E = 0	E = 0	SN = 0	SN = 0
SE = 0	SE = 0	SE = 0	SP = 0.184[a]	SP = 0
SS = 0.180[a]	SS = 0	SS = 0.154[c]	SH = 0	SH = 0
R^2 = 0.10[a]	R^2 = 0	R^2 = 0.02[c]	SB = 0	SB = 0
Self-Progress	Self-Future	Self-Best	A = 0	A = 0.098[d]
			WS = 0	WS = 0
			E = 0	E = 0
A = –0.218[a]	A = 0	A = –0.169[c]	SE = 0	SE = 0
WS = 0.179[b]	WS = 0	WS = 0.120[d]	SS = 0	SS = 0.187[a]
E = 0	E = 0	E = 0.172[c]	R^2 = 0.38[a]	SW = 0.353[a]
SE = –0.138[c]	SE= 0	SE = 0		R^2 = 0.46[a]
SS = 0	SS = 0	SS = 0		N = 290
R^2 = 0.06[a]	R^2= 0	R^2 = 0.04[b]		
		Females		
Self-Others	Self-Deserved	Self-Needs	Self-Wants	Satisfaction
A = 0	A = 0	A = –0.121[d]	SO = 0.295[a]	SO = 0.275[a]
WS = 0	WS = 0	WS = 0	SD = 0	SD = 0
E = 0	E = 0	E = 0.167[b]	SN = 0.218[a]	SN = 0
SE = 0	SE = 0	SE = 0	SP = 0	SP = 0.183[a]
SS = 0.116[d]	SS = 0	SS = 0	SH = 0	SH = 0
R^2 = 0.01[d]	R^2 = 0	R^2= 0.02[e]	SB = 0.236[a]	SB = 0
Self-Progress	Self-Future	Self-Best	A = 0.102[d]	A = 0
			WS = 0	WS = 0
			E = 0	E = 0
A = –0.214[a]	A = –0.106[d]	A = 0	SE = 0	SE = 0.111[c]
WS = 0	WS = 0	WS = 0	SS = 0	SS = 0.117[c]
E = 0.152[c]	E = 0	E = 0	R^2 = 0.36[a]	SW = 0.301[a]
SE = 0	SE = 0	SE = 0		R^2 = 0.44[a]
SS = 0	SS = 0.127[d]	SS = 0		N = 341
R^2 = 0.04[a]	R^2 = 0.02[c]	R^2 = 0		

"class-differentiated value system". Although I suspect it is misleading to describe perceptual limitations as some kind of an expanded range of values, I think we would all agree on the fuzziness of perceived discrepancies.

It may also have been noticed that, while all of the discrepancy measures are designed to run from the relatively unattractive (=1) to the attractive (=7), sometimes a score of 4 indicates a point of congruence and sometimes not. For example,

Table 3.35 Satisfaction with area lived in

		Males		
Self-Others	Self-Deserved	Self-Needs	Self-Wants	Satisfaction
A = –0.118[d]	A = –0.200[a]	A = –0.188[b]	SO = 0.257[a]	SO = 0.228[a]
WS = 0	WS = 0.120[d]	WS = 0.141[d]	SD = 0	SD = 0.125[c]
E = 0	E = 0	E = 0	SN = 0.215[a]	SN = 0
SE = 0	SE = 0	SE = 0	SP = 0.275[a]	SP = 0
SS = 0.121[d]	SS = 0	SS = 0	SH = –0.095[d]	SH = 0
R^2 = 0.03[c]	R^2 = 0.04[b]	R^2 = 0.04[b]	SB = 0	SB = 0
Self-Progress	Self-Future	Self-Best	A = 0	A = 0
			WS = 0	WS = 0
			E = 0	E = 0
A = –0.176[b]	A = 0	A = 0	SE = 0	SE = 0
WS = 0	WS = –0.120[d]	WS = 0	SS = 0	SS = 0.225[a]
E = 0	E = 0	E = 0	R^2 = 0.35[a]	SW = 0.420[a]
SE = 0	SE = 0	SE = 0		R^2 = 0.49[a]
SS = 0	SS = 0	SS = 0.125[d]		*N* =291
R^2 = 0.03[b]	R^2= 0.01[d]	R^2 = 0.01[d]		
		Females		
Self-Others	Self-Deserved	Self-Needs	Self-Wants	Satisfaction
A = 0	A = 0	A = 0	SO = 0.208[a]	SO = 0.235[a]
WS = 0	WS = 0	WS = 0	SD= 0	SD = 0
E = 0.125[d]	E = 0	E = 0	SN = 0.217[a]	SN = 0
SE = 0.125[d]	SE = 0	SE = 0	SP = 0	SP = 0.136[b]
SS = 0	SS = 0	SS = 0	SH = –0.171[a]	SH = 0
R^2 = 0.03[b]	R^2 = 0	R^2 = 0	SB = 0.352[a]	SB = 0
Self-Progress	Self-Future	Self-Best	A = 0	A = 0
			WS = 0	WS = 0
			E = 0	E = 0
A = –0.178[b]	A = –0.145[c]	A = 0	SE = 0	SE = 0
WS = 0	WS = 0	WS = 0	SS = 0	SS = 0.176[a]
E = 0.138[d]	E = 0	E = 0	R^2 = 0.41[a]	SW = 0.417[a]
SE = 0	SE = 0	SE = 0		R^2 = 0.46[a]
SS = 0	SS = 0.114[d]	SS = 0		*N* = 343
R^2 = 0.03[b]	R^2 = 0.03[b]	R^2 = 0		

for the self-wants measure 4 indicates "half as well as what you want" and for the self-deserved measure 4 indicates "matches exactly what is deserved". At this point, I don't know if these differences are important or not. However, at least for the self-deserved measure, it is important to have the congruence point at 4 in order to see what happens when people get more than they think they deserve. Examining cross-tabulations and a variety of measures of association between satisfaction and

Table 3.36 Satisfaction with recreation activity

Males				
Self-Others	Self-Deserved	Self-Needs	Self-Wants	Satisfaction
A = 0	A = 0	A = 0	SO = 0.386[a]	SO = 0.355[a]
WS = 0	WS = 0	WS = 0	SD = 0.190[a]	SD = 0
E = 0	E = 0	E = 0	SN = 0	SN = 0
SE = 0.200[a]	SE = 0.215[a]	SE = 0.171[b]	SP = 0.154[c]	SP = 0
SS = 0.171[b]	SS = 0	SS = 0	SH = 0	SH = 0
R^2 = 0.09[a]	R^2 = 0.04[a]	R^2 = 0.03[b]	SB = 0.111[d]	SB = 0
Self-Progress	Self-Future	Self-Best	A = 0	A = 0
			WS = 0	WS = 0
			E = 0	E = 0
A = 0	A = 0	A = 0	SE = 0	SE = 0.113[c]
WS = –0.120[d]	WS = 0	WS = 0	SS = 0	SS = 0.111[c]
E = 0	E = 0	E = 0	R^2 = 0.47[a]	SW = 0.377[a]
SE = 0.155[c]	SE = 0	SE = 0		R^2 = 0.53[a]
SS = 0	SS = 0	SS = 0		N = 295
R^2 = 0.03[b]	R^2 = 0	R^2 = 0		
Females				
Self-Others	Self-Deserved	Self-Needs	Self-Wants	Satisfaction
A = 0	A = 0	A = 0	SO = 0.394[a]	SO = 0.200[a]
WS = 0	WS = 0	WS = 0	SD = 0	SD = 0
E = 0.151[b]	E = 0	E = 0	SN = 0.124[c]	SN = 0.136[b]
SE = 0.161[b]	SE = 0	SE = 0	SP = 0.121[d]	SP = 0
SS = 0.231[a]	SS = 0.228[a]	SS = 0.241[a]	SH = 0	SH = 0
R^2 = 0.13[a]	R^2 = 0.05[a]	R^2 = 0.06[a]	SB = 0.180[a]	SB = 0
Self-Progress	Self-Future	Self-Best	A = 0	A = 0
			WS = 0	WS = 0
			E = 0	E = 0
A = 0	A = –0.111[d]	A = 0	SE = 0.170[a]	SE = 0
WS = 0	WS = 0	WS = 0	SS = 0	SS = 0.136[a]
E = 0	E = 0	E = 0	R^2 = 0.52[a]	SW = 0.478[a]
SE = 0.176[b]	SE = 0	SE = 0		R^2 = 0.58[a]
SS = 0.164[b]	SS = 0.109[d]	SS = 0.234[a]		N = 341
R^2 = 0.07[a]	R^2 = 0.02[c]	R^2 = 0.05[a]		

self-deserved discrepancy scores, I found no evidence of a U-shaped relationship. In particular, there was no evidence that satisfaction decreased as one perceived that one was getting more than one deserved. This is contrary to some results cited by Walster et al. (1976).

Just as no evidence of a U-shaped relationship appeared, there was no evidence that what I call "conditioning variables" function as moderating variables as the latter is understood in LaRocco et al. (1980) and Zedeck (1971). Examination of

Table 3.37 Satisfaction with religion

		Males		
Self-Others	Self-Deserved	Self-Needs	Self-Wants	Satisfaction
A = 0	A = 0	A = 0	SO = 0.433[a]	SO = 0.327[a]
WS = 0	WS = 0	WS = 0	SD = 0	SD = 0
E = 0	E = 0	E = 0	SN = 0.332[a]	SN = –0.152[c]
SE = 0	SE = 0	SE = 0.260[a]	SP = 0	SP = 0
SS = 0.212[b]	SS = 0	SS = 0	SH = 0	SH = 0
R^2 = 0.04[b]	R^2 = 0	R^2 = 0.06[a]	SB = 0	SB = 0.189[a]
Self-Progress	Self-Future	Self-Best	A = 0	A = 0
			WS = 0	WS = 0
			E = 0	E = 0.105[c]
A = 0	A = 0	A = 0	SE = 0	SE = 0.108[c]
WS = 0	WS = 0	WS = 0	SS = 0.135[d]	SS = 0
E = 0	E = 0	E = 0	R^2 = 0.45[a]	SW = 0.531[a]
SE = 0	SE = 0	SE = 0		R^2 = 0.70[a]
SS = 0.149[d]	SS = 0	SS = 0.207[b]		N = 173
R^2 = 0.02[d]	R^2 = 0	R^2 = 0.04[b]		
		Females		
Self-Others	Self-Deserved	Self-Needs	Self-Wants	Satisfaction
A = 0	A = 0	A = 0	SO = 0.259[a]	SO = 0.400[a]
WS = 0	WS = 0	WS = 0	SD = 0	SD = 0
E = 0	E = 0	E = 0	SN = 0.241[a]	SN = 0
SE = 0.275[a]	SE = 0	SE = 0	SP = 0	SP = 0.165[b]
SS = 0	SS = 0.184[b]	SS = 0.167[c]	SH = 0	SH = 0
R^2 = 0.07[a]	R^2 = 0.03[b]	R^2 = 0.02[c]	SB = 0.239[a]	SB = 0
Self-Progress	Self-Future	Self-Best	A = 0	A = 0
			WS = 0	WS = 0
			E = 0	E = –0.111[c]
A = 0	A = –0.142[d]	A = 0	SE = 0.184[a]	SE = 0.127[c]
WS = 0	WS = 0	WS = 0	SS = 0	SS = 0.103[d]
E = 0	E = 0	E = 0	R^2 = 0.45[a]	SW = 0.248[a]
SE = 0.157[d]	SE = 0	SE = 0		R^2 = 0.58[a]
SS = 0.165[c]	SS = 0	SS = 0.179[b]		N = 219
R^2 = 0.06[a]	R^2 = 0.02[d]	R^2 = 0.03[b]		

over 1700 pairs of equations including one with and one without a conditioning variable in the form of a product term revealed no significant changes in the predictive power of the equations. For example, the predictive strength of self-others discrepancy scores and age was the same as that of self-others scores, age and the product of self- others scores and age.

Table 3.38 Satisfaction with self-esteem

		Males		
Self-Others	Self-Deserved	Self-Needs	Self-Wants	Satisfaction
A = 0	A = 0	A = 0	SO = 0.438[a]	SO = 0.228[a]
WS = 0	WS = 0	WS = 0	SD = 0.131[d]	SD = 0.170[a]
E = 0	E = 0	E = 0	SN = 0.151[d]	SN = 0
SS = 0.227[a]	SS = 0.134[d]	SS = 0.223[a]	SP = 0	SP = 0
R^2 = 0.05[a]	R^2 = 0.02[d]	R^2 = 0.05[a]	SH = 0	SH = –0.096[d]
Self-Progress	Self-Future	Self-Best	SB = 0	SB = 0
			A = 0	A = 0
			WS = 0	WS = 0
A = 0	A = 0	A = 0	E = 0	E = 0
WS = 0	WS = –0.134[d]	WS = 0	SS = 0.094[d]	SS = 0.160[a]
E = 0	E = 0	E = 0	R^2 = 0.42[a]	SW = 0.400[a]
SS = 0.156[c]	SS = 0	SS = 0.174[b]		R^2 = 0.54[a]
R^2 = 0.02[c]	R^2 = 0.02[d]	R^2 = 0.03[b]		N = 293
		Females		
Self-Others	Self-Deserved	Self-Needs	Self-Wants	Satisfaction
A = 0	A = 0	A = 0	SO = 0.247[a]	SO = 0.305[a]
WS = 0	WS = 0	WS = –0.123[d]	SD = 0.143[d]	SD = 0
E = 0	E = 0	E = 0	SN = 0.314[a]	SN = 0
SS = 0.294[a]	SS = 0.198[a]	SS = 0.276[a]	SP = 0	SP = 0
R^2 = 0.08[a]	R^2 = 0.04[a]	R^2 = 0.08[a]	SH = 0	SH = 0
Self-Progress	Self-Future	Self-Best	SB = 0.154[a]	SB = 0
			A = 0.146[a]	A = 0
			WS = 0	WS = 0
A = 0	A = 0	A = 0.129[c]	E = 0	E = 0
WS = 0	WS = 0	WS = 0	SS = 0.089[d]	SS = 0.115[b]
E = 0	E = –0.134[c]	E = 0	R^2 = 0.54[a]	SW = 0.491[a]
SS = 0.291[a]	SS = 0.140[c]	SS = 0.285[a]		R^2 = 0.61[a]
R^2 = 0.08[a]	R^2 = 0.03[b]	R^2 = 0.09[a]		N = 340

In correspondence concerning earlier work, Aubrey McKennell suggested that satisfaction and self-want discrepancy variables might merely be two measures of the same thing. Using the strategy recommended by Zeller and Carmines (1980) to distinguish method artifacts from substantive dimensions when factor analysis produces two factors from a data-set, it is possible to test this suggestion. The crux of Zeller and Carmines' argument is the simple observation that if two variables are measuring the same thing, then they ought to have similar relations to other "theoretically relevant external variables… in terms of direction, strength, and consistency" (Zeller and Carmines 1980, p. 97). Since this data-set includes 952 cases in which a satisfaction and a self-want discrepancy variable are related to a common third "theoretically relevant external variable", there are plenty of opportunities to

Table 3.39 Satisfaction with transportation

		Males		
Self-Others	Self-Deserved	Self-Needs	Self-Wants	Satisfaction
A = – 0.213[a]	A = 0	A = 0.193[a]	SO = 0.258[a]	SO = 0.282[a]
WS = 0.188[b]	WS = 0.160[c]	WS= 0.222[a]	SD = 0	SD = 0
E = 0	E = 0	E = 0	SN = 0.230[a]	SN = 0.176[b]
SE = 0	SE = 0	SE = 0	SP = 0.168[b]	SP = 0
SS = 0	SS = 0	SS = 0	SH = 0	SH = 0
R^2= 0.05[a]	R^2 = 0.02[c]	R^2 = 0.06[a]	SB = 0.205[a]	SB = 0
Self-Progress	Self-Future	Self-Best	A = 0.103[d]	A = 0.083[d]
			WS = 0	WS = 0
			E = 0	E = 0
A = – 0.244[a]	A = 0	A = – 0.276[a]	SE = 0	SE = 0.117[b]
WS = 0.119[d]	WS = –0.133[d]	WS = 0.213[a]	SS = 0	SS = 0
E = 0	E = 0	E = 0	R^2 = 0.48[a]	SW = 0.377[a]
SE = 0	SE = 0	SE = 0		R^2 = 0.52[a]
SS = 0	SS = 0	SS = 0		N = 285
R^2 = 0.05[a]	R^2 = 0.01[d]	R^2 = 0.08[a]		
		Females		
Self-Others	Self-Deserved	Self-Needs	Self-Wants	Satisfaction
A = 0	A = 0	A = 0	SO = 0.247[a]	SO = 0.305[a]
WS = 0	WS = 0	WS = 0	SD = 0.143[d]	SD = 0.177[a]
E = 0	E = 0	E = 0	SN = 0.314[a]	SN = 0
SE = 0	SE = –0.119[d]	SE = –0.157[b]	SP = 0	SP = 0
SS =0	SS = 0	SS = 0	SH = 0	SH = 0
R^2 = 0	R^2 = 0.01[d]	R^2 = 0.02[b]	SB = 0.154[a]	SB = 0
Self-Progress	Self-Future	Self-Best	A = 0.146[a]	A = 0.092[c]
			WS = 0	WS = 0
			E = 0	E = 0
A = 0	A = 0	A = 0	SE = 0.089[d]	SE = 0.169[a]
WS = 0	WS = 0	WS = 0.130[e]	SS = 0	SS = 0
E = 0	E = 0	E = 0	R 2 = 0.54[a]	SW = 0.415[a]
SE = 0	SE = 0	SE = 0		R^2 = 0.57 a
SS = 0	SS = 0.174[a]	SS = 0		N = 336
R^2 = 0	R^2 = 0.03[a]	R^2 = 0.01[c]		

apply the Zeller and Carmines test. I looked at every one of these triples, counting the relations as similar if the satisfaction and self-want variables both had significant associations to the third variable in the set (whether the associations were positive or negative), and counting the relations as different only if one of the former variables had a significant relation to the third. Clearly, my criterion of similarity of relations is easier to satisfy than that proposed by Zeller and Carmines.

Table 3.40 Satisfaction with education

Males				
Self-Others	Self-Deserved	Self-Needs	Self-Wants	Satisfaction
A = 0	A = 0	A = 0	SO = 0.218[a]	SO = 0.158[b]
WS = 0	WS = 0	WS = 0	SD = 0	SD = 0
E = 0.172[b]	E = 0	E = 0	SN = 0.291[a]	SN = 0
SE = 0.178[b]	SE = 0	SE = 0	SP = 0	SP = 0
SS = 0	SS = 0.15S[c]	SS = 0.149[c]	SH = 0	SH = 0
R^2 = 0.06[a]	R^1 = 0.02[c]	R^2 = 0.02[c]	SB = 0.191[a]	SB = 0.205[a]
Self-Progress	Self-Future	Self-Best	A = 0	A = 0
			WS = 0	WS = 0
			E = 0	E = 0
A = 0	A = 0	A = 0	SE = 0	SE = 0
WS = 0	WS = –0.239[a]	WS = 0	SS = 0	SS = 0.251[a]
E = 0	E = 0	E = 0	R^2 = 0.26[a]	SW= 0.286[a]
SE = 0	SE = 0	SE = 0		R^2 = 0.34[a]
SS = 0.130[d]	SS = 0	SS = 0.130[d]		*N* =295
R^2 = 0.01[d]	R^2 = 0.05[a]	R^2 = 0.01[d]		
Females				
Self-Others	Self-Deserved	Self-Needs	Self-Wants	Satisfaction
A = 0	A = 0	A = 0	SO = 0.151[b]	SO = 0.209[a]
WS = 0	WS = 0	WS = 0	SD = 0.183[b]	SD = 0
E = 0.191[a]	E = 0	E = 0	SN = 0.310[a]	SN = 0.130[c]
SE = 0.232[a]	SE = 0	SE = 0	SP = 0	SP = 0.111[d]
SS = 0	SS = 0	SS = 0.112[d]	SH = 0	SH = 0
R^2 = 0.09[a]	R^2 = 0	R^2 = 0.01[d]	SB = 0	SB = 0.153[b]
Self-Progress	Self-Future	Self-Best	A = 0	A = 0
			ws=o	WS = 0.095[c]
			E = 0	E = 0
A = 0	A = 0	A = 0	SE = 0.149[b]	SE = 0
WS = 0	WS = 0	WS = 0	SS = 0	SS = 0.092[d]
E = 0	E = 0	E = 0	R^2 = 0.28[a]	SW = 0.258[a]
SE = 0	SE = 0	SE = 0		R^2 = 0.37[a]
SS = 0	SS = 0	SS = 0		*N* = 341
R^2 = 0	R^2 = 0	R^2 = 0		

[a] $P \leqslant 0.001$
[b] $P \leqslant 0.005$
[c] $P \leqslant 0.01$
[d] $P \leqslant 0.05$
0 Significance level too low to enter equation

Nevertheless, similar relations were found in only 304 (32%) of the 952 sets of triples. I conclude, therefore, that the satisfaction and self-want discrepancy variables are not merely two measures of the same thing.

As indicated earlier, the predictive success and explanatory power of theories constitute reasonable and minimal measures of adequacy. Unfortunately, they do not constitute unambiguous measures. For example, one might be more interested in the comparative than in the absolute predictive success ratio of a theory. Does the theory have a success ratio better than chance, better than alternative available theories, or better than any logically possible alternatives? If one says success ratios should be better than chance, does that mean each prediction should have at most a 5% probability of success merely as a result of chance (i.e., the standard assumption about minimal statistical significance when testing particular hypotheses), that each prediction should have at least a 50% probability of success or, perhaps, that the total batting average of the theory, considering all the predictions derived from it, should be at least 50%? Exactly how should the infamous Principle of Indifference be applied here, if at all? I and others have shed enough ink on such questions in other places to allow me to neglect lengthy comment now. However, because I adopted the relatively naive adequacy measure of Reichenbach (1949) and there is so much more to be said about such things, at least this one paragraph seems warranted. (Interested readers can find my most relevant views on these issues in Michalos 1969, 1971, 1976, 1980b, 1980c, 1983b.)

In an extremely provocative article, Zajonc (1980, p. 151) claimed that,

Affect is considered by most contemporary theories to be postcognitive, that is, to occur only after considerable cognitive operations have been accomplished. Yet… [he concludes] that affect and cognition are under the control of separate and partially independent systems that can influence each other in a variety of ways, and that both constitute independent sources of effects in information processing.

Although I have scrupulously tried to avoid any direct reference to affect and its relations to cognition, a few words are in order. (I will have a detailed discussion of these issues in my book on *A Pragmatic Theory of Value.*)

Basically, I believe that *affect* is an *effect* of cognitive and, more precisely, conative operations, as well as a *cause* of a variety of actions broadly construed (i.e., including cognition). This is suggested by Figs. 3.1 and 3.2, but it is not made explicit. The perceptual core of MDT that is illustrated in Fig. 3.2 shows net satisfaction as the effect of several antecedents, while the full theory illustrated in Fig. 3.1 shows net satisfaction as the cause of action. My unstated assumption is that the causal antecedents specified in the basic hypotheses of MDT, H1-H6, are sufficient to produce any effects that are logically entailed by the concepts of satisfaction and happiness. Because any plausible conceptual analysis of net satisfaction and happiness would have to entail some reference to positive and negative affect, it follows that the working assumption of MDT is that any affective experiences connected to satisfaction and happiness are also caused by the antecedents specified in the theory.

Strictly speaking, then, the formulation of MDT that has guided this research is an oversimplification of my views about the relations between cognition, conation and affect. At this point my views are not entirely clear and it is, therefore, impossible for me to make MDT more precise. On the one hand, affect is a *signal* of previous cognition and conation; it is the felt aspect of thinking, wanting, needing and so on. On the other hand, affect is a *motivating force*; it is the felt aspect of attention, interest, purposiveness and so on. Research like that of Schwarz and Clore (1983) and Wills (1981) focuses on the motivating or causal nature of affect, while most of my research, including the present paper, has focused on the causal antecedents of affect insofar as affect is implied by satisfaction and happiness.

In his *magnum opus*, *The Principles of Psychology,* William James (1890) clearly recognized that cognitions are virtually always found fused with feelings and interests. So, theories that boldly (or naively) try to assign some priority to one or the other are almost certainly engaged in some sort of scientific oversimplification. James, of course, would have been the first to allow such speculation, for his view of theories was that "none is absolutely a transcript of reality, but any of them may be useful. Their great use is to summarize old facts and to lead to new ones." (From James' *Pragmatism* (1907) according to Barzun 1983, p. 86). It is in this spirit that MDT has been proposed, with its relatively primitive view of the relation between cognition and affect.

Finally, some mention should be made of the voluntarism which is at the heart of MDT and my own brand of pragmatic philosophy. It is a familiar fact of everyone's experience and a well-documented fact of psychological research that people can be persuaded or can persuade themselves to be more or less satisfied or happy with a wide variety of features of their lives (Diener 1984; Schwarz and Clore 1983; Fordyce 1983; Michalos 1985). At a minimum that implies that in some circumstances, some kind of cognitive activity has some kind of priority over some kind of affect. The particular kinds of cognitive activities and the resulting affective states posited by MDT have already been explained. What must be emphasized now is the immense practical significance of the proposed causal sequence. Insofar as MDT is a reliable and valid representation of reality, the idea of *managing* satisfaction and happiness is plausible. This, of course, has a bright as well as a dark side.

On the bright side, MDT provides a moderately confirmed theoretical justification for education and rational persuasion. After all, if peoples' satisfaction and happiness are functions of how they perceive and think about their own and others wants, needs, deserts, status, etc., then there is a fundamental role to be played by all (informal and formal) education institutions. People's satisfaction and happiness can be more or less cognitively well-founded, and reasonable people will want to be sure that they are essentially well-founded.

On the darker side, however, MDT provides the same moderately confirmed theoretical justification for those who are inclined, wittingly or not, to pernicious manipulation. Enough has been written about misleading advertising (Michalos 1980d) and the role of freedom of information in democracies (Galnoor 1977), to allow us to add nothing here. For our purposes, the important point is that the very same psychological processes that make it possible to rightly persuade people of things that are true, good and beautiful, also make it possible to wrongly persuade people of their opposites, falsehoods, evil and ugliness. Wills (1981) reviews a depressingly long list of studies showing that people's satisfaction can be increased by making "downward comparisons" with less fortunate others. It would be sad if this sort of satisfaction and happiness management caught on, and instead of trying to improve the world, most people merely tried to make themselves feel good by either actively inflicting or acquiescing while others inflicted hardship on relatively defenseless people. Wills' research suggests that this scenario is far from fantastic. Clearly, then, besides having a socio-psychological theory that assures us that people's satisfaction and happiness can be managed, we must have a theory of value and a moral theory to help us identify *good management* in the broadest sense of these terms. These latter theories I hope to provide in my treatise on value. The present version of MDT is a first installment.

Summary

In this article I have introduced a fairly thorough account of multiple discrepancies theory (MDT), briefly reviewed its historical antecedents and submitted it to some empirical testing. The tests were made on a sample of 700 undergraduate students from the University of Guelph's 1984 summer term. The main results were as follows:

(a) Of 2184 predictions made from MDT, 771 (35%) were successful;
(b) Of a subset of 528 predictions involving only effects of perceived discrepancies, 289 (55%) were successful;
(c) MDT explained 49% of the variance in reported happiness scores for the whole group, 53% in global satisfaction and 50% or more in seven out of twelve domain satisfaction scores;
(d) MDT was most successful in accounting for the variance in satisfaction with financial security (58%), paid employment (59%), recreation activity (56%), religion (62%) and self-esteem (58%);
(e) Prediction success rates from six discrepancy variables to the selfwants variable were higher than the rates from the same six variables to satisfaction and happiness, indicating that the impact of the six variables on our main dependent variables is most often indirect rather than direct;
(f) On average, the global satisfaction and happiness of females was influenced by satisfaction in more domains than that of males;
(g) In five out of six cases, MDT explained more of the variance in happiness and global satisfaction than an analytic model positing global well-being as a linear function of domain satisfactions;
(h) Some evidence was produced suggesting that in terms of relative explanatory power, a rank ordering may be formed with aspiration theory at the top, followed by the theories of social comparison, equity, person-environment fit and finally cognitive dissonance;

(i) The voluntaristic, pragmatic philosophy underlying MDT was emphasized, including its immense practical significance for good or evil.

Acknowledgements I would like to thank the following people for their help with various aspects of the research presented in this paper: all the instructors who let me use their class time to administer my questionnaire, F.M. Andrews, A. Dyer, H. Esser, W. Glatzer, H.J. Krupp. D.C. Poff, U.E. Simonis, and W. Zapf. Earlier versions were presented at the University of Mannheim, J.W. Goethe-University of Frankfurt and the International Institute for Environment and Society at the Wissenschaftszentrum Berlin. In all these places, I received helpful comments from people attending the seminars, for which I am very grateful.

Appendix A

See Tables 3.27, 3.28, 3.29, 3.30, 3.31, 3.32, 3.33, 3.34, 3.35, 3.36, 3.37, 3.38, 3.39, 3.40.

Appendix B

Definitions	
Health	The present state of your general, overall health (relatively free of common and chronic illnesses)
Financial security	How well your income (including investments, property, etc.) takes care of your daily needs and provides funds for unexpected or unplanned expenses
Family relations	Kind of contact and frequency of contact you have with your family members. This includes personal contact, phone calls, and letters
Paid employment	Any work for wages, salaries or fees
Friendship	Kind of contact and frequency of contact you have with your friends. This includes personal contact, phone calls, and letters
Housing	The present type, atmosphere and state of the home you live in at the time. Suitability of the home (e.g., apartment, house, farm, room, etc.)
Area you live in	The general place in which you live, including climate, location and lifestyle
Recreation activity	Personal recreation activities you engage in for pure pleasure when you are not doing normal daily chores or some type of work. This includes relaxing, reading, T.V., regular get togethers, church activities, arts and crafts, exercises, trips, etc.
Religion	Your spiritual fulfillment
Self-Esteem	How good you feel about yourself; your sense of self-respect
Transportation	In general, how well public and private transportation meets your needs (e.g., convenience, expense)

(continued)

(continued)

Definitions	
Education	Your formal education as provided in the university you are presently attending
No opinion	This is a catch-all box covering not applicable, can't remember, no comment, etc

References

Abbey, A., & Andrews, F. M. (1985). Modeling the psychological determinants of life quality. *Social Indicators Research, 16,* 1–34.

Abelson, R. P., et al. (eds.). (1968). *Theories of cognitive consistency: A sourcebook.* Chicago: Rand McNally and Co.

Adams, J. S. (1965). Inequity in social exchange. In L. Berkowitz (Ed.), *Advances in experimental social psychology* (pp. 267–300). New York: Academic Press.

Adams, J. S., & Freedman, S. (1976). Equity theory revisited: Comments and annotated bibliography. In L. Berkowitz, & E. Walster (Eds.), *Advances in experimental social psychology* (pp. 43–90). New York: Academic Press.

Anderson, A. B., Basilevski, A., & Hum, D. P. J. (1983). Measurement: Theory ́and techniques. In P. H. Rossi, J. D. Wright, & A. B. Anderson (Eds.), *Handbook of survey research* (pp. 231–287). New York: Academic Press.

Andrews, F. M., & Withey, S. B. (1976). *Social indicators of well-being.* New York: Plenum Press.

Appelgryn, A. E., & Plug, C. (1981). Application of the theory of relative deprivation to occupational discrimination against women. *South African Journal of Psychology, 11,* 143–147.

Barnett, L. R., & Nietzel, M. T. (1979). Relationship of instrumental and affectional behaviors and self-esteem to marital satisfaction in distressed and nondistressed couples. *Journal of Consulting and Clinical Psychology, 47,* 946–957.

Barzun, J. (1983). *A stroll with William James.* Chicago: University of Chicago Press.

Berkowitz, L. (1968). The study of urban violence: Some implications of laboratory studies of frustration and aggression. *American Behavioral Scientist, 11,* 14–17.

Bledsoe, J. C., Mullen, D. J., & Hobbs, G. J. (1980). Validity of the Mullen diagnostic survey for leadership improvement. *Perceptual and Motor Skills, 59,* 838–846.

Booth, R. F., McNally, M. S., & Berry, N. H. (1979). Hospital corpsmen perceptions of working in a fleet Marine force environment. *Military Medicine, 144,* 31–34.

Campbell, A. P., Converse, P. E., & Rodgers, W. L. (1976). *The quality of American life.* New York: Russell Sage Foundation.

Canter, D., & Rees, K. (1982). A multivariate model of housing satisfaction. *International Review of Applied Psychology, 31,* 185–208.

Caplan, R. D. (1979). Social support, person-environment fit, and coping. In L. A. Ferman, & J. P. Gordus (Eds.), *Mental health and the economy* (pp. 89–137). Kalamazoo, Michigan: Upjohn Institute.

Caplan, R. D. (1983). Person-environment fit: Past, present, and future. In C. L. Cooper (Ed.), *Stress research* (pp. 35–77). New York: Wiley.

Cherrington, D. J., & England, J. L. (1980). The desire for an enriched job as a moderator of the enrichment-satisfaction relationship. *Organizational Behavior and Human Performance, 25,* 139–159.

Cook, K. S. (1975). Expectations, evaluations, arid equity. *American Sociological Review, 40,* 372–388.
Crosby, F. (1976). A model of egoistical relative deprivation. *Psychological Review, 83,* 85–113.
Crosby, F. J. (1982). *Relative deprivation and working women.* New York: Oxford University Press.
Davis, J. A. (1959). A formal interpretation of the theory of relative deprivation. *Sociometry, 22,* 280–296.
Diener, E. (1984). Subjective well-being. *Psychological Bulletin, 95,* 542–575.
Duncan, O. D. (1975). Does money buy satisfaction? *Social Indicators Research, 2,* 267–274.
Edwards, W., & Tversky, A. (1967). *Decision making*. Middlesex: Penguin Books.
Festinger, L. (1957). *A theory of cognitive dissonance.* Stanford, California: Stanford University Press.
Fordyce, M. W. (1983). A program to increase happiness: Further studies. *Journal of Counseling Psychology, 30,* 483–498.
Galnoor, I. (ed.). (1977). *Government secrecy in democracies.* New York: Harper & Row, Publishers.
Glenn, N. D. (1981). The well-being of persons remarried after divorce. *Journal of Family Issues, 2,* 61–75.
Goodman, P. S. (1966). *A study of time perspective: Measurement and correlates (Doctoral Disseration, Cornell University).*
Goodman, P. S. (1974). An examination of referents used in the evaluation of pay. *Organizational Behavior and Human Performance, 12,* 170–195.
Goodman, P. S., & Friedman, A. (1971). An examination of Adams' theory of inequity. *Administrative Science Quarterly, 16,* 271–288.
Gottlieb, B. H. (1984). *Social support and the study of personal relationships.* Paper Presented at the Second International Conference on Personal Relationships, July 22–27, 1984, in Madison, WI.
Gurr, T. R. (1970). *Why men rebel.* Princeton, N.J: Princeton University Press.
Harrison, R. V. (1978). Person-environment fit and job stress. In C. L. Cooper. & R. Payne, (Eds.) *Stress at work* (pp. 175–205). New York: Wiley.
Harrison, R. V. (1983). The person-environment fit model and the study of job stress. In T. A. Beehr, & R. S. Bhagat (Eds.), *Human stress and cognition in organizations: An integrated perspective.* New York: Wiley.
Hatfield, E., Greenberger, D., Traupmann, J., & Lambert, P. (1982). Equity and sexual satisfaction in recently married couples. *Journal of Sex Research, 18,* 18–32.
Hatfield, J. D., & Huseman, R. C. (1982). Perceptual congruence about communication as related to satisfaction: Moderating effects of individual characteristics. *Academy of Management Journal, 25,* 349–358.
Harsanyi, J. C. (1982). Morality and the theory of rational behaviour. In A. Sen, & B. Williams, *Utilitarianism and beyond* (pp. 39–62). Cambridge: Cambridge University Press.
James, W. (1890). *The principles of psychology.* New York: Dover Publications. (reprinted 1950).
Kauder, E. (1965). *A history of marginal utility theory.* Princeton, NJ: Princeton Press.
Kuhn, A. (1974). *The logic of social systems.* San Francisco: Jossey-Bass.
Kurella, S. (1979). The social needs of patients and their satisfaction with medical care: a survey of medical inpatients in the community hospitals of the German Democratic Republic. *Academy Postgraduate Medical Education, 13A,* 737–742.
Land, K. C. (1969). Principles of path analysis. In E. F. Borgatta, & G. W. Bohrnstedt (Eds.), *Sociological methodology* (pp. 3–37). San Francisco: Jossey-Bass.
LaRocco, J. M., House, J. S., & French, J. R. P. (1980). Social support, occupational stress, and health. *Journal of Health and Social Behaviour, 21,* 202–218.
Lewin, K. et al. (1944). Level of aspiration. In J. McV. Hunt (Ed.), *Personality and behaviour disorders* (pp. 333–378). New York: Ronald Press Co.
Luce, R. D., & Raiffa, H. (1957). *Games and Decisions.* New York: John Wiley and Sons.

Merton, R. K., & A. S. Kitt, (1950). Contributions to the theory of reference group behavior. In R. K. Merton, & P. F. Lazarsfeld (Eds.), *Continuities in social research* (pp. 40–105).
Michalos, A. C. (1967). Postulates of rational preference. *Philosophy of Science, 34,* 18–22.
Michalos, A. C. (1969). *Principles of Logic*. Englewood Cliffs: Prentice-Hall.
Michalos, A. C. (1971). *The popper-carnap controversy*. Hague: Martinus Nijhoff.
Michalos, A. C. (1976). The morality of cognitive decision-making. In M. Brand, & D. Walton (Eds.), *Action theory* (pp. 325–340). Dordrecht: D. Reidel.
Michalos, A. C. (1978). *Foundations of decision-making*. Ottawa: Canadian Library of Philosophy.
Michalos, A. C. (1980a). Satisfaction and happiness. *Social Indicators Research, 8,* 385–422.
Michalos, A. C. (1980b), Philosophy of science: Historical, social and value aspects. In P. T. Durbin (Ed.), *A guide to the culture of science, technology and medicine* (pp. 197–281). New York: The Free Press.
Michalos, A. C. (1980b). A reconsideration of the idea of a science court. *Research in Philosophy and Technology, 3,* 10–28.
Michalos, A. C. (1980d) Advertising: Its logic, ethics and economics. In J. A. Blair, & R. H. Johnson (Eds.), *Informal logic,* (pp. 93–111). Inverness, CA: Edgepress.
Michalos, A. C. (1982a). The satisfaction and happiness of some senior citizens in rural Ontario. *Social Indicators Research, 11,* 1–30.
Michalos, A. C. (1982b). North American social report. *Economics, religion, and morality* (Vol. V). Dordrecht: D. Reidel.
Michalos, A. C. (1983a). Satisfaction and happiness in a rural northern resource community. *Social Indicators Research, 13,* 224–252.
Michalos, A. C. (1983b). Technology assessment, facts and values. In P. T. Durbin, & F. Rapp (Eds.), *Philosophy and technology* (pp. 59–81). Dordrecht: D. Reidel Publishing Co.
Michalos, A. C. (1985). Job satisfaction, marital satisfaction and the quality of life: A review and a preview. In F. M. Andrews (Ed.), *Research on the quality of life*. Ann Arbor: University of Michigan Press.
Oldham, G. R., et al. (1982). The selection and consequences of job comparisons. *Organizational Behavior and Human Performance, 29,* 84–111.
Oldham, G. R., & Miller, H. E. (1979). The effect of significant other's job complexity on employee reactions to work. *Human Relations, 32,* 247–260.
Oliver, R. L. (1980). A cognitive model of the antecedents and consequences of satisfaction decisions. *Journal of Marketing Research, 17,* 460–469.
Patchen, M. (1961). *The choice of wage comparisons*. Englewood Cliffs, N.J.: Prentice-Hall.
Reichenbach, H. (1949). *Theory of probability* (2nd ed.). Berkeley: University of California Press.
Reis, H. T. (1982). An introduction to the use of structural equations: Prospects and problems. *Review of Personality and Social Psychology, 3,* 255–287.
Rhyne, D. (1981). Bases of marital satisfaction among men and women. *Journal of Marriage and the Family, 43,* 941–955.
Rodman, H. (1963). The lower-class value stretch. *Social Forces, 42,* 205–215.
Ross, C. E., Mirowsky, J., & Duff, R. S. (1982). Physician status characteristics and client satisfaction in two types of medical practice. *Journal of Health and Social Behavior, 23,* 317–329.
Runciman, W. G. (1966). *Relative deprivation and social justice*. Berkeley: University of California Press.
Schuessler, K. F. (1982). *Measuring social life feelings*. San Francisco: Jossey-Bass Pub.
Schwarz, N., & Clore, G. L. (1983). Mood, misattribution, and judgments of well-being: Informative and directive functions of affective states. *Journal of Personality and Social Psychology, 45,* 513–523.
Shaftesbury, L. (1711). *An inquiry concerning virtue and merit (London).*
Suls, J., & Sanders, G. S. (1982). Self-evaluations through social comparison: A developmental analysis. *Review of Personality and Social Psychology, 3,* 171–197.

Turner, R. J., Frankel, B. G., & Levin, D. M. (1983). Social support: Conceptualization, measurements, and implications for mental health. *Research in Community and Mental Health, 3,* 67–111.

Veenhoven, R. (1984). *Conditions of Happiness*. Dordrecht: D. Reidel Pub. Co.

Walster, E., Berscheid, E., & Walster, G. W. (1976). New directions in equity research. In L. Berkowitz, & E. Walster (Eds.), *Advances in experimental social psychology* (pp. 1–42). New York: Academic Press.

Weaver, C. N. (1980). Job satisfaction in the United States in the 1970s. *Journal of Applied Psychology, 65,* 364–367.

Weintraub, Z. (1981). The relationship between job satisfaction and work performance. *Revista de Psihologia, 27,* 59–67.

Williams, Jr., R. M. (1975). Relative deprivation. In L. A. Coser (Ed.), *The idea of social structure: Papers in Honor of Robert K. Merton* (pp. 355–378). New York: Harcourt Brace Jovanovich.

Wills, T. A. (1981). Downward comparison principles in social psychology. *Psychological Bulletin, 90,* 245–271.

Wills, T. A. (1983). Social comparison in coping and help-seeking. In B. M. DePaulo, A. Nadler, & J. D. Fisher (Eds.), *New directions in helping, Volume 2: Help-seeking* (pp. 109–141). New York: Academic Press.

Zajonc, R. B. (1980). Feeling and thinking: Preferences need no inferences. *American Psychologist, 35,* 151–175.

Zedeck, S. (1971). Problems with the use of 'moderator' variables. *Psychological Bulletin, 76,* 295–310.

Zeller, R. A., & Carmines, E. G. (1980). *Measurement in the social sciences: the link between theory and data.* Cambridge: Cambridge University Press.

Chapter 4
A Feminist View of Women and Development

Alex C. Michalos

When I tell people I'm a feminist, they generally respond with a look of complete bewilderment. It's as if I had just told them I wear pantyhose. I don't. The world being as it is, the response is understandable. My impression is that most people, including most women, seem to think that feminists are relatively unattractive females who wish they were males. If this is the view of most people, then most people are wrong. Since feminism is, among other things, a political movement and a philosophy existing in some form in all parts of the globe and in all periods of recorded history, it would be silly for me to try to write on behalf of all feminists. Hence, as my title indicates, I will present a feminist view.

For me, feminism consists of a positive vision of the future, and a negative assessment of the present and past. Taking the bad news first, I think that to be a feminist one has to have taken a historical and contemporary look at societies around the world and come to the conclusion that women have been and are systematically oppressed by men. Virtually all of our basic institutions have been designed, more or less wittingly, to restrict the growth and development of women. This is true of education, science, religion, law and social custom. This is not the place for a lengthy bibliography, but it will be useful to mention some basic information.

Michalos, A.C.: 1988. A feminist view of women and development. Worldscape, 2, pp. 5–7.

A.C. Michalos (✉)
University of Northern British Columbia, Prince George, BC, Canada
e-mail: michalos@brandonu.ca

A.C. Michalos, *Development of Quality of Life Theory and Its Instruments*,
DOI 10.1007/978-3-319-51149-8_4

In 1983 the United Nations reported that "women do two-thirds of the world's work, receive only 10% of earnings paid and own only 1% of its property"[1] They also make up two-thirds of the world's illiterates.[2] Rough as such international statistics must be, these are shocking figures. However, in the context of other international and national data, they are believable. In the last issue of *Worldscape*, Dr. George Sorger[3] informed us of the great disparity in land ownership in Latin America. If the countries of the world are divided along a North-South axis, "the North constitutes less than one third of the world's population, [but] it possesses and disposes of more than 70% of the world's wealth".[4] The United States has only about 6% of the world's population, consumes over 40% of the world's resources and produces nearly half of the world's pollution.[5] In Canada today the richest fifth of our population owns about 70% of the total wealth.[6] In 1985, 13% of all Canadian families were classified in the low income or povertystricken category. "Families headed by female lone parents have by far the highest incidence of low income of all family types. Nearly half (48%) of all lone-parent families headed by women had low incomes in 1985".[7] Clearly, the wealth and resources of the world are distributed very unequally, heaping great benefits on relatively few people and great costs on relatively many people. In this context, the UN figures regarding the poorest of the poor are believable. The feminization of poverty that has been documented for Canadian women is part of a global phenomenon.

Many factors have contributed to the current impoverished status of women, but I only want to call your attention to a few items in support of my claim above regarding the contribution of institutionalised sexism. Louise Michelle Newman put together a collection of papers called *Men's Ideas/Women's Realities*.[8] It's a set of articles taken from *Popular Science Monthly* from about 1870–1915 documenting the scientific and literary climate that women faced during the Progressive Era as they struggled to be admitted to universities, to practice law and medicine, to vote

[1]National Action Committee on the Status of Women (1985): "The persistence of inequality", in D. Drache and D. Cameron (eds.), *The Other Macdonald Report*, (Toronto: James Lorimer, 1985), p. 98.

[2]*MATCH* Newspaper, November 1987.

[3]G. Sorger, "The problem of global hunger: examining two hypotheses, resources versus distribution", *Worldscape*, Vol. 1, Fall 1987, pp. 4–7.

[4]O. Adeniji, Presentation to the Third Working Session, *Symposium on Global Security for the Twenty-First Century*, (New York: United Nations, 1987), p. 109.

[5]A.C. Michalos, *North American Social Report*, Vol. 4, (D. Reidel, Dordrecht, 1981), p. 6.

[6]A.C. Michalos, "A Case for a progressive annual net wealth tax", *Public Affairs Quarterly*, (1988), forthcoming.

[7]S. Methot, "Low Income in Canada", *Canadian Social Trends*, (Spring, 1987), p. 2.

[8]L.M. Newman (ed.), *Men's ideas/Women's Realities*, New York: Pergamon Press, 1985), passim.

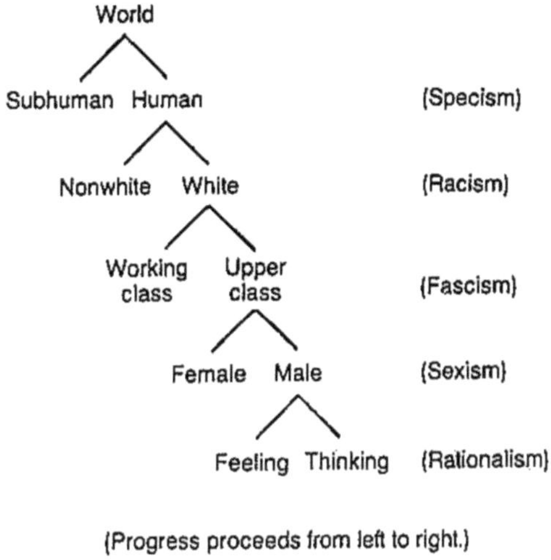

Fig. 4.1 Sun city plan of human development

and to get equal opportunities to work in all fields for the same wages as men. One really has to read the outrageous rationalisations of "the other side" to appreciate the battle, but brief mention of a couple of leading theories of the period might help.

The sociologist, Herbert Spencer—whose work most decidedly influenced ideas on progress and development—published a famous paper in 1873 called "Psychology of the Sexes".[9] The thesis was perfectly straightforward and directly devastating for women. Briefly, Spencer claimed that human growth and development required energy, and that any energy used in the development of female reproductive systems could not be used in the development of brains. Hence, women could be either completely developed females and intellectually dull, or they could be intellectually bright but incompletely developed females. Although the Church Fathers managed to think of Jesus of Nazareth as "fully God and fully man", the Fathers of science could not manage to think of females as "fully women and fully smart". Presumably, it was no accident that such doctrines came from the Fathers.

Those who hadn't heard of Spencer, the sociologist, had probably heard of Charles Darwin, the biologist, whose theories of evolution Spencer vulgarised. The theory of evolution generally attributed to Darwin (which is not to say every theory of evolution), with the help of such sources as the Bible, the works of Aristotle and Spencer may be regarded as a blueprint for what I have come to call *The Sun City Plan of Human Development* (see Fig. 4.1). In the Plan, there is a place for everything and everyone in a hierarchical scheme that leaves women exactly where Spencer left them. First, the world is divided into subhumans and humans, with the latter being obviously superior to the former. Nowadays, we call this *specism.* Within the class of humans, white people are supposed to be superior to nonwhite

[9]Reprinted in Newman, *op. cit.*, pp. 17–25.

people. Nowadays, we call this *racism*. Within the class of white folks, however, the working classes are not as good as the upper classes. That's the stuff of *fascism*. Within the upper classes, women are plainly inferior to men. That's *sexism*. Finally, the Plan asserts that among the fine upper class white men, some are "softheaded" and others are "hardheaded". (A nice metaphor that!) Since thinking is clearly superior to feeling, the hardheads, as the thinkers, are clearly superior to the softheads. That's the view philosophers call *rationalism*. Once one arrives at the lofty position of thorough rationalism, of course, one is home free. One's theory becomes completely impervious (I resist impenetrable) to the brute "facts of life".

Armed with the sociology and social psychology of Spencer and the biology of Darwin, the anti-progressives of the Progressive Era could boast that they had the support of the very latest and best science. Anti-progressives today do not have such clear sailing, but they are not totally adrift. Today the apparent heirs of the Spencerian-Darwinian metaphysical legacy are defending a new synthesis called sociobiology.[10] Although there never was, nor will be a person developed without any social and environmental influences, the heirs continue to publish their errors.

In summary, the negative case shows that because women have been oppressed by institutionalised male-dominated education, science, religion, law and social custom, I think it is imperative to acknowledge this fact. This is a necessary condition for developing a feminist consciousness in people, and the latter is necessary for improving the human condition of men and women.

To move on to the positive view of feminism, I should say first of all that all of my research on personal satisfaction and happiness indicates that the pursuit of achievable goals is absolutely necessary.[11] People must have a vision of the good life, of what they want out of life, in order to be happy or satisfied. To a significant extent, personal satisfaction and happiness with one's job, marriage, housing, social status, etc., is a function of realising one's goals. Thus, it is vitally important to have a vision of the good life, for ourselves and those around us.

My feminist vision is that of a future society where men and women live together as equals, equals in the workplace and at home. It is a society in which women and men are granted equal status as human beings and equal opportunities for growth and development. In the end, it is a society where feeling is granted equal status with thinking, and where people care about other people in much the same way that they care about themselves. It is beyond the Great Society of Lyndon Johnson and the Just Society of Pierre Trudeau. It is a vision of a compassionate society.

As a matter of fact, this feminist vision of a good life and a compassionate society is consistent with the visions articulated by several UN sponsored commissions. At least since the beginning of the 1980s, the links between development,

---

[10]E.O. Wilson, *Sociobiology: The New Synthesis*, (Cambridge: Harvard University Press, 1975), *passim*.

[11]For example, see A.C. Michalos, *Integrated Development Planning Using Socio-Economic and Quality of Life Indicators*, (Paris: UNESCO, 1986).

disarmament, environment and global security have been well-known. For example, see the 1981 report of the UN Expert Group on the Relationship between Disarmament and Development (the Thorsson Commission) or the 1980 report of the Independent Commission on International Development Issues (the Brandt Commission). The Chairperson of the World Commission on Environment and Development (the Brundtland Commission) wrote that

> the 'environment' is where we all live, and 'development' is what we all do in attempting to improve our lot within that abode. The two are inseparable. Furthermore, development issues must be seen as crucial by the political leaders who feel that their countries have reached a plateau towards which other nations must strive. Many of the development paths of the industrialised nations are clearly unsustainable… Many critical survival issues are related to uneven development, poverty, and population growth…. What is needed now is a new era of economic growth—growth that is forceful and at the same time socially and environmentally sustainable.[12]

Emphasizing a standard feminist theme, the new growth and development called for in these international commissions rejects the Hobbesian view of the state of nature as one of all against all, and the natural necessity for competition, dominance and control. "True peace", Maharajakrishna Rasgotra wrote, "is the product of a general state of tranquillity among nations. It is a quest for justice, friendship and co-operation among nations. Such peace cannot come from competition for power and dominance—and that is what the arms race is all about. The era of peace will be inaugurated when the race for nuclear arms is halted".[13]

A former chairperson of Great Britain's Campaign for Nuclear Disarmament, Joan Ruddock, has pulled the various threads of this discussion together as follows:

> 1. If we want to promote peace, we have to find it in ourselves. This means rejecting militarism, racism, sexism, nationalism and elitism among leaders. It means working nonviolently and co-operatively.
> 2. We must make clear the links between the arms race, which is led and marketed by the developed world, and the poverty and starvation which prevail in the underdeveloped world.
> 3. We must take the trouble to maintain international links, providing crucial communications channels within the peace movement.
> 4. We must never hesitate to act because our action seems too small. We must never put aside anger and emotion, but instead channel them wisely.[14]

Having presented my negative assessment and positive vision in fairly global and abstract terms, it remains to outline some more concrete steps that might be taken in Canada to help create a world compatible with that vision. Briefly, I would

---

[12]World Commission on Environment and Development, "Chairperson's Forward", in Our Common Future, (Oxford: Oxford University Press, 1987), pp. xi–xii.

[13]M. Rosgotra, Presentation to the Third Working Session, *Symposium on Global Security for the Twenty-First Century*, loc. cit., p. 131.

[14]J. Ruddock, "Unilateral Initiatives: Theory and Practice", in T.L. Perry and J.G. Foulks (eds.), *End the Arms Race: Fund Human Needs*, (Vancouver: Gordon Soules Publishers, 1986), p. 206.

recommend, for example, the necessity of prioritizing women's issues at the municipal, provincial and federal levels of government including equal pay for work of equal value, abortion rights, day care, wife and child abuse, concern over the arms race and so forth, in order to bring women's issues and the vision of a compassionate society into the mainstream of Canadian politics and economics. We must recognize that women's role in society is not just as mother, wife and secondary income earner. Until government agencies and officials, men and even women realize that women, regardless of class, play productive roles in society and not just "proper" roles suited to a male-oriented world view, and that women should inherently have the same socioeconomic and political rights and considerations as their male counterparts, development for women will not be accomplished. *The Sun City Plan of Human Development* will only be further reinforced with detrimental results for society as a whole.

Chapter 5
Highlights of Four Volume Global Report on Student Well-Being

Alex C. Michalos

This research project began in 1983 with a grant from the Social Sciences and Humanities Research Council of Canada to test a theory I invented to explain human satisfaction and happiness.

The research ended in 1993 with the publication of the final volumes of *Global Report on Student Well-Being*, Michalos (1991a, b, 1993a, b).

Multiple Discrepancies Theory (MDT) posits that people's satisfaction and happiness with life as a whole and 12 specific domains of life (health, finances, family, job, friends, housing, living partner, recreation, religion, self-esteem, transportation and education) are functions of 7 perceived gaps; e.g., the gap between what people have and what they want to have, between what they have and what they think their neighbours have, what they have and think they need, what they have and think they deserve, what they have and expected to have by now, what they have and hope to have in the future, what they have and the best they ever had before.

I surveyed a sample of over 18,000 university students in 39 countries, requiring translation of my questionnaire into 22 languages.

This was the largest world survey of students ever undertaken by anyone, anywhere when it was taken.

At the time, about 80% of all research in social psychology was done using student samples and generally results with students are very similar to results with average citizens. In fact, it was possible to compare some of my results with national probability samples for Canada, the USA, Japan and 13 western European countries, and I found many similarities.

Michalos, A.C.: Highlights of four volume Global Report on Student Well-Being.

A.C. Michalos (✉)
University of Northern British Columbia, Prince George, BC, Canada
e-mail: michalos@brandonu.ca

A.C. Michalos, *Development of Quality of Life Theory and Its Instruments*,
DOI 10.1007/978-3-319-51149-8_5

On average, men and women reported highest levels of satisfaction from family relations and living partners, and lowest levels of satisfaction from their finances and transportation.

On average, people in relatively developed countries reported higher levels of satisfaction than people in less developed countries, for interpersonal relationships as well as material goods satisfaction.

On average, for 12 specific domains of life, women had higher levels of satisfaction than men.

On average, for 12 domains of living, the top 10% of countries were Bahrain, Finland, Netherlands and Philippines; the bottom 10% were Cameroon, Turkey, Japan and Korea.

Canada and the USA were in the top half of the 39 countries.

The USA had higher average satisfaction scores than Canada in 12 of 14 areas of life, including life as a whole.

Canada had a higher average satisfaction score than the USA only in the domain of living partner.

On average, MDT was most successful at explaining satisfaction with living partners, jobs and religion, and least successful at explaining overall happiness with life.

On average, MDT explained about 55% of the variation in reported satisfaction and happiness scores, reaching as high as 71% for living partner satisfaction and as low as 41% for overall happiness with life.

MDT was slightly more successful explaining satisfaction in relatively developed than in less developed countries, though it was very successful over a wide variety of countries such as Finland, Bangladesh, Korea, New Zealand and Tanzania.

On average, only about 2% of the variation in reported satisfaction scores could be explained by culture, ethnicity or country of birth.

On average, for 12 domains of living and life as a whole, the most influential predictors of satisfaction and happiness were the gaps between what one has and wants (goal achievement), and the gap between what one has and one's neighbours have (social comparison).

For men, social comparison was most important; for women, goal achievement was most important.

For men and women, following goal achievement and social comparisons, considerations of need was more important than considerations of equity, though women gave more weight to need and men gave more weight to equity.

In 8 of 14 areas, the most influential predictors of satisfaction and happiness for Canadians were the goal achievement gaps followed by social comparison.

In 10 of 14 areas, the most influential predictors of satisfaction and happiness for Americans were the social comparison gaps followed by goal achievement.

In 14 of 14 areas, Finns were more influenced by goal achievement than by social comparison.

In 11 of 14 areas, Japanese were more influenced by goal achievement than by social comparison.

Regarding the 12 specific domains of life studied, for students who were unmarried and unemployed, the satisfaction they got from their university education was the most influential predictor of their satisfaction with life as a whole.

Regarding the 12 specific domains of life for married and/or full-time employed students, both males and females, satisfaction with their living partner contributed most to their happiness.

A detailed summary of some points from the 4 volumes follows below. Some examples will make the tables clear.

Table 5.1 provides summaries of results for the highest scoring countries in all four volumes. We begin with Volume 4 because the display was easiest to organize from that perspective. The first column under Religion, "Egy 6.5 O > W" is short for "On a 7-point satisfaction scale running from 1 = the most dissatisfying to 7 = the most satisfying, the Egyptian sample average was 6.5 and the most influential predictor was the social comparison gap (O) followed by the goal achievement gap (W)".

In the same column,

MIV	T	M	F
	O	O	W
	W	W	O

means that the Most Influential Predictor Variable (MIV) for the Total sample (T) and for Males (M) reading down was social comparison (O) followed by goal achievement (W), while for Females (F) reading down it was goal achievement (W) followed by social comparison (O). Where the equals (=) sign appears, the scores were the same. The letters 'na' mean no figures are available.

Results for Canada and the USA are given for each domain because most Canadians are probably most interested in comparing these 2 countries.

Of the 39 countries in my study, the only names listed below are those with average satisfaction scores in the top 10% for all countries.

The country abbreviations are:

Bah = Bahrain	Tai = Taiwan	Jor = Jordan
Tan = Tanzania	Phi = Philippines	Fin = Finland
PR = Puerto Rico[a]	US = USA	Can = Canada
Net = Netherlands	Gre = Greece	Por = Portugal
Bra = Brazil	NZ = New Zealand	Swe = Sweden
Bel = Belgium	Col = Colombia	Ban = Bangladesh
Isr = Israel	Egy = Egypt	Mex = Mexico

[a]Puerto Rico is Strictly a US protectorate

Table 5.1 Summary of top 10% country results for all domains and global variables, averages for total samples and most influential predictors

Volume 4			
Religion	Education	Recreation	Health
Egy 6.5 O > W	Tan 5.5 W > O	Por 5.5 O > W	Bra 5.9 W > O
Bah 6.4 W > O	Phi 5.4 W > O	Fin 5.4 W > O	Fin 5.8 W > O
Tai 6.2 O > W	PR 5.4 W > O	Net 5.3 W > O	Gre 5.8 O > W
Jor 5.9 O > W	US 5.3 W > O	Phi 5.3 O > W	Bah 5.6 W > O
			Net 5.6 W > O
			PR 5.6 W > O
MIV-T M F	MIV-T M F	MIV-T M F	MIV-T M F
O O W	W W W	W W =	W W W
W W O	O O O	O O =	O O O
Can 4.7 O > W	Can 5.1 W > O	Can 5.0 W > O	Can 5.5 W = O
US 4.9 O > W	US 5.3 W > O	US 5.2 O > W	US 5.5 W > O
Volume 3			
Employment	Finances	Housing	Transportation
Tai 6.6 W > O	Bah 5.1 O > W	Bra 5.4 O > W	Fin 4.8 W > O
Fin 5.0 W > O	Fin 4.8 W > O	Fin 5.4 W > O	US 4.8 W > O
Por 4.9 W > O	Phi 4.7 O > W	PR 5.4 W > O	NZ 4.7 W > O
Swe 4.8 na		Bah 5.3 O > W	Por 4.7 W > O
		Bel 5.3 O > W	Swe 4.7 W > O
		Col 5.3 na	
MIV-T M F	MIV-T M F	MIV-T M F	MIV-T M F
O O W	O O =	O O O	W O W
W W O	W W =	W W W	O W O
Can 3.8 O > W	Can 4.0 O > W	Can 5.1 W > O	Can 4.6 O > W
US 4.3 O > W	US 4.3 O > W	US 5.2 W > O	US 4.8 W > O
Volume 2			
Family	Friends	Partner	Self-esteem
Bah 5.8 O > W	Bah 5.7 W > O	Fin 6.1 W > O	Bra 5.8 O > W
Fin 5.7 W > O	Phil 5.7 O > W	Bah 5.9 na	Bah 5.7 O > W
Jor 5.7 O > W	US 5.6 O > W	Tai 5.9 W > O	Jor 5.6 O > W
Ban 5.6 W > O	Can 5.5 W > O		
Bra 5.6 W > O	Bel 5.5 na		
Isr 5.6 O > W	Egy 5.5 O > W		
	Jor 5.5 O > W		
MIV-T M F	MIV-T M F	MIV-T M F	MIV-T M F
O O O	O O W	O O O	O O O
W W W	W W O	W W W	W W W
Can 5.4 W > O	Can 5.5 W > O	Can 5.4 O > W	Can 5.1 O > W
US 5.5 O > W	US 5.6 O > W	US 5.3 W > O	US 5.2 O > W

(continued)

Table 5.1 (continued)

Volume 1			
Life Satisfaction	Happiness	12 Variable Averages	
Fin 5.4 W > O	US 5.3 O > W	Bah 5.4	Can 4.9
US 5.3 O > W	Net 5.2 W > O	Fin 5.3	US 5.1
UK 5.2 O > W	Swe 5.2 W > O	Net 5.2	
Net 5.2 W > O	UK 5.2 O > W	Phi 5.2	
PR 5.2 W > O	Mex 5.2 W > O		
		14 Dependent Variables	
MIV-T M F	MIV-T M F	MIV-T M F	
W W W	O O O	= O W	
O O O	W W W	= W O	
Can 5.1 W > O	Can 5.1 W > O	Can 8/14 W > O	
US 5.3 O > W	US 5.3 O > W	US 10/14 O > W	

Table 5.2 lists all the participating countries' mean and standard deviation scores for satisfaction and happiness with life as a whole, and Pearson correlations among the scores. Table 5.3 lists the percent of variance explained in life satisfaction and happiness scores by MDT for all the countries, totals, males and females.

Table 5.2 Participating countries' mean and standard deviation scores for satisfaction and happiness with life as whole, and Pearson correlations

Country	Satisfaction		Happiness		Pearson correlation between satisfaction and happiness[b]
	Mean	SD	Mean		
Austria	4.92	1.01	4.48	1.12	0.65
Bahrain	4.96	1.22	4.86	1.30	0.55
Bangladesh[a]	4.31	1.10	5.00	1.16	0.68
Belgium	5.21	0.80	4.99	1.07	0.62
Brazil	4.94	1.02	5.04	1.11	0.59
Cameroon	4.12	0.90	4.02	0.96	0.34
Canada	5.11	0.94	5.06	1.20	0.67
Chile	4.97	0.84	4.70	1.03	0.49
Colombia	5.12	0.86	5.02	1.10	0.60
Egypt[a]	4.55	1.06	4.44	1.12	0.52
Finland	5.44	0.99	5.01	1.16	0.67
Germany	4.84	0.96	4.97	1.11	0.61
Greece	4.83	0.90	4.42	0.92	0.53

(continued)

Table 5.2 (continued)

Country	Satisfaction		Happiness		Pearson correlation between satisfaction and happiness[b]
	Mean	SD	Mean		
Hungary	4.77	0.72	4.52	0.96	0.63
India[a]	4.72	1.09	4.82	1.43	0.48
Israel	4.98	0.85	4.58	1.39	0.50
Japan	4.09	1.05	4.49	1.11	0.49
Jordan	4.49	1.12	4.53	1.19	0.52
Kenya[a]	4.46	1.01	4.46	1.11	0.58
Korea	4.21	1.50	4.38	1.17	0.57
Mexico	5.12	0.79	5.17	1.09	0.52
Netherlands	5.17	1.02	5.23	1.08	0.72
New Zealand	5.06	0.96	5.07	1.22	0.69
Norway	5.14	0.89	4.96	1.02	0.53
Philippines	5.02	0.92	4.90	1.11	0.55
Portugal	3.26	1.52	2.25	1.66	na
Puerto Rico	5.18	0.94	5.02	1.17	0.56
Singapore	4.76	0.95	4.73	1.00	0.65
S. Africa	4.53	1.14	4.37	1.17	0.49
Spain	4.55	0.89	4.52	0.94	0.48
Sweden	4.96	1.09	5.19	1.21	0.67
Switzerland	5.08	0.83	4.95	1.06	0.67
Taiwan	4.35	0.95	4.56	1.21	0.50
Tanzania[a]	4.97	1.23	4.95	1.22	0.65
Thailand	4.61	0.94	4.07	1.05	na
Turkey[a]	4.21	1.02	4.61	1.09	0.63
U. Kingdom	5.20	0.87	5.22	1.11	0.65
USA	5.28	1.00	5.27	1.20	0.67
Yugoslavia	4.70	1.14	4.54	1.22	0.62
Total Mean	4.77	1.00	4.70	1.14	0.58
Dev.C. Mean	4.82	0.99	4.70	1.13	0.58
L.D.C. Mean	4.54	1.09	4.71	1.19	0.59
World	4.76	1.11	4.71	1.27	0.59

[a]Below 142-country median on per capita GNP and literacy rate
[b]$p < 0.001$
Source Michalos (1991a)

Table 5.3 Percent of variance explained by MDT in life satisfaction and happiness

Country	Satisfaction			Happiness		
	Total	Males	Females	Total	Males	Females
Austria	56	58	57	46	57	38
Bahrain	37	–	33	47	–	44
Bangladesh[a]	54	54	50	57	58	56
Belgium	40	–	–	31	–	
Brazil	42	–	45	32	28	34
Cameroon	31	29	–	33	35	–
Canada	42	44	41	45	48	44
Chile	39	37	39	31	34	33
Colombia	–	–	–	–	–	–
Egypt[a]	33	35	36	37	42	32
Finland	67	72	64	42	34	46
Germany	39	41	38	38	43	33
Greece	32	–	28	29	–	29
Hungary	35	–	30	44	–	41
India[a]	36	30	–	46	46	–
Israel	32	37	28	32	26	40
Japan	41	41	40	36	35	33
Jordan	39	40	–	40	41	–
Kenya[a]	52	49	56	54	61	50
Korea	30	29	–	32	29	–
Mexico	38	37	–	33	26	–
Netherlands	48	39	55	52	57	49
New Zealand	47	29	55	41	24	50
Norway	38	–	33	36	–	35
Philippines	35	46	29	30	38	26
Portugal	43	40	–	13	19	–
Puerto Rico	44	37	49	46	35	49
Singapore	49	–	47	58	–	57
S. Africa	33	37	28	32	45	25
Spain	39	39	37	37	48	28
Sweden	56	65	43	46	56	34
Switzerland	50	54	44	48	49	46
Taiwan	34	37	32	35	36	35
Tanzania[a]	65	69	–	74	73	–
Thailand	30	34	27	32	21	43
Turkey[a]	45	44	–	43	39	–
U. Kingdom	34	35	30	37	35	33
USA	48	43	50	43	46	41
Yugoslavia	40	38	48	41	25	61

(continued)

Table 5.3 (continued)

Country	Satisfaction			Happiness		
	Total	Males	Females	Total	Males	Females
Total Mean	42	43	41	40	40	40
Dev.C.Mean	41	42	39	37	37	40
L.D.C.Mean	48	47	48	52	53	46
World	45	47	44	42	41	44

[a]Below 142-country median on per capita GNP and literacy rate
Source Michalos (1991a)

References

Michalos, A.C. (1991a). *Global report on student well-being, Volume 1: Life satisfaction and happiness*. New York: Springer.
Michalos, A.C. (1991b). *Global report on student well-being, Volume 2: Family, friends, living partner and self-esteem*. New York: Springer.
Michalos, A.C. (1993a). *Global report on student well-being, Volume 3: Employment, finances, housing and transportation*. New York: Springer.
Michalos, A.C. (1993b). *Global report on student well-being, Volume 4: Religion, education, recreation and health*. New York: Springer.

Chapter 6
Comments on Papers for the Special Issue on Global Report on Student Well-Being

Alex C. Michalos

All of the papers published in this issue of *Social Indicators Research* have some relation to my four-volume *Global Report on Student Well-Being* Michalos (1991a, b, 1993a, b), and the papers are followed by brief reviews of each volume. Below I will make some comments on each paper. The only comment I want to make about the reviews concerns the fact that no summaries of Multiple Discrepancies Theory (MDT) or the data-collection methodology appear in the final three volumes of the treatise. Since the reviewers of each of these volumes independently reached the conclusion that such summaries were needed, I can only conclude that they were right. Even though it took me four volumes to tell my story, I was seriously pressed for space. I thought that most readers of the volumes would be familiar with MDT while very few readers would have seen the global data-set and the hundreds of results cranked out of it. Apart from my own material, I wanted to provide a thorough review of the most recent work on satisfaction with life as a whole and the 12 specific domains of life that I examined. I tried but failed to think of a brief way to present appropriate summaries. Now I wish I had tried harder.

The entire data-set for 39 countries and over 18,000 undergraduates is available at nominal cost from me on 13 diskettes. It is also archived at the University of Alberta's population data-bank, which can be accessed directly through Internet. I would be glad to provide parts of the data-set in case anyone has a particular interest in one or only a few of the countries studied. Besides the data, I have copies of my original English questionnaire translated into 22 languages. For people interested in cross-cultural research on subjective well-being (SWB) or objective

Michalos, A.C.: 1995. Comments on papers for the Special Issue on Global Report on Student Well-Being. Social Indicators Research, 34, pp. 1–6. © Kluwer Academic Publishers 1995.

A.C. Michalos (✉)
University of Northern British Columbia, Prince George, BC, Canada
e-mail: michalos@brandonu.ca

A.C. Michalos, *Development of Quality of Life Theory and Its Instruments*,
DOI 10.1007/978-3-319-51149-8_6

well-being (OWB), these translations can provide a good starting point for new projects.

Finally, I want to thank all the contributors to this issue, including my Book Review Editor, Doh C. Shin, who managed to get all the reviews in on relatively short notice.

In Vol. 1 (pp. 87, 124–125) I mentioned the problem that several other researchers had also found regarding the relatively lower SWB scores of Japanese samples compared to American samples in the presence of relatively similar OWB scores measured by per capita income. The paper by Diener, Suh, Smith and Shao addresses this problem in considerable detail using my samples of undergraduates in two Pacific Rim countries (South Korea and Japan) and the United States, and new samples of undergraduates in these countries plus the People's Republic of China. To my knowledge, these researchers examine more alternative possible explanations of the phenomena in question than any other researchers to date. To some extent, among many other things, their results support the general cognitivist view of SWB because they found that norms for both feeling and expressing SWB were good predictors of reported SWB. They correctly wrote that "we cannot be certain from the present data about the causal direction between the norms and the affect which is experienced. The question of whether the norms cause levels of SWB, or follow from them, is an extremely important one." As usual, I think it would be wise to suppose that the causal arrows go in both directions, and to design models and tests for that assumption. We already have evidence showing that the causal arrows run in both directions for job satisfaction (Vol. 1: pp. 55–56; Vol. 3: pp. 5–6) and satisfaction with one's own health (Vol. 4: pp. 11–15).

The paper by Veenhoven compares the performance of three types of explanatory theories (comparison-theory, folklore-theory and livability-theory) using my undergraduate data-set for 38 countries and a general population data-set drawn from several studies in 28 countries. Although he tells us that, according to his definition, comparison-theories "are one-sided cognitive theories of happiness that ignore the affective-motivational part of human nature", I think he would classify MDT with such theories. That is anomalous since MDT explicitly takes account of the "affective-motivational part of human nature" in its use of goal/achievement or self/wants comparisons, but this is a minor issue. However, there are a couple major issues about which we disagree.

First, Veenhoven assumes that human needs can be specified in some relatively objective way that makes them a relatively better basis than personal perceptions for comparing the quality of people's lives. To put this in a slightly different way, he thinks people's OWB is a better predictor of SWB than any of their subjective/judgmental features. In Michalos (1978) I argued that the specification of human needs suffers from the same value-laden problems as the specification of human wants, and therefore needs do not provide any more objective basis than wants for studying the quality of life.

Veenhoven and I agree that theories should be tested by examining their predictive success, among other things of course. What I found most interesting about his paper is his approach to such examination. In my *Global Report* I measured predictive success by calculating the ratio of successful to total individual predictions from MDT. Veenhoven's approach is to select a salient subset of logical consequences of the alternative theories and to compare the predictive success of each theory for that set of consequences. The result of this approach is that livability-theory appears to perform better than the other two theories. This implies that people's OWB is a better predictor of SWB than any of their comparison judgments, and that is anomalous because we have mountains of evidence showing precisely the opposite. In the vast majority of studies, relatively subjective features are much better predictors of happiness than relatively objective features.

I am not sure about the best way to dispose of this apparent discrepancy between our two approaches. I have some doubts about relying on zero-order comparisons as much as Veenhoven's approach requires and I certainly prefer multiple regression as a general technique for measuring the relative impact of different predictors. But some of Veenhoven's analyses seem too straightforward to be challenged by such doubts and preferences. Perhaps the best way to eliminate the discrepancy is to challenge his assumption that comparison-theory implies that "reference is random". This assumption is contrary to every particular articulation of such a theory and every empirical test that I have seen. Most people see themselves or their situations as at least as good as average others, and most people do not select comparison groups at random. For examples, see Vol. 1: pp. 50–51, 124–125; Vol. 2: pp. 8–13; Vol. 3: pp. 6–7, 20; Vol. 4: pp. 13–14. If this assumption is abandoned, then comparison-theory does not have most of the consequences Veenhoven derived from it.

The paper by Lance, Clack and Michalos provides the most extensive direct test ever made of three familiar alternative models of the relationships between domain satisfaction and satisfaction with life as a whole. The traditional Bottom-Up (BU) model posits life satisfaction as a linear function of the satisfaction obtained in diverse domains of life (health, family relations, etc.). The Top-Down (TD) model posits satisfaction obtained in diverse domains as a linear function of life satisfaction, and the Bidirectional (BD) model posits causal arrows running in both directions. The analysis was based on the American undergraduate data-set drawn for my *Global Report* and eleven domains of life were considered. Generally speaking, the paper shows that TD performed better than BU and that BD performed best of all. The relative performance of TD compared to BU is remarkable given the vast literature confirming our hypothesis that overall life satisfaction must be some sort of summary of the satisfaction people get from various domains of living. Now we know that much more attention must be paid to causal influences running in the opposite direction, and better still, to bidirectional models.

I would like to make two cautionary observations about this paper. First, while it is true that MDT posits perceived discrepancies as a function of objective discrepancies (i.e., what is in our heads as a function of what is outside in the "real" world), there is an important loop in the theory that indicates that the "real" world is to some extent a function of and constructed by human action. This is explained in some detail in Vol. 1: pp 54–58. Second, while the paper refers to traits, dispositions and heredity as possible mechanisms to explain people's overall satisfaction with life as a whole, for reasons explained in Vol. 1: pp. 16–17, I do not have much confidence in such hypotheses. I have more confidence in the sort of halo effect hypotheses suggested in the paragraph immediately following the one mentioning traits and so on. In particular, I suspect that people's cognitive, affective and conative states are mixed together in a kind of psychological stew, and that what we see depends on the particular instruments used to sample it. Again, however, unlike ordinary soup spoons that simply scoop up whatever is in the pot, I think the sampling devices we use partially construct what is in the pot.

The paper by Staats, Armstrong-Stassen and Partlo compares American and Canadian samples of undergraduates from the original data-set in 1984 with a new data-set in 1992. "In general," they wrote, "student perceptions of well-being seem poorer now than in the past." This paper is especially important because it provides additional support for the hypothesized relationships between the predictors self-esteem and social support in the context of the total configuration of MDT's predictors, and satisfaction and happiness. Besides this, the paper continues the pioneering work Staats has done developing a measure of hopefulness and applying it to studies of SWB.

The paper by Osseiran-Waines compares the Bahraini undergraduate sample drawn for my *Global Report* with a 1992 sample drawn from the same university. Originally I hoped to have papers like this one for each of the countries in my global sample. I knew that my appreciation of the cultures and current events in many of my undergraduate samples was very limited, and I was sure that scholars on the scene would be able to provide information and insights that I just did not have. Osseirian-Waines has proved that I was right and she provided precisely the sort of information I hoped to see. It was good to see that MDT still performed well on the new Bahraini sample, but even better to see the more detailed information about student attitudes toward religion and the impact of religious beliefs on SWB. Because MDT includes only predictors that have usually shown a fairly consistent impact on SWB across a variety of populations, it does not include any measure of religious commitment among its conditioners. This paper reminds us that for some populations it would be very helpful to include such a conditioner.

The paper by Schulz compares the explanatory power of MDT to that of resource theory, using the Austrian undergraduate data-set from my *Global Report*. Like the previous paper by Osseirian-Waines, this paper provides additional information about a variety of features of students' lives, features that are not considered in MDT. Like the Veenhoven paper, this one also tends to expect more from relatively objectively measurable features of people's lives than anything postulated by MDT. MDT outperforms resource theory in this paper, given the latter's current set of specified resources. However, Schulz correctly points out that the latter's current set of predictors may be expanded in ways that increase its explanatory power.

References

Michalos, A. C. (1978). *Foundations of decision-making*. Ottawa: Canadian Library of Philosophy.
Michalos, A. C. (1991a). *Global report on student well-being, Volume 1: Life satisfaction and happiness*. New York: Springer.
Michalos, A. C. (1991b). *Global report on student well-being, Volume 2: Family, friends, living partner and self-esteem*. New York: Springer.
Michalos, A. C. (1993a). *Global report on student well-being, Volume 3: Employment, finances, housing and transportation*. New York: Springer.
Michalos, A. C. (1993b). *Global report on student well-being, Volume 4: Religion, education, recreation and health*. New York: Springer.

Chapter 7
Aspects of the Quality of Life in Prince George: A Case Study in Canada

Alex C. Michalos

Introduction

In September 1994, Canada opened its first new university in 25 years, the University of Northern British Columbia, at Prince George. This unique event provided the opportunity to try to assess the impact of a new university on the quality of life of residents in the host community. Thus, in the summer of 1994 the author undertook a survey in order to obtain baseline data that some future researcher might want to use as the "before" part of a before and after investigation. This paper reports the results of that survey. As the author was himself a new arrival in the community, most of the items used in the survey were of a general sort that had been used in other community surveys.

Measuring Tools and Sampling Procedure

Two thousand 8-page questionnaires were mailed to a systematically selected sample of Prince George's 72,000 residents in June 1994, roughly every 18th household listed in the local telephone book.

Michalos, A.C.: 1996. Aspects of the quality of life in Prince George. South Asian Journal of Psychology, 1, pp. 45–70.

A.C. Michalos (✉)
University of Northern British Columbia, Prince George, BC, Canada
e-mail: michalos@brandonu.ca

A.C. Michalos, *Development of Quality of Life Theory and Its Instruments*,
DOI 10.1007/978-3-319-51149-8_7

The first page contained a general question designed to measure the extent to which respondents' or their family members used 23 different public services. The response categories were "not at all = 1 point", "sometimes = 2" and "often = 3".

That was followed by a Question designed to measure the extent to which respondents would like to see "less = 1 point", "the same = 2" or "more = 3" of their tax dollars spent on each of the same 23 services.

The third and fourth pages listed 54 "things affecting people today", including the previously mentioned public services plus more personal things like family relations, health, jobs and so on. The extent to which people were satisfied with these things was measured on a 7-point Likert scale with response categories ranging from "very dissatisfied = 1 point", through "an even balance = 4", to "very satisfied = 7".

Following these questions, there was a 7-point question designed to measure the extent to which people were happy with their lives as a whole, ranging from "very unhappy 1 point", through "an even balance = 4", to "very happy = 7".

This was followed by two open-ended questions asking respondents, first, to describe the "best thing about living in this community", and then "the worst thing". Respondents were then asked, "If you could change anything about this community to improve the quality of life here, what would that change be?".

The fifth page of the questionnaire had 18 statements about which respondents were asked to indicate the extent of their agreement, with five response categories ranging from "strongly disagree = 1 point", through "don't know = 3", to "strongly agree = 5".

Following two pages of demographic questions, there was a page designed for people who had moved to Prince George "within the last 5 years". For each of 17 things, respondents were asked if they had any thoughts about it prior to moving. If they answered affirmatively, they were then asked if they expected things to be better and then they were asked if things actually were better.

By the end of July, 501 (25%) useable questionnaires were returned, which form the working data-set for the survey. Respondents included 299 (60%) females and 202 (40%) males. Three hundred and fifty (70%) were now married and living with their spouse. The average age was 43, with a range from 14 to 85. Four hundred and twenty-six (85%) owned or were in the process of buying their home. A full 234 (47%) had some university education, with 128 (26%) holding a university degree. The first language of 467 (93%) respondents was English. Two hundred and eighty one (56%) were employed full-time and 70 (14%) part-time. Two hundred and seventy-seven (55%) had total family incomes of $50,000 or more, with an average from $95,000 to $99,999. Three hundred and fifty-one (71%) had been living in Prince George over 5 years, with an average residence of 22 years. Of the 141 (29%) saying they moved to the city within the last 5 years, 138 came from somewhere in Canada. (Only 492 people answered the mobility question).

According to the 1991 census, 49% of the city's adult residents were female, 40% were married and living with their spouse, 68% owned or were in the process of buying their home and 87% had English as their first language. Broadly speaking, then, our working sample represents relatively long-term residents, with women and the upper half of the socio-economic spectrum over-represented.

Results and Discussion

The results of the present study are presented in the Tables 7.1, 7.2, 7.3, 7.4, 7.5, 7.6, 7.7, 7.8, 7.9, 7.10, 7.11, 7.12 and 7.13.

Table 7.1 lists the percent of respondents who personally or whose families used or contacted agencies often. The most frequently used community services (out of 23) within the last year were the municipal water system (91%), garbage collection (86%), sewage system (84%), parks and recreation (52%) and libraries (45%).

The least frequently used or contacted services were those of the departments of corrections, highways and fire (<l%), the ambulance service (1%). Police, public housing, elderly care and planning (2%).

Table 7.2 lists the percent of respondents asserting that less, the same or more tax dollars should be spent on each of the public services listed in Table 7.1. By far more people preferred to see more spending in the health field than anywhere else. Eighty-two percent wanted more tax money spent on local hospitals and clinics, and next to that 58% wanted more money spent on the public health service. Fifty-six percent wanted more money spent on police protection. Following these items 48% wanted more tax money spent on elementary and secondary education, and elderly care service.

Table 7.1 Percent of respondents who personally or whose families used or contacted agencies often (N = 491)

Used libraries	45
Used parks and recreation	52
Used hospitals and clinics	16
Used ambulance	1
Used elementary education	31
Used secondary education	22
Used College of New Caledonia	15
Used University of Northern B.C.	3
Used garbage collection	86
Used water system	91
Used sewage system	84
Used public housing	2
Used public welfare services	3
Contacted police department	2
Contacted fire department	<1
Contacted correctional dept	<1
Contacted highway dept	<1
Used elderly care service	2
Used child care service	−8
Contacted planning officials	2
Contacted federal gov. officials	3
Contacted provincial gov. off.	5
Contacted local gov. officials	3

Table 7.2 Percent of respondents asserting that less, more or the same amount of tax money should be spent on various services (N = 491)

	Less	Same	More
Libraries	6	76	18
Parks and recreation	4	65	31
Hospitals and clinics	2	16	82
Ambulance	2	74	24
Elementary education	6	46	48
Secondary education	6	47	48
College of New Caledonia	5	63	31
University of Northern B.C.	6	62	33
Garbage collection	10	86	5
Water system	3	87	9
Sewage system	3	88	8
Public housing	27	59	14
Public welfare services	60	33	7
Police protection	3	41	56
Fire protection	3	78	19
Correctional programs	38	51	12
Highways, streets and roads	3	51	46
Elderly care service	2	50	48
Child care service	15	54	32
Community planning	18	64	18
Federal gov. administration	76	23	1
Provincial gov. administration	75	24	1
Local gov. administration	62	35	3
Public health service	4	38	58

Percentages may not sum to 100 as a result of rounding figures

By far more people preferred to see less spending for federal (76%) and provincial (75%) government administration than for anything else, with local government administration (62%) and public welfare services (60%) close behind.

There was general agreement that spending was about right for the most frequently used public services; sewage (88%), water (87%) and garbage collection (86%), and nearly as much agreement that spending was about right for one of the least frequently used services, namely, that of the fire department (78%).

Table 7.3 lists the percent of respondents reporting that they were "very" or "somewhat dissatisfied" versus "very" or "somewhat satisfied" with 54 things affecting their lives, and mean satisfaction scores for these things. Highest mean levels of satisfaction were reported for satisfaction with respondents' living partners and spouses (6.1), followed closely by satisfaction with their family relations (5.9), friendships (5.8) and their housing (5.8). The relatively high levels of satisfaction with living partners, family and friends is typical of many studies around the world (Michalos 1991a, 1993a).

Table 7.3 Percent of respondents reporting that they are very or somewhat dissatisfied versus very or somewhat satisfied with some things affecting their lives, and mean satisfaction scores (N = 485 unless indicated)

	Very or somewhat dissatisfied	Very or somewhat satisfied	Mean
Your family relations	2	71	5.9
Your living partner/spouse (N = 453)	5	79	6.1
Your job (N = 471)	6	59	5.4
Job opportunities	18	23	4.1
Your friendships	1	69	5.8
Your health	3	63	5.6
Your religion or spiritual fulfillment	2	52	5.4
Your standard of living	5	60	5.5
Your own house, apartment	3	68	5.8
Your neighbourhood	5	65	5.7
Friendliness of your neighbours	3	48	5.2
Your financial security	11	38	4.7
Your recreation activities	3	40	5.0
Your accomplishments	5	49	5.2
Your self-esteem	3	69	5.5
Your life as a whole	3	63	5.6
Your overall quality of life	1	63	5.7
Your overall happiness	2	67	5.6
City of Prince George	3	58	5.5
The beauty of Prince George	16	25	4.2
Parks and recreation	4	33	4.9
Prince George's location	8	34	4.7
Average weather here	8	24	4.4
Elementary education	16	18	4.0
College of New Caledonia	4	24	4.6
University of Northern B.C. (N = 469)	5	31	4.7
Libraries	4	48	5.3
Hospitals and clinics	28	14	3.6
Public health service	9	18	4.3
Ambulance service	4	24	4.5
Planning/zoning regulations	13	13	4.0
Public transportation in P.G.	19	16	3.9
Street lighting	13	17	4.1
Traffic congestion	5	30	4.6

(continued)

Table 7.3 (continued)

	Very or somewhat dissatisfied	Very or somewhat satisfied	Mean
Number of motor vehicle accidents	36	2	2.9
Highways, streets and roads	21	9	3.6
Sidewalks and pedestrian walkways	12	23	4.2
Noise levels here	9	18	4.2
Local housing conditions	6	19	4.4
Public housing (N = 474)	8	6	3.9
Garbage collection	2	41	5.1
Quality of water	12	35	4.6
Sewage system	2	35	4.9
Children's play areas	7	27	4.6
Child care service (N = 481)	10	9	4.0
Elderly care service (N = 480)	15	8	3.8
Shopping facilities	21	22	4.0
Amount of taxes you pay	43	8	2.9
Judicial services	31	6	3.2
Police protection	9	25	4.4
Correctional programs	14	10	3.8
Drug and alcohol abuse here	51	1	2.5
Federal gov. officials	35	4	3.0
Provincial gov. officials	36	4	3.0
Local gov. officials	22	9	3.5

The average scores for the 7-point scales of happiness and satisfaction with life as a whole were the same 5.6, indicating most people were a little to somewhat happy and satisfied with their lives. Using the same happiness scale in 1985 on 18,000 university undergraduates in 39 countries, the average score was 4.7 (Michalos 1991a, b). For Canadian undergraduates, the average was 5.1, compared to 5.0 for students in Bangladesh, 4.8 in India, 4.7 in Singapore and 4.1 in Thailand (Michalos 1991a, b). For an adult sample from the Town of Cochrane, Ontario in 1982, it was 5.3 (Michalos 1983). For a sample of Ontario rural seniors in 1981, it was 5.3 (Michalos 1982). For a sample of the University of Guelph office, clerical and technical staff in 1979, it was 5.4 (Michalos 1980). Compared to all the other groups, then, the PG sample was happier on average, which is what one would have expected, given the over representation of the relatively well-off segment of PG and other studies of the modest but positive association between income and a variety of measures of subjective well-being (Michalos 1991a, b).

The average score for the 7-point scale regarding people's satisfaction with the overall quality of their lives was 5.7. As Table 7.7 shows, the three global subjective well-being measures were fairly well correlated at the 99% level of confidence: life satisfaction with the quality of life (r = 0.59) and with happiness (r = 0.43), and happiness with the quality of life (r = 0.46).

Highest levels of reported dissatisfaction were given for drug and alcohol abuse in the city (2.5), number of motor vehicle accidents and amount of taxes paid (2.9), and federal and provincial government officials (3.0).

Table 7.4 lists the results of correlating scores (Pearson product-moment correlations) for usage of public services, spending preferences and levels of satisfaction. Because relatively higher levels of use, preferences for more spending and higher levels of satisfaction are all indicated by larger numbers, positive correlations among these things indicate that they are directly related and negative correlations indicate that they are inversely related. The first thing to be noticed about these correlations is that on average their absolute values are fairly small. The average correlation between use and spending scores was r = 0.12, between

Table 7.4 Correlations among scores for usage of public services, spending preferences and levels of satisfaction

	Use/spend	Spend/sat	Use/sat
Used libraries	0.26	ns	0.26
Used parks and recreation	0.17	−0.18	0.04
Used hospitals and clinics	0.16	−0.28	−0.06
Used ambulance	0.12	−0.18	ns
Used elementary education	0.29	−0.17	−0.06
Used secondary education	0.17	na	na
Used College of New Calendonia	0.20	0.08	0.11
Used University of Northern B.C.	0.11	0.21	0.06
Used garbage collection	0.07	−0.07	0.11
Used water system	0.02	−0.24	−0.06
Used sewage system	−0.07	−0.19	0.20
Used public housing	0.14	−0.12	−0.06
Used public welfare services	0.25	na	na
Contacted police department	0.06	−0.19	−0.03
Contacted fire department	−0.03	na	na
Contacted correctional dept.	0.13	0.14	0.02
Contacted highway dept.	0.05	−0.51	−0.07
Used elderly care service	0.06	−0.35	0.03
Used child care service	0.18	−0.36	0.03
Contacted planning officials	0.09	0.01	0.05
Contacted federal gov. officials	0.02	0.29	0.03
Contacted provincial gov. off.	0.07	0.35	0.12
Contacted local gov. officials	0.06	0.25	0.11

$P < 0.01$, *ns* not statistically significant, *na* not available for analysis. Generally, relatively higher levels of use. Preferences for more spending and higher levels of satisfaction are all indicated by larger numbers. So positive correlations indicate these things are directly related and negative correlations indicate these things are inversely related

spending and satisfaction r = 0.21, and between use and satisfaction r = 0.08. Even in the strongest case, then, only about 4% of the variance in spending preferences can be explained by satisfaction with the service. If this relationship is so weak, one wonders what exactly does motivate spending preferences for public service.

While the average correlations are modest, they are often interesting. For example, while only 16% of respondents reported any use of hospitals and clinics, 28% were very or somewhat dissatisfied with them and 82% thought more tax money should be spent on them. The spending and satisfaction figures were negatively associated (r = −0.28), indicating that as respondents' levels of satisfaction went down, their willingness to spend more on the service went up. The spending and use figures were positively associated (r = 0.16), indicating that their willingness to spend more increased slightly with increased usage of the service.

Considering provincial government officials, only 5% of respondents reported that they contacted them often, 62% reported that less tax money should be spent on them and 36% were very or somewhat dissatisfied with them. The spending and use figures were slightly positively correlated (r = 0.07), indicating that willingness to spend more on such officials was only slightly related to the actual experience of making use of them. However, the spending and satisfaction figures were more strongly positively associated (r = 0.35), indicating that the more satisfied respondents were with their provincial officials, the more they were inclined to favour spending more tax money on them. Still, since only about 12% of the variance in spending preferences could be explained by satisfaction with the officials that means that 88% has to be accounted for by something other than satisfaction with officials' performance. Exactly what that 'something' might be would be worth exploring in the future.

Table 7.5 provides some comparative figures resulting from regressing mean life satisfaction scores on mean scores for satisfaction with various domains of life. The simple linear model used to obtain these figures was one of the first models applied by social indicators researchers and it is still one of the most frequently used models (Michalos 1991a, b). Since the model merely explains overall life (global) satisfaction in terms of the (domain) satisfaction one gets from one's job, family relations and so on, it is useless for explaining satisfaction in the generic sense. For the latter, one would require something other than satisfaction to do the explanatory work. For example, in multiple discrepancies theory satisfaction is posited as the effect of things like the perceived discrepancies between what one has and wants, and between what one has and others have (Michalos 1985). Nevertheless, although the simple linear model is not deep, it does allow one to measure the impact of satisfaction with various domains of life on one's perceived overall satisfaction with life. Here we will also apply the model to explain happiness with life as a whole and satisfaction with the quality of one's life.

On average, for the six samples represented in Table 7.5, we were able to explain 54% of the variance in reported life satisfaction from some subset of the 14 predictor variables listed in the table. Our best success came from the Prince George sample (column F), at 60%. When all variables are standardized to have means of zero and standard deviations of one, the standardized regression coefficients (Betas)

Table 7.5 Comparison of life satisfaction regressions for university clerical staff, rural seniors, eastern northern community, Guelph students, world sample of students and Prince George residents

	1979 A[a]	1981 B	1982 C	1984 D	1985/86 E	1994 F
Percent of variance explained in life satisfaction	57	49	53	53	49	60
Predictors satisfaction with	Standardized regression coefficients					
Health	0.11	0.18	0.17	0.12	0.11	b
Financial security	0.15	−0.01	0.24	0.11	0.16	b
Family relations	0.35	0.10	0.10	0.13	0.06	b
Job	0.10	c	b	0.09	b	0.08
Friendships	0.20	0.08	0.07	0.17	0.08	0.13
Housing	−0.5	0.21	0.10	0.12	0.12	0.14
Area lived in	b	0.01	0.13	b	c	b
Recreation activity	0.08	0.08	0.05	0.12	0.13	b
Religion	c	0.13	0.07	b	b	b
Self-esteem	0.13	0.17	0.19	0.31	0.19	0.50
Transportation	0.09	0.05	0.06	b	0.05	b
Gov. services	c	0.13	0.04	c	c	0.13
Living partner	c	0.06	c	c	0.15	0.09
Education	−0.03	c	c	0.16	0.19	b

$P < 0.01$

[a]A = Clerical staff (N = 312), B = seniors (N = 273), C = East northerners (N = 328), D = Guelph students (N = 296), E = world students (N = 5107), F = Prince George residents (N = 430)

[b]Significance level too low to enter equation

[c]Not in questionnaire

measure the percent of movement in the dependent variable when a predictor variable moves one full unit and every other predictor in the set is held constant. For example, under column F one finds that the Beta value for self-esteem is B = 0.50, which means that for every full unit increase in satisfaction with one's own self-esteem, one's life satisfaction increases half a unit. Inspection of the other figures in that column reveals that satisfaction in no other domain had as great an impact on overall life satisfaction for the 430 Prince George respondents.

Reading across the row to the left from 50, one sees that satisfaction with one's own self-esteem was also the strongest predictor of life satisfaction for the sample of 296 University of Guelph students (column D), at B = 0.31. The Guelph sample was a part of the global student sample whose results are listed in column E. Inspection of that column shows that satisfaction with one's own self-esteem tied with satisfaction with one's university education as the strongest predictors of life satisfaction for the 5107 students in the global sample.

For the other three samples, satisfaction with one's self-esteem was not as powerful a predictor as (had less explanatory power than) satisfaction with one or more other domains. For the 312 sampled members of the office, clerical and technical staff of the University of Guelph (column A), satisfaction with one's family relations had the greatest explanatory power (B = 0.35), followed by satisfaction with one's friendships (B = 0.20), satisfaction with one's financial security (B = 0.15) and then satisfaction with one's self-esteem (B = 0.13). For the 273 sampled rural seniors (column B), satisfaction with their housing had the strongest predictive strength (B = 0.21), followed by satisfaction with their health (B = 0.18) and then with their self-esteem (B = 0.17). For the 328 eastern northerners (column C), satisfaction with their financial security had the greatest explanatory power (B = 0.24), followed by satisfaction with self-esteem (B = 0.19).

The figures just reviewed clearly illustrate the fact that different groups of people with different life circumstances, resources and constraints use different mixtures of ingredients to determine their life satisfaction. The explanatory model used here allowed the groups represented in Table 7.5 to draw satisfaction from roughly the same set of 14 domains. Analytically speaking, some groups used more and some used fewer of these domains to build their life satisfaction. The Prince George group used only six of the 14 possibilities, while the rural senior group used all 12 of the 12 possibilities available to them. In other research (Michalos 1985), it was noticed that women tend to draw satisfaction from more domains than men, but it was never noticed that elderly people also draw satisfaction from more domains than younger people. That would be worth exploring in the future.

Table 7.6 provides some comparative figures resulting from regressing mean happiness scores on mean scores for satisfaction with various domains of life. On average, for the six samples represented in this Table, we were able to explain 35% of the variance in reported happiness with life as a whole from some subset of the 14 predictor variables listed in the Table. Our best success came from the clerical staff sample from the University of Guelph (column A), at 45%. The strongest explanatory variable for that sample was satisfaction with family relations, which had a Beta value of B = 0.38. Thus, figuratively speaking, for every full-step increase in satisfaction with their family relations the overall happiness of these respondents increased 38% of a step.

As one moves across the columns of Table 7.6, one finds that the strongest explanatory variable for the rural seniors group was satisfaction with their friendships (B = 0.23), satisfaction with their financial security was the strongest predictor for the eastern northern group (B = 0.21), satisfaction with self-esteem for the Guelph students (B = 26), and satisfaction with living partners for the world student sample (B = 0.18) and the Prince George sample (B = 0.22). As in the case of-life satisfaction, different groups built up their overall happiness with different mixtures of ingredients and some groups drew upon more domains than others.

In order to be able to make rough comparisons among the six groups considered in Tables 7.5 and 7.6, it was necessary to use a relatively small and consistent set of 14 predictors, However, in the interest of discovering some additional explanatory variables, more regressions were run testing many more (nearly 40) predictors that were available in the Prince George survey. As things turned out, in the presence of

Table 7.6 Comparison of happiness regressions for university clerical staff, rural seniors, Eastern northern community, Guelph students, world sample of students and Prince George residents

	1979	1981	1982	1984	1985/86	1994
	A	B	C	D	E	F
Percent of variance explained in happiness	45	32	36	39	28	27
Predicators satisfaction with	Standardized regression coefficients					
Health	0.12	0.12	0.18	0.17	0.09	b
Financial security	0.09	0.06	0.21	b	0.13	b
Family relations	0.38	−0.03	0.09	0.14	0.06	b
Job	0.03	c	0.09	0.18	b	0.10
Friendships	0.23	0.23	0.01	0.21	0.10	0.10
Housing	0.01	−0.01	0.10	b	0.07	b
Area lived in	b	0.01	0.05	b	c	b
Recreation activity	0.03	0.04	0.05	b	0.07	0.13
Religion	c	0.01	0.03	b	b	b
Self-esteem	0.07	0.09	0.14	0.26	0.13	0.21
Transportation	0.05	0.05	b	b	b	b
Gov. services	c	0.08	0.03	c	c	b
Living partner	c	0.30	c	c	0.18	0.22
Education	−0.03	c	c	b	0.10	b

$P < 0.01$
[a]A = Clerical staff (N = 312), B = Seniors (N = 273), C = East northerners (N = 328), D = Guelph students (N = 296), E = world students (N = 5036), F = Prince George residents (N = 412)
[b]Significance level too low to enter equation
[c]Not in questionnaire

some new variables, the explanatory power of some of those in the older set was significantly reduced.

Table 7.7 contains the correlation matrix of the 13 surviving predictors plus the three dependent variables, satisfaction with one's life as a whole and. with the quality of one's life, and happiness with life as a whole.

Table 7.8 gives the results of regressing the three dependent variables on the 13 predictors. We were able to explain 63% of the variance in reported life satisfaction, 57% of the variance in reported satisfaction with the quality of life and 29% of the variance in reported happiness. So, our ability to explain life satisfaction increased by 3% points and our ability to explain happiness increased by 2% points, This was very modest improvement considering the additional number of explanatory variables tested. My guess would be that the improvement was modest because we are reaching the reliability limits of our single item dependent variables (Carmines and Zeller 1979) and because life satisfaction, happiness and the quality of life are not merely the sum of the satisfaction one gets from particular domains of life.

Table 7.7 Correlation matrix for regression variables (decimal points omitted)

Var.	Variable number															
	1	2	3	4	5	6	7	8	9	10	11	12	13	14	15	16
2	23															
3	25	48														
4	26	25	15													
5	25	39	28	44												
6	26	34	26	26	41											
7	24	24	21	32	41	36										
8	40	20	16	40	28	31	31									
9	27	27	22	26	33	36	35	37								
10	37	37	32	47	40	40	33	39	42							
11	42	39	35	45	49	40	29	40	36	72						
12	14	16	14	19	19	16	32	23	30	32	36					
13	15	15	13	22	20	15	21	17	29	19	18	42				
14	ns	ns	ns	ns	17	ns	ns	12	18	22	23	34	24			
15	41	33	32	46	47	29	21	48	44	53	59	34	21	16		
16	26	32	36	31	35	29	17	29	33	43	43	20	17	15	46	

$P < 0.01$, *ns* = Not Significant, N = 374

Var. 1 = satisfaction with one's own home, 2 = sat. with family relations, 3 = sat. with partner or spouse, 4 = sat. with job, 5 = sat. with friends, 6 = sat. with health, 7 = sat. with religion, 8 = sat. with financial security, 9 = sat. with recreation activities, 10 = sat. with self-esteem, 11 = sat. with, life as a whole, 12 = sat. with police protection, 13 = sat with public transportation, 14 = sat. with University of Northern British Columbia, 15 = sat with quality of life, 16 = happiness with life as a whole

Perhaps the most interesting discovery from these regressions is the fact that only two predictors, satisfaction with one's own self-esteem and satisfaction with one's accomplishments, have roles to play in explaining all three dependent variables and the roles are different in each case. Regarding satisfaction with life as a whole, satisfaction with one's own self-esteem dominates the other four predictors. The latter's Beta value of B = 0.52 is over three times as great as its next competitor, satisfaction with one's standard of living (B = 0.16). Satisfaction with one's accomplishments has an even smaller impact (B = 0.14) on life satisfaction in the presence of the other predictors in that set.

Regarding happiness with life as a whole, satisfaction with one's own self-esteem ranks third in explanatory power (B = 0.16), behind satisfaction with one's living partner (B = 0.24) and satisfaction with the weather (B = 0.17). Satisfaction with one's accomplishments (B = 0.14) is in fourth place.

For satisfaction with the quality of life, satisfaction with self-esteem is fourth in the race for explanatory power (B = 0.15), falling behind the first placed satisfaction with one's standard of living (B = 0.28), with the local libraries (B = 0.22) and accomplishments (B = 0.21).

Table 7.8 Multiple regression of life satisfaction, happiness and quality of life on domain satisfaction

Predicators satisfaction with	Standardized regression confidents ($p < 0.01$)
Self-esteem	0.52
Living standard	0.16
Police protection	0.11
Accomplishments	0.14
Family relations	0.09
Variance explained in satisfaction with life as a whole satisfaction with	63% (N = 488)
Self-esteem	0.16
Living partner	0.24
Weather	0.17
Accomplishments	0.14
Friends	0.10
Variance explained in happiness with life as a whole satisfaction with	29% (N = 426)
Accomplishments	0.21
Living standard	0.28
Libraries	0.22
Self-esteem	0.15
City of Prince George	0.11
Living partner	0.12
Weather	0.09
Variance explained in perceived quality of life	57% (N = 442)

Reflecting on the list of variables predicting satisfaction with the quality of life in Prince George. It is clear that the concept of "quality of life" captures a somewhat broader range of things than those captured by 'life satisfaction' and 'happiness'. In particular, among other things, the quality of life in Prince George seems to be connected to something like the general ambiance of the city and the cultural opportunities provided by its libraries. As we turn to the results from the open-ended questions in the survey, additional light will be thrown on our respondents' views of the quality of their lives.

Table 7.9 lists the numbers and percentages of respondents indicating "the best thing about living in Prince George". For our respondents, the most frequently mentioned best thing about living in Prince George was the "friendly and good people here". As a matter of fact, that seems to be the best thing about living in most cities according to their residents (Michalos 1993b). Following this response by a quarter of our sample, people mentioned the city's proximity to nature (14.1%), accessible amenities (13.7%), the size of the community (13.3) opportunities for year round recreation (12.5) and for jobs (9.5). Of the dozen things listed in this table five are directly related to the natural environment.

Table 7.9 Numbers and percentages of respondents indicating the best thing about living in Prince George

Best thing	Number	Percent
Friendly, good people	127	25.2
Proximity to nature	71	14.1
Accessible to amenities	69	13.7
Size of the community	67	13.3
Year round recreation	63	12.5
Job opportunity	48	9.5
Country life style	39	7.7
Reasonable cost of living	34	6.8
Beauty of the area	17	3.4
Growing community	12	2.4
Geographic location	11	2.2
Space/elbow room	11	2.2
38 other things each cited by		
Fewer than 2% of respondents		

Table 7.10 lists the numbers and percentages of respondents indicating "the worst thing about living in Prince George". The most frequently mentioned worst thing about living here was the winter season, which was described as "too long and cold" by 20.7% of our sample. Following this, 15.7% mentioned crime and violence, 13.5% mentioned the smell and air pollution (from our pulp and paper mills), 13.1% mentioned the city's isolated location and 9.5% mentioned the ugliness of our city centre.

Table 7.10 Numbers and percentages of respondents indicating the worst thing about living in Prince George

Worst thing	Number	Percent
Winter too long and cold	104	20.7
Crime and violence	79	15.7
Smell and air pollution	68	13.5
Isolated location	66	13.1
Ugly centre city area	48	9.5
Weather	36	7.1
Poor shopping areas	33	6.6
Social problems	29	5.8
Inadequate health services	28	5.6
Cost/distance from things	24	4.8
City lacks entertainment	18	3.6
Prov. gov. lack of concern with		
Health care	11	2.2
61 other things each cited by fewer than 2% of respondents		

Having determined the things about life in Prince George that were especially good and especially bad, we wanted to find out what respondents "would change to improve the quality of life here." Table 7.11 lists the most frequently mentioned changes, beginning with beautifying the central city area (17.7%). Following that, 10.1% mentioned reducing crime and 8.5% mentioned eliminating air pollution. It is interesting that the top three candidates for things to change are included in the top five worst things about living here. Even more interesting is the fact that the two remaining of the five most frequently mentioned worst things about living here are beyond human manipulation, namely, the winter season and the geographic location of the city. Presumably our respondents would change these things too if they could.

One might have thought that given people's levels of dissatisfaction with federal and provincial government officials, there should have been large numbers of people calling for a change of these officials themselves or a change in their behaviour. However, recalling the results of the regressions listed in Table 7.8, it is clear that our respondents' satisfaction or dissatisfaction with their elected officials had no statistically significant impact on their reported life satisfaction happiness or satisfaction with the quality of their lives, Given their levels of dissatisfaction, may be they are lucky that there is no connection. On the other hand, if there were a strong and visible connection between their views about their lives and their elected officials, maybe they would be motivated to mobilize for progressive change.

Table 7.12 lists the percentages of people indicating disagreement or strong disagreement versus agreement or strong agreement to a set of statements about various aspects of their community and their lives. The statement receiving the greatest support (96%) was the one affirming that "Good communities require high

Table 7.11 Numbers and percentages of respondents indicating the thing they would change to improve the quality of life in Prince George

Thing to change	Number	Percent
Beautify central city	89	17.7
Reduce crime	51	10.1
Eliminate air pollution	43	8.5
Improve shopping areas	42	8.3
Improve recreation facilities	32	6.3
Improve health care	22	4.4
Increase city events	20	4.0
Create arts, cultural programs	19	3.8
Reduce social problems	16	3.2
Improve policing	16	3.2
Create more safe recreation for youth	13	2.6
Solve hospital problems	12	2.4
Increase secondary industries 82 other things each cited by fewer than 1.8% of respondents	9	1.8

Table 7.12 Aspects about the community and life with which people disagree or disagree strongly versus agree or agree strongly (N = 497)

Statement	Disagree or strongly disagree	Agree or strongly agree	Mean
Unemployment is a serious problem in this community	17.5	68.7	3.7
I don't think local public officials care much about what I think	34.3	40.0	3.2
This community needs more co-operative planning for development	11.6	61.1	3.6
I would rate my current physical health as excellent	22.1	72.5	3.7
I don't think provincial officials care much about what I think	16.9	64.0	3.7
Good communities require high levels of co-operation	1.0	96.0	4.4
My home needs some major repairs	64.5	31.4	2.6
There is someone in this community I can always count on for good advice	11.7	65.6	3.7
This community needs more industry	14.6	67.9	3.7
I would leave this community if I had the opportunity	56.4	22.4	2.5
I don't think federal public officials care much about what I think	10.2	70.4	3.9
Good communities require high levels of competition	21.6	54.2	3.4
The College of New Caledonia is a major asset to this community	3.6	91.8	4.21
I know someone in this community who sincerely cares about my well-being	5.6	84.1	4.2
I believe this community is a better place to live than it was 5 years ago	21.6	58.1	3.5
The University of Northern B.C. is a major asset to this community	2.0	90.8	4.5
Continued growth will hurt the quality of life in this community	71.1	12.2	2.2
I believe this community will be a better place to live 5 years from mow than it is today	9.8	55.4	3.6

levels of co-operation". This was contrasted with 54% affirming that "Good communities require high levels of competition". Given the past decade of bombardment with right-wing propaganda about the need for and virtues of competition (Michalos 1995), it was encouraging to see that the co-operative spirit was relatively strong in Prince George.

The next two statements receiving the highest levels of support were those that mentioned the city's two post-secondary institutions. Ninety-two percent of respondents agreed that the local community college Is “a major asset” to the community and 91% felt the same way about the university.

While 70% affirmed that federal public officials did not “care much” about what they thought, 64% felt that way about provincial officials and only 40% felt that way about local officials. On the other hand, where public officials failed, others were apparently successful. Eighty-four percent of the sample affirmed that “someone in the community” sincerely cares about their well-being and 66% agreed that there was someone in the community that they “can always count on for good advice”.

It was encouraging to see that while 68% of respondents believed that the “community needs more industry”, only 12% believed that “continued growth will hurt the quality of life” here. If large numbers believed continued growth would destroy the quality of their lives, that would have suggested that there would be conflicts over possible industrial growth in the future.

Responses to all of the 18 statements were entered into regression equations along with the previously predictively successful domain satisfaction scores as predictors of life satisfaction, happiness and satisfaction with the quality of life. Interestingly it was found that, regarding the prediction of life satisfaction, only one statement had any explanatory power in the presence of the domain satisfaction scores, namely, the statement that “there is someone in this community I can always count on for good advice”. This statement had a Beta value of B = 0.06. Regarding happiness, none of the 18 statements had any statistically significant predictive power. For satisfaction with the quality of life, the good advice statement had a Beta value of B = 0.13, the statement “I don t think provincial public officials care much about what I think” had a value of B = 0.09, and the statement “I believe this community is a better place to live than it was 5 years ago” had a value of B = 0.08. Perhaps even more interestingly, in the case of all three variables, the addition of these predictors had a depressive effect (of about 2% points) on the percent of variance explained in each of the three global dependent variables. So, my attempt to boost our capacity to explain the global variable scores with the help of some of these statement scores was counter-productive.

At the end of our questionnaire, the focus was on the 141 respondents who had moved to Prince George “within the last 5 years”. From other research (Michalos 1994) it was known that most people move because of job changes or changed housing needs. The most frequently mentioned reasons for leaving their prior place of residence at all (of 16) were that the respondent or a spouse found a new job (27%) or they thought there would be more job opportunities elsewhere (20%) or there simply were no available jobs in their previous residential area (17%).

The most frequently mentioned reasons for moving to Prince George were that they found work here (63%) or they had family here (11%). Six percent moved here to further their education.

Table 7.13 lists the results of asking these relatively new members of our community what particular things they thought about prior to moving, whether they expected those things to be better and whether they were in fact better. Before they moved, 86% of these respondents thought about the jobs they would have here, 79% of those who thought about their jobs thought things would be better here and 71%

Table 7.13 Respondents who had moved to Prince George within the last 5 years: Things they thought about expected to be better and perceived outcomes (N = 141)

Issue thought about	Percent thinking	Percent expecting things to be better	Percent thinking things are better
Their job	86	79	71
Some family member's job	53	78	71
Cost of housing	76	60	50
Cost of living	73	55	38
PG for retirement	12	42	56
Quality of life in PG	83	58	67
Friendliness of people in PG	64	53	74
Public safety	46	59	22
Health care	48	56	27
Family relations	57	69	75
Outdoor recreation	61	69	83
Quality of Schools	38	53	47
College of CNC	27	60	56
University of NBC	26	68	76
Shopping areas	66	59	38
Natural environment	54	63	58
Weather	64	41	39

of the latter thought things actually are better. Eighty-three percent had thought about the quality of life here before they moved 58% of those people thought it would be better here than it was in their previous place of residence and 67% of the latter thought it is better. Seventy-six percent thought about the cost of housing here before they moved, 60% thought it would be better here and 50% thought it is better.

Fewer than half of the relatively new arrivals (46%) thought about public safety here before they moved, and while 59% of those thought it would be better here than in their previous place of residence, only 22% thought it is better. Forty eight percent thought about health care here before they moved and 56% of those thought it would be better although unfortunately only 27% thought it is better.

Conclusion

The main aim of this research was to provide some baseline data that could serve as the "before" part of a before and after analysis that some future researcher might want to undertake to determine the impact of a new university on a small city.

Accordingly, we explored people's use of public services, their spending preferences for tax revenues, satisfaction with a wide variety of aspects of their community and their lives, and correlations among these things. Open-ended questions were used to discover in the respondents' own words the best things about living in Prince George, the worst things and the things they would change first, to improve the quality of their lives. A simple linear mode was used to explain life satisfaction, happiness 'and satisfaction with the quality of respondents' lives on the basis of satisfaction they received in specific domains of their lives, like job satisfaction and satisfaction with their family relations, This model was able to account for 63% of the variance in life satisfaction scores, 57% of the variance in satisfaction with the quality of life scores and 29% of the variance in happiness scores.

The much more difficult task of sorting out the impact of the new university from the impacts of all the other changes in the community over the next few years has been left to some future researcher. The author and those who worked on this survey tried to provide enough information to make a before and after analysis possible. Unfortunately it was beyond our ability to make it easy.

References

Carmines, E. G., & Zeller, R. A. (1979). *Reliability and validity assessment.* Beverly Hills: Sage Publications.

Michalos, A. C. (1980). Satisfaction and happiness. *Social Indicators Research, 8,* 385–422.

Michalos, A. C. (1982). The satisfaction and happiness of some senior citizens in rural Ontario. *Social Indicators Research, 11,* 1–30.

Michalos, A. C. (1983). The satisfaction and happiness in a rural northern resource community. *Soctal Indicators Research, 13,* 224–252.

Michalos, A. C. (1985). Multiple discrepancies theory (MDT). *Social Indicators Research, 16,* 347–413.

Michalos, A.C. (1991a). *Global report on student well-being, Volume 1: Life satisfaction and happiness.* New York: Springer.

Michalos, A. C. (1991b). *Global report on student well-being, Volume 2: Family friends, living partner and self-esteem.* New York: Springer.

Michalos, A. C. (1993a). *Global report on student well-being, Volume 3:* Employment, finances, housing and transportation. New York: Springer.

Michalos, A. C. (1993b). *Global report on student well-being, Volume 4: Religion, education, recreation and health.* New York: Springer.

Michalos, A. C. (1994). Goal formation, achievement and their consequences for residential satisfaction and mobility. In J. Cecora (Ed.), *Changing values and attitudes in family households with rural peer groups, social networks, and action spaces* (pp. 31–40). Bonn: Society for Agricultural Policy Research and Rural Sociology.

Michalos, A. C. (1995). *A pragmatic approach to business ethics.* Thousand Oaks: Sage Publications.

Chapter 8
Quality of Life in Jasper, Alberta

Bruno D. Zumbo and Alex C. Michalos

Introduction

In this essay, we report on the results of a survey of citizen beliefs and attitudes about the quality of life in Jasper, Alberta, Canada in the summer of 1997. The town of Jasper is inside Jasper National Park, which is one of Canada's most beautiful and famous park areas. At the time of the survey, the town was governed by the Jasper Improvement District Council and there was considerable debate about moving to self-government. The District does not have all the powers that a municipal government would have. It has the authority and responsibility for taxation, culture and recreation, family and community support services, library services and protective services (e.g., ambulance). Parks Canada has the authority for municipal services such as water, streets, protective services (e.g., fire department), bylaws and bylaw enforcement, sewage and development (e.g., building permits, business licences).

It seemed to be a perfect time to obtain a broad-based assessment of the perceived quality of life of permanent residents of the town, as well as an assessment of views about the future development of the town and the likely impact of self-government. Some comparisons made with similar surveys taken in other communities were also made (e.g., Michalos 1996).

Zumbo, B.C., & Michalos, A.C.: 2000. Quality of life in Jasper, Alberta. Social Indicators Research, 49(2), pp. 121–145.

A.C. Michalos (✉)
University of Northern British Columbia, Prince George, BC, Canada
e-mail: michalos@brandonu.ca

B.D. Zumbo
College of Arts, Social and Health Sciences, University of Northern British Columbia, Prince George, BC, Canada

A.C. Michalos, *Development of Quality of Life Theory and Its Instruments*,
DOI 10.1007/978-3-319-51149-8_8

The structure of the essay is as follows. In the next section "Sampling Technique and Questionnaire", we describe our sampling technique and questionnaire. Then we move to a description of our sample section "Sample Characteristics" and descriptive statistics regarding satisfaction levels for a variety of public services and other aspects of life section "Satisfaction". Section "Best Things, Worst Things and Things to Change" summarizes responses to our open-ended questions about the best and worst things about living in Jasper, and things to change to improve the quality of life there. This is followed by a section "User-Fees and Government Value for Tax Dollars" in which we review respondents' attitudes toward user-fees and the value received from tax dollars. In the next section "Agreements and Disagreements", we discuss the most salient responses to a set of 21 statements about which we asked respondents to express agreement or disagreement. We then section "Reduction of Satisfaction Items to Indices" create 15 indices out of the 93 satisfaction items reviewed in section "Satisfaction", which we use to help explain our three global dependent variable scores in section "Explaining Life Satisfaction, Happiness and Satisfaction with the Quality of Life from Selected Satisfaction Items and Indices". In section "Explaining Life Satisfaction, Happiness and Overall Satisfaction with the Quality of Life from Selected Domain Satisfaction Items", we explain the three global dependent variable scores from a limited set of 14 variables, which allows us to compare our Jasper results with results from seven other surveys taken over nearly 20 years. In section "Relative Importance of the Predictor Variables" we apply a new statistical method for ordering the predictor variables from the regressions reported in sections "Explaining Life Satisfaction, Happiness and Overall Satisfaction with the Quality of Life from Selected Domain Satisfaction Items" and "Explaining Life Satisfaction, Happiness and Satisfaction with the Quality of Life from Selected Satisfaction Items and Indices" in terms of their relative importance in each regression model (Thomas et al. 1998). The final section "Conclusion" is a brief conclusion.

Sampling Technique and Questionnaire

Questionnaires were hand-delivered by volunteers to 1200 housing units in Jasper in June and July 1997, covering all of the town's 1669 households. Respondents were given a plastic bag in which to deposit their completed questionnaires, which were later picked up or dropped off in some boxes conveniently located in the community.

The first three pages of the questionnaire listed 95 "services and other things affecting people today", including such things as family support services, snow removal, the cost of local housing, family relations, health, jobs and so on. The extent to which people were satisfied with these things was measured on a 7-point Likert scale with response categories ranging from "very dissatisfied = 1 point", through "an even balance = 4", to "very satisfied = 7".

Following these questions, there was a 7-point question designed to measure the extent to which people were happy with their lives as a whole, ranging from "very unhappy = 1 point", through "an even balance = 4", to "very happy = 7".

These were followed by a page containing a general question designed to measure the extent to which respondents felt that 26 particular public services should be controlled more or less by Parks Canada rather than by the local Jasper Improvement District Council. The response categories were "less = 1", "same = 2" and "more = 3".

The next two pages of the questionnaire had 21 statements about which respondents were asked to indicate the extent of their agreement, with five response categories ranging from "strongly disagree = 1 point", through "don't know = 3", to "strongly agree = 5".

This was followed by two open-ended questions asking respondents, first, to describe the "best thing about living in this community", and then "the worst thing". Respondents were then asked, "If you could change anything about this community to improve the quality of life here, what would that change be?"

We then raised the question: "Do you think that more public services should be supported by user-fees instead of by general taxes?" The response options were simply "yes" or "no".

Finally, we asked respondents to tell us whether they thought they got poor or good value for their tax dollars from federal, provincial and District governments. The options for each sort of government were "poor value = 1", "average value = 2" and "good value = 3".

Sample Characteristics

By the end of July, 447 (37%) useable questionnaires were returned, which form the working data-set for the survey. Respondents included 241 (55%) females and 197 (45%) males. Two-hundred and sixty-six (61%) were now married and living with their spouse. The average age was 44, with a range from 17 to 82. Two hundred and eighty-nine (67%) owned or were in the process of buying their home. One hundred and sixty-five (37%) had some university education, with 95 (21%) holding a university degree. The first language of 375 (84%) respondents was English. Two hundred and thirty-nine (54%) were employed full-time and 78 (17%) part-time. One hundred and forty-seven (35%) had total family incomes of from $40,000 to $69,999 CDN.

According to the 1996 census, which is the last official full population count available from Statistics Canada, there were 1669 private households in the Improvement District (mostly living in Jasper) and 48% (1511) of the Improvement District's permanent adult residents aged 15 years or older were female. Unfortunately, no other figures from that census are available. However, from the 1991 census we know that there were also 48% female, 38% were married and living with their spouse, 22% had some university education, 8% held a university degree, 49% owned or were in the process of buying their home, 43% were employed full-time and 42% were employed part-time, 30% had total family incomes of from $40,000 to $69,999 CDN, and 87% had English as their first language. Broadly speaking, then, it is likely that our working sample has a few more females, married people, home owners, university educated and full-time employed people than the total population from which it was drawn.

Satisfaction

Table 8.1 lists the mean scores for the 95 satisfaction items and the one happiness item. The most satisfying aspects of people's lives were satisfaction with the physical beauty of Jasper (*mean* = 6.6), friendships, recreation activities and the quality of drinking water (6.0), Jasper as a place to live, life as a whole and the overall quality of life (5.9), family relations, personal health and self-esteem (5.8). The mean score for happiness with life as a whole was also 5.8.

The mean score for satisfaction with the physical beauty of Jasper is remarkable because it is so much higher than the usual mean scores of roughly 6 points for satisfaction items and because it so clearly dominates family and living partner satisfaction which usually dominate such lists (Michalos 1991b). Clearly, the spectacular beauty of the area is deeply appreciated by its permanent residents.

Highest levels of dissatisfaction were expressed for infant community operated child care (0.9), infant home-based operated child care and school-age home-based child care (1.0), pre-school home-based child care (1.2), school-age community operated child care (1.4), relief time family caregivers of the elderly (1.6), and preschool community operated child care (1.9). The fact that 47% of the sampled households had at least one child under 17 years of age living at home does not help us understand why so much dissatisfaction surrounded the issue of child care. Presumably, there are many families in need of such care.

Best Things, Worst Things and Things to Change

For our respondents, the most frequently mentioned "best thing about living in Jasper" was a physical collage described by the phrases "the beauty of the surroundings", "the scenery", "the mountains", "the environment" and "being in a national park". One hundred and ninety-five (44%) of our respondents mentioned such things. Second, 96 (21%) mentioned the "friendly people" which, as a matter of fact, seems to be what most people in most cities around the world regard as the best thing about living in them (Michalos 1993). Following these responses, the people in our sample mentioned the town's outdoor opportunities (20%) and its small town atmosphere (19%).

The most frequently mentioned "worst thing about living in Jasper" was "the high cost of living". One hundred and sixty-one (36%) of respondents mentioned this feature. Second, 73 (16%) said they "did not like park management". Following

Table 8.1 Mean satisfaction and happiness levels

Satisfaction with	Mean	N
Your house, apartment or mobile home	5.7	440
Your neighbourhood as a place to live	5.7	441
Jasper as a place to live	5.9	439
Your family relations, generally	5.8	441
Your living partner	5.4	435
Your job	4.6	435
Your pay level	4.3	433
Your work schedule	4.6	434
Your friendships	6.0	443
Your health	5.8	441
Your religion or spiritual fulfilment	4.5	441
Your overall standard of living	5.7	441
Your financial security	4.9	440
The physical beauty of Jasper	6.6	443
Your recreation opportunities	6.0	441
What you are accomplishing in life	5.4	439
Your self-esteem	5.8	439
How you feel about life as a whole	5.9	439
Police protection services	5.5	443
Public transportation services	2.8	434
Public highways, streets and roads	4.0	441
Street lighting	4.9	443
Play areas for children	4.2	441
Elementary education	3.2	438
Junior/Senior high school education	2.2	436
Availability of post-secondary education	2.2	435
Y.R.E.C.	2.9	408
Seton General Hospital	4.7	439
Clinics	5.1	442
Counselling services	2.5	436
Maternity public health services	2.0	439
School public health services	2.4	436
Availability of local housing	2.5	426
Cost of local housing	2.1	432
Density of local housing	2.9	431
The friendliness of neighbours	5.5	442
Ambulance service	4.6	436
Parks Canada officials	3.5	438
I.D. staff and councillors	3.5	428
Federal M.P.	3.0	434
Provincial M.L.A.	3.0	426
Local parks and recreation facilities	5.4	434

(continued)

Table 8.1 (continued)

Satisfaction with	Mean	N
Grocery shopping facilities	3.8	440
Clothing shopping facilities	2.4	440
Household supplies shopping facilities	2.8	436
The amount of taxes you pay	2.1	436
Recycling	5.2	438
Domestic animal control and enforcement	3.6	438
Pre-school community operated child care	1.9	434
Pre-school home-based child care	1.2	431
School-age community operated child care	1.4	432
School-age home-based child care	1.0	431
Infant community operated child care	0.9	429
Infant home-based operated child care	1.0	426
The library	5.4	436
Your overall quality of life	5.9	441
Job opportunities	3.6	435
Traffic congestion	3.5	432
Sewage system	4.2	426
Garbage system	5.2	438
Sidewalks and pedestrian walkways	4.6	436
Planning and zoning regulations	2.6	432
Correctional services	2.0	428
Judicial services	2.7	426
Noise levels here	4.4	436
Drug and alcohol abuse	2.6	429
The number of motor vehicle accidents	3.6	428
The weather most of the time	4.4	439
Jasper's geographical location	5.6	439
Number of sports related injuries	2.5	427
Health promotion education	3.9	430
Services for the disabled	2.5	432
Institutional elderly care services	2.5	437
Home care elderly care services	2.4	439
Relief time family care givers of the elderly	1.6	432
Arts opportunities	3.8	432
Cultural opportunities	3.8	432
Snow removal	3.4	441
Conditions of sidewalks during winter	3.0	441
Cleanliness of the town	5.1	442
Cleanliness of the back alleys	4.0	442
Quality of the drinking water	6.0	440
Services for workers in tourism industry	3.3	433

(continued)

Table 8.1 (continued)

Satisfaction with	Mean	N
Youth services	2.5	438
Family support services	3.2	437
Employment services	2.9	435
Wildlife management	4.3	438
Domestic animal management	3.6	435
The use of local housing	3.0	426
Amount of Federal taxes you pay	2.5	433
Amount of Provincial taxes you pay	2.5	436
Amount of District taxes you pay	2.2	433
Amount of education taxes you pay	2.0	435
Organized athletics	4.0	431
Public performances of music/theatre	3.8	437
Overall happiness	5.8	405

these things, 36 (8%) felt that there was a lack of shopping facilities "for everyday needs" and that taxes were too high.

Having determined the things about life in Jasper that were especially good and especially bad, we wanted to find out what respondents "would change to improve the quality of life" there. First, 81 (18%) respondents said they would lower their cost of living, and following that, 65 (15%) said they would move toward self-government. After these things, 53 (12%) said they would slow down development of the town, 30 (7%) would reduce taxes, 26 (6%) would increase the number of stores with "everyday needs", and 16 (4%) would "get rid of the elk in the townsite".

User-Fees and Government Value for Tax Dollars

Regarding user-fees, of 427 people who answered the question, 162 (36%) claimed that the town should, 179 (40%) claimed that the town should not raise more money from this source and 78 (17%) had no opinion. Assuming the sampling error margins were about 5% points for our survey results, the support for user-fees might be as low as 31% and the opposition might be as high as 45%. Since our sample had a disproportionate number of property owners in it, one might assume some bias in favour of user-fees. So, it is probably fair to say that in the whole community there is more opposition than support for the idea of increasing the use of user-fees as a source of public revenue.

Table 8.2 gives the percents of people indicating that they got poor, average or good value for their tax dollars from each of the three levels of government. Ten percent asserted that they got good value from the District government, compared to only 3% from the provincial government and 7% from the federal government. On

Table 8.2 Percent saying they get poor, average or good value for their tax dollars

Spent by the	Poor value		Average value		Good value		Don't know	
	N	%	N	%	N	%	N	%
Federal Government	200	47	155	37	29	7	39	9
Provincial Government	196	46	165	39	14	3	47	11
District Government	126	30	176	42	43	10	71	17

the other hand, 47% thought they got poor value from the federal government, 46% thought they got poor value from the provincial government, but only 30% thought they got poor value from the District government. These figures are of course completely consistent with respondents' reported preferences for self-government.

In the light of the figures reported in the previous paragraph, one might have expected to find some significant correlation between respondents' reported levels of agreement with the statement "I believe this community would be best served by having its own municipal government" and their reported levels of satisfaction with life as a whole and their overall quality of life, or with their overall happiness. In fact, there is no significant correlation at all between the former and the latter scores.

Agreements and Disagreements

Table 8.3 lists the percentages of people indicating disagreement or strong disagreement versus agreement or strong agreement with a set of 21 statements about various aspects of their community and their lives. The statement receiving the greatest support (96%) was the one affirming that "Good communities require high levels of co-operation". This was contrasted with 34% affirming that "Good communities require high levels of competition". Given the past decade of bombardment with right-wing propaganda about the need for and virtues of competition (Michalos 1995) and the traditional Albertan support for relatively conservative governments, it was interesting to see that the co-operative spirit was relatively strong in Jasper. In fact, 79% supported the statement that "This community needs more co-operative planning for development".

The statement receiving the second highest level of support (89%) was the one affirming that the "Cost of living is a serious problem in this community". Immediately following this one, there were two statements indicating social support. The statements were "I know someone in this community who sincerely cares about my well-being" (85%) and "There is someone in this community I can always count on for good advice" (82%).

The statement receiving the greatest disagreement (79%) was the one affirming that "This community needs more business development". That was followed by

Table 8.3 Aspects about the community and life with which people disagree or disagree strongly versus agree or agree strongly (N = 431)

Statement	Disagree or strongly disagree	Agree or strongly agree	No opinion
Too many people in this community are over-qualified for the jobs they have	26	30	44
We need more full time and fewer parttime jobs	21	57	22
Unemployment is a serious problem in this community	57	23	21
I don't think local public officials care much about what I think	32	51	1
This community needs more co-operative planning for development	12	79	10
I would rate my current physical health as excellent	17	75	8
I don't think provincial officials care much about what I think	10	74	17
Good communities require high levels of co-operation	1	96	3
My home needs some major repairs	67	26	6
There is someone in this community I can always count on for good advice	12	82	17
This community needs more business development	79	16	7
I would leave this community if I had the opportunity	61	20	19
I don't think Parks Canada officials care much about what I think	16	72	12
Good communities require high levels of competition	45	34	20
I know someone in this community who sincerely cares about my well-being	3	85	11
I believe this community is a better place to live than it was 5 years ago	54	22	23
Continued growth will hurt the quality of life in this community	25	64	12
I believe this community will be a better place to live 5 years from now than it is today	37	15	48
Downsizing is a serious problem in this community	32	37	31
Cost of living is a serious problem in this community	9	89	3
I believe this community would be best served by having its own municipal government	22	50	29

"My home needs some major repairs", with 67% disagreeing and "I would leave this community if I had the opportunity", with 61% disagreeing.

While 72% affirmed that "I don't think Parks Canada officials care much about what I think", 74% felt that way about "provincial public officials" and 51% felt that way about "local public officials". Responses to these three items are also consistent with the general support for self-government. Fifty percent agreed with the statement "I believe this community would be best served by having its own municipal government".

Reduction of Satisfaction Items to Indices

Given 93 satisfaction items, it seemed reasonable to undertake some data-reduction strategies in order to get a more manageable set of variables to explain and predict our three global indicator scores (life satisfaction, satisfaction with overall quality of life, and happiness). After several attempts to cluster items using various factor-analytic techniques produced largely incoherent factors, we became convinced that such techniques were simply not useful for constructing indices from the great number and variety of available items. Instead, we proceeded to conceptually analyze our items, sort them into clusters and then create coherent indices on the basis of acceptable Cronbach alpha values. The 15 indices with their constituent items resulting from these exercises are listed in Table 8.4.

Briefly, we created indices for general satisfaction with taxes (alpha = 0.89), child care services (0.89), elderly and disabled care services (0.91), health, hospitals and clinics (0.88), recreation opportunities (0.85), human services (0.84), shopping facilities (0.80), personal worth (0.79), sanitation and waste removal services (0.78), finances (0.76), house and neighbourhood (0.74), job (0.73), government (0.71), educational opportunities (0.68), and interpersonal relations (0.67). Since these indices pertain to fundamental aspects of people's lives, we think other researchers will find these especially useful.

Explaining Life Satisfaction, Happiness and Overall Satisfaction with the Quality of Life from Selected Domain Satisfaction Items

Table 8.5 provides some comparative figures resulting from regressing mean life satisfaction scores on mean scores for satisfaction with various domains of life. The simple linear model used to obtain these figures was one of the first models applied by social indicators researchers and it is still one of the most frequently used models (Michalos 1991a). Since the model merely explains overall life (global) satisfaction in terms of the (domain) satisfaction one gets from one's job, family relations and

Table 8.4 Items in satisfaction indices, with alpha values

Satisfaction with elderly/disabled care: Alpha = 0.91
Services for the disabled
Institutional elderly care services
Home care elderly care services
Relief time family care givers of the elderly
Satisfaction with taxes: A = 0.89
Amount of Federal taxes you pay
Amount of Provincial taxes you pay
Amount of District taxes you pay
Amount of education taxes you pay
The amount of taxes you pay
Satisfaction with child care: A = 0.89
Pre-school community operated child care
Pre-school home-based child care
School-age community operated child care
School-age home-based child care
Infant community operated child care
Infant home-based operated child care
Satisfaction with health/hospitals: A = 0.88
Seton General Hospital
Clinics
Counselling services
Maternity public health services
School public health services
Ambulance service
Satisfaction with recreation: A = 0.85
Your recreation activities
Play areas for children
Y.R.E.C.
Local parks and recreation facilities
The library
Arts opportunities
Cultural opportunities
Organized athletics
Public performances of music/theatre
Satisfaction with human services: A = 0.84
Services for workers in tourism industry
Youth services
Family support services
Employment services
Satisfaction with shopping: A = 0.80
Grocery shopping facilities

(continued)

Table 8.4 (continued)

Clothing shopping facilities
Household supplies shopping facilities
Satisfaction with personal worth: A = 0.79
What you are accomplishing in life
Your self-esteem
Satisfaction with sanitation/waste management: A = 0.78
Snow removal
Conditions of sidewalks during winter
Cleanliness of the town
Cleanliness of the back alleys
Wildlife management
Domestic animal management
Satisfaction with finances: A = 0.76
Your overall standard of living
Your financial security
Satisfaction with house/neighborhood: A = 0.74
Your house, apartment or mobile home
Your neighbourhood as a place to live
Availability of local housing
Cost of local housing
Density of local housing
Use of local housing
Satisfaction with your job: A = 0.73
Your job
Your pay level
Your work schedule
Satisfaction with government: A = 0.71
Parks Canada officials
I.D. staff and councillors
Federal M.P.
Provincial M.L.A.
Satisfaction with educational opportunities: A = 0.68
Elementary education
Junior/senior high school education
Availability of post-secondary education
Satisfaction with interpersonal relations: A = 0.67
Your family relations generally
Your living partner
Your friendships

so on, it is not useful for explaining satisfaction in the generic sense. For the latter, one would require something other than satisfaction to do the explanatory work. For example, in multiple discrepancies theory (MDT) satisfaction is posited as the effect

Table 8.5 Comparison of life satisfaction regressions from 8 surveys

	1979	1981	1982	1984	1985/86	1994	1997	1997
	A[a]	B	C	D	E	F	G	H
Percent of variance explained in life satisfaction	57	49	53	53	49	60	64	65
Predictors satisfaction with:	Standardized regression coefficients							
Health	0.11	0.18	0.17	0.12	0.11	b	b	0.17
Financial security	0.15	−0.01	0.24	0.11	0.16	b	0.09	b
Family relations	0.35	0.10	0.10	0.13	0.06	b	0.09	0.16
Job	0.10	c	b	0.09	b	0.08	0.08	0.11
Friendships	0.20	0.08	0.07	0.17	0.08	0.13	0.07	b
Housing	−0.05	0.21	0.10	0.12	0.12	0.14	b	b
Area lived in	b	0.01	0.13	b	c	b	b	b
Recreation activity	0.08	0.08	0.05	0.12	0.13	b	b	b
Religion	c	0.13	0.07	b	b	b	b	b
Self-esteem	0.13	0.17	0.19	0.31	0.19	0.50	0.57	0.57
Transportation	0.09	0.05	0.06	b	0.05	b	b	c
Gov. services	c	0.13	0.04	c	c	0.13	b	b
Living partner	c	0.06	c	c	0.15	0.09	0.13	b
Education	−0.03	c	c	0.16	0.19	b	c	c

$P < 0.01$, [a]A = Clerical staff (N = 312), B = Seniors (N = 273), C = East. northerners (N = 328), D = Guelph students (N = 296), E = world students (N = 5107), F = Prince George residents in 1994 (N = 430), G = Prince George residents in 1997 (N = 512), H = Jasper residents in 1997 (N = 229). [b]Significance level too low to enter equation. [c]Not in questionnaire

of such things as the perceived discrepancies between what one has and wants, between what one has and others have, and so on (Michalos 1985, 1991a). Nevertheless, although the simple linear model does not explain satisfaction in the generic sense, it does allow one to measure the impact of satisfaction with various domains of life on one's perceived overall satisfaction with life. In this section we will also apply the model to explain happiness with life as a whole and satisfaction with the overall quality of life.

On average, for the eight samples represented in Table 8.5, we were able to explain 56% of the variance in reported life satisfaction from some subset of the 14 predictor variables listed in the table. Our best success came from the Jasper sample in 1997 (column H), at 65%. When all variables are standardized to have means of zero and standard deviations of one, the standardized regression coefficients (Betas) measure the percent of movement in the dependent variable when a predictor variable moves one full unit and every other predictor in the set is held constant. For example, under column H one finds that the Beta value for self-esteem is $B = 0.57$, which means that for every full standard deviation increase in satisfaction with one's own self-esteem, one's life satisfaction increases a bit over half a standard deviation. Inspection of the other figures in that column reveals that satisfaction in no other domain had as great an impact on overall life satisfaction for the 229 Jasper respondents.

It should be noted that the presence of correlation among the predictor variables affects the magnitude of the standardized regression coefficients. Therefore, it is not recommended that standardized regression coefficients be interpreted as reflecting the importance of the predictor. Thus far in this essay we are not interpreting the importance of the predictors, per se, but rather we use the standardized regression coefficients, in part, to help us make comparisons across samples. In section ("Relative Importance of the Predictor Variables") we will come back to these regression models and consider the relative importance of the predictor variables.

Reading across the row to the left from 0.57, one sees that satisfaction with one's own self-esteem was also the strongest predictor of life satisfaction for the 512 Prince George residents in the 1997 sample (column G, $B = 0.57$), for the 430 residents in the 1994 Prince George sample (column F, $B = 0.50$) and for the sample of 296 University of Guelph students (column D), at $B = 0.31$. That Guelph sample was part of the global student sample whose results are listed in column E. Inspection of that column shows that satisfaction with one's own self-esteem tied with satisfaction with one's university education as the strongest predictors of life satisfaction for the 5107 students in the global sample.

For the other three samples, satisfaction with one's self-esteem was not as powerful a predictor as (had less explanatory power than) satisfaction with one or more other domains. For the 312 sampled members of the office, clerical and technical staff of the University of Guelph (column A), satisfaction with one's family relations had the greatest explanatory power ($B = 0.35$). For the 273 sampled rural seniors (column B), satisfaction with their housing had the strongest predictive strength ($B = 0.21$) and for the 328 eastern northerners (column C), satisfaction with their financial security had the greatest explanatory power ($B = 0.24$).

The figures just reviewed clearly illustrate the fact that different groups of people with different life circumstances, resources and constraints use different mixtures of ingredients to determine their life satisfaction. The explanatory model used here allowed the groups represented in Table 8.5 to draw satisfaction from roughly the same set of 14 domains. Analytically speaking, some groups used more and some used fewer of these domains to build their life satisfaction. The Jasper group used only 4 of the 12 possibilities open to them. Besides making use of only 4 domains all together, they drew more overall life satisfaction from satisfaction with their own self-esteem than they did from the other three domains combined, i.e., satisfaction with their health ($B = 0.17$), family relations ($B = 0.16$) and job ($B = 0.11$).

Table 8.6 provides some comparative figures resulting from regressing mean happiness scores on mean scores for satisfaction with various domains of life. On average, for the eight samples represented in this table, we were able to explain 34% of the variance in reported happiness with life as a whole from some subset of the 14 predictor variables listed in the table. Our best success came from the clerical staff sample from the University of Guelph (column A), at 45%. The strongest

Table 8.6 Comparison of happiness regressions from 8 surveys

	1979	1981	1982	1984	1985/86	1994	1997	1997
	A[a]	B	C	D	E	F	G	H
Percent of variance explained in life satisfaction	45	32	36	39	28	27	38	27
Predictors satisfaction with:	Standardized regression coefficients							
Health	0.12	0.12	0.18	0.17	0.09	[b]	[b]	[b]
Financial security	0.09	0.06	0.21	[b]	0.13	[b]	0.14	0.19
Family relations	0.38	−0.03	0.09	0.14	0.06	[b]	0.14	[b]
Job	0.03	[c]	0.09	0.18	[b]	0.10	[b]	[b]
Friendships	0.23	0.23	0.01	0.21	0.10	0.10	0.09	[b]
Housing	0.01	−0.01	0.10	[b]	0.07	[b]	[b]	[b]
Area lived in	[b]	0.01	0.05	[b]	[c]	[b]	[b]	[b]
Recreation activity	0.03	0.04	0.05	[b]	0.07	0.13	[b]	[b]
Religion	[c]	0.01	0.03	[b]	[b]	[b]	[b]	[b]
Self-esteem	0.07	0.09	0.14	0.26	0.13	0.21	0.27	0.25
Transportation	0.05	0.05	[b]	[b]	[b]	[b]	[b]	[c]
Gov. services	[c]	0.08	0.03	[c]	[c]	[b]	0.09	[b]
Living partner	[c]	0.30	[c]	[c]	0.18	0.22	0.22	0.22
Education	−0.03	[c]	[c]	[b]	0.10	[b]	[c]	[c]

$P < 0.01$, [a]A = Clerical staff (N = 312), B = Seniors (N = 273), C = East. Northerners (N = 328), D = Guelph students (N = 296), E = world students (N = 5036), F = Prince George residents (N = 412), G = Prince George residents in 1997 (N = 466), H = Jasper residents in 1997 (N = 210). [b]Significance level too low to enter equation. [c]Not in questionnaire

explanatory variable for that sample was satisfaction with family relations, which had a Beta value of $B = 0.38$. Thus, figuratively speaking, for every full-step increase in satisfaction with their family relations, the overall happiness of these respondents increased 38% of a step.

As one moves across the columns of Table 8.6, one finds that the strongest explanatory variable for the rural seniors group was satisfaction with their friendships ($B = 0.23$), satisfaction with their financial security was the strongest predictor for the eastern northern group ($B = 0.21$), satisfaction with self-esteem for the Guelph students ($B = 0.26$), the 1997 Prince George sample ($B = 0.27$) and the Jasper sample ($B = 0.25$), and satisfaction with living partners for the world student sample ($B = 0.18$) and the 1994 Prince George sample ($B = 0.22$). As in the case of life satisfaction, different groups built up their overall happiness with different mixtures of ingredients and some groups drew upon more domains than others. The Jasper sample used only 3 of the 12 possibilities open to them, with satisfaction with living partners ($B = 0.22$) and financial security ($B = 0.19$) having almost as much influence as satisfaction with self-esteem.

When we examined the impact of the same domain satisfaction scores on satisfaction with the overall quality of life in Jasper, we found that there were five statistically significant predictors which collectively accounted for 44% of the variation in the global indicator scores (N = 229). Again, satisfaction with one's own selfesteem was the strongest predictor (*B* = 0.30). Following that, there was a cluster containing satisfaction with local recreation opportunities (*B* = 0.18), Jasper as a place to live (*B* = 0.18), religion (*B* = 0.17) and financial security (*B* = 0.16). The most interesting thing about the cluster was that three of the items had no significant impact on life satisfaction or happiness. Clearly, respondents are conceptualizing their overall quality of life in a way that distinguishes it to some extent from overall life satisfaction and happiness.

Explaining Life Satisfaction, Happiness and Satisfaction with the Quality of Life from Selected Satisfaction Items and Indices

Table 8.7 gives the results of regressing the three dependent global variables on the 15 indices plus some individual items. We were able to explain 37% of the variance in reported overall happiness, 63% of the variance in reported satisfaction with life as a whole and 44% of the variance in reported satisfaction with the overall quality of life.

Perhaps the most interesting discovery from these regressions is the fact that only the indices of personal worth and finances have a role to play in explaining all three dependent variables. Regarding happiness (*B* = 0.36), satisfaction with life as a whole (*B* = 0.56) and with the overall quality of life (*B* = 0.40), the index of personal worth is more influential than any of the other predictors. For overall happiness, after the index of personal worth, there is satisfaction with one's finances (*B* = 0.22), interpersonal relations (*B* = 0.16) and recycling (*B* = 0.10). For satisfaction with life as a whole, after the index of personal worth, there is a cluster containing satisfaction with interpersonal relations (*B* = 0.17), finances (*B* = 0.15) and police protection (*B* = 0.13), followed by satisfaction with the weather (*B* = 0.08). For satisfaction with the quality of life, after the index of personal worth, there is satisfaction with finances (*B* = 0.24), and a cluster containing satisfaction with Jasper as a place to live (*B* = 0.12), sanitation and waste management (*B* = 0.10) and recycling (*B* = 0.09). The latter cluster presents an interesting set of quality-of-life predictors for respondents living in a beautiful national park.

Given the great number and variety of items and indices available in these regressions, it seems remarkable to us that satisfaction with recycling emerged as a modest but statistically significant predictor of happiness and satisfaction with the overall quality of life in Jasper.

Table 8.7 Explanations of happiness, satisfaction with life as a whole and satisfaction with the quality of life

	Beta
Happiness	
Predictors satisfaction with:	
Personal worth	0.36
Finances	0.22
Interpersonal relations	0.16
Recycling	0.10
Variance explained	37% (N = 285)
Life satisfaction	
Predictors satisfaction with:	
Personal worth	0.56
Interpersonal relations	0.17
Finances	0.15
Police protection	0.13
Weather	0.08
Variance explained	63% (N = 306)
Satisfaction with quality of life	
Predictors satisfaction with:	
Personal worth	0.40
Finances	0.24
Jasper as a place to live	0.12
Sanitation/waste mgt.	0.10
Recycling	0.09
Variance explained	44% (N = 309)

Relative Importance of the Predictor Variables

Keeping in mind the caveat we provided in section "Explaining Life Satisfaction, Happiness and Overall Satisfaction with the Quality of Life from Selected Domain Satisfaction Items" about interpreting the relative importance of predictor variables based on the magnitude of the Beta coefficient, Thomas et al. (1998) presented a new statistical method for ordering predictor variables in a linear model in terms of their importance in the model. The Thomas, Hughes, and Zumbo method proceeds by defining importance as the relative proportion (percentage) of the resultant model R-squared that can be attributed to each predictor variable. Said another way, their method additively partitions the R-squared value so that one can attribute a certain proportion of the R-squared to each predictor variable. The computation of this new statistic is straightforward: multiply the Beta coefficient by the simple correlation of the predictor and dependent variable, and then divide this quantity by the model R-squared. One simply performs these computations for each predictor variable in a model.

Table 8.8 lists the results for each of the linear regression models reported in this essay. As an example of how to interpret these new methods let us focus on the

Table 8.8 Variable-ordering for the models in Table 8.5 through Table 8.7

	% of the R-squared attributed to the predictor
Life satisfaction (Table 8.5)	
Satisfaction with:	
Health	14
Family relations	12
Job	8
Self-esteem	66
Happiness (Table 8.6)	
Satisfaction with:	
Financial security	25
Self-esteem	42
Living partner	33
Happiness (Table 8.7)	
Satisfaction with:	
Personal worth	52
Finances	28
Interpersonal relations	15
Recycling	5
Life satisfaction (Table 8.7)	
Satisfaction with:	
Personal worth	66
Interpersonal relations	12
Finances	12
Police protection	7
Weather	3
Satisfaction with quality of life (Table 8.7)	
Satisfaction with:	
Personal worth	52
Finances	29
Jasper as a place to live	10
Sanitation/waste mgt.	5
Recycling	4

Jasper model reported in Table 8.5. From Table 8.8 we can see that 66% of the explained variation in life satisfaction is attributable to satisfaction with self-esteem whereas 26% of the explained variation is attributable to health and family relations together, and the remaining 8% to job satisfaction. This sort of analysis is possible because of additive properties of the Thomas-Hughes-Zumbo method. Furthermore, self-esteem is clearly the most important predictor in that model whereas health and family relations are tied for second most important and job satisfaction the least important.

Some noteworthy findings in Table 8.8 are: (a) 75% of the explained variation in happiness (Table 8.6) is attributable to satisfaction with self-esteem and satisfaction with living partner together, (b) with reference to the regressions reported in Table 8.7, satisfaction with personal worth is not only clearly the most important predictor, but for each model over 50% of the explained variation is attributable to satisfaction with personal worth.

Conclusion

The main aim of this research was to discover and explain citizen beliefs and attitudes about the quality of life in Jasper, Alberta in the summer of 1997. We explored people's satisfaction with a wide variety of aspects of their community and their lives. In the respondents' own words, we discovered the best and worst things about living in Jasper, and the things they would change first to improve the quality of their lives. We found relatively less support for increasing the use of use-fees than one might have expected and roughly just what one would have expected about citizen views of the value received from tax dollars. We created 15 indices of satisfaction with fundamental aspects of people's lives, which should be very useful to other researchers. Then we explained happiness, life satisfaction and overall satisfaction with the quality of life from a limited set of 14 variables, which allowed us to compare our Jasper results with results from seven other surveys taken over nearly 20 years. Finally, we used a simple linear model to account for 63% of the variance in life satisfaction scores, 44% of the variance in satisfaction with the quality of life scores and 37% of the variance in happiness scores.

Acknowledgements The authors would like to express their appreciation to Toni Fletcher, George Krefting, Wendy Marks, Joanne Matthews, Shelley Rennick and Kathleen Waxer for the help they gave us in the development, administration, analysis and reporting of the survey.

References

Michalos, A. C. (1985). Multiple discrepancies theory (MDT). *Social Indicators Research, 16,* 347–413.

Michalos, A. C. (1991a). *Global report on student well-being. Volume 1: Life satisfaction and happiness*. New York: Springer.

Michalos, A. C. (1991b). *Global report on student well-being. Volume 2: Family, friends, living partner and self-esteem*. New York: Springer.

Michalos, A. C. (1993). *Global report on student well-being. Volume 3: Employment, finances, housing and transportation*. New York: Springer.

Michalos, A. C. (1995). *A pragmatic approach to business ethics*. Thousand Oaks: Sage Publications.

Michalos, A. C. (1996). Aspects of the quality of life in Prince George: A case study in Canada. *South Asian Journal of Psychology, 1,* 45–70.

Thomas, D. R., Hughes, E., & Zumbo, B. D. (1998). On variable importance in linear regression. *Social Indicators Research.*

Chapter 9
British Columbians' Expectations and Attitudes Going into the Third Millennium

Alex C. Michalos and Bruno D. Zumbo

Introduction

In the spring of 1999 researchers at the Institute for Social Research and Evaluation, University of Northern British Columbia, formed a partnership with the *Prince George Citizen* to undertake a survey of the expectations and attitudes of British Columbians as we left the second and entered the first hundred years of the third millennium. The general plan was to divide the province somewhat arbitrarily into a southern and a northern part, and to compare the views of residents in the two parts. The town of Hundred Mile House was selected as the demarcation point, with households located in or south of town designated as southern residents and households located north of town designated as northern residents. Besides creating a description of residents' expectations and attitudes toward the future, we assessed the current quality of their lives using a battery of measures that have been used by us and others in a wide variety of places at different times over the past 25 years (e.g., Michalos and Zumbo 1999).

The structure of the essay is as follows. In the next section "Sampling Technique and Questionnaire", we describe our sampling technique and questionnaire, and then we describe our sample (section "Sample Characteristics"). In section "Expectations and Attitudes" we provide descriptive statistics regarding

Michalos, A.C., & Zumbo, B.C.: 2000. British Columbians' expectations and Attitudes going into the third millennium.

A.C. Michalos (✉)
University of Northern British Columbia, Prince George, BC, Canada
e-mail: michalos@brandonu.ca; michalos@unbc.ca

B.D. Zumbo
Institute for Social Research and Evaluation, University of Northern British Columbia, Prince George, BC V2N 4Z9, Canada

A.C. Michalos, *Development of Quality of Life Theory and Its Instruments*,
DOI 10.1007/978-3-319-51149-8_9

respondents' expectations and attitudes toward events that may occur in the next 100 years, as well as satisfaction levels for a variety of aspects of life. In section "Health", we compare respondents' self-reported health with the self-reported health of 142,674 Americans from the 50 states of the USA in 1998. Section "Fears, Hopes and Things to Change" summarizes responses to our open-ended questions about respondents' greatest fears, hopes and things they would change to improve the quality of their lives. In section "Explaining Life Satisfaction, Happiness and Overall Satisfaction with the Quality of Life from Domain Satisfaction Items", we explain respondents' satisfaction with life as a whole, happiness and satisfaction with the overall quality of life from a limited set of 16 variables, which allows us to compare our British Columbian results with results from seven other surveys taken over nearly 20 years. In section "Relative Importance of the Predictor Variables" we apply a new statistical method for ordering the predictor variables from the regressions reported in section "Explaining Life Satisfaction, Happiness and Overall Satisfaction with the Quality of Life from Domain Satisfaction Items" in terms of their relative importance to global assessments of life in each regression model (Thomas et al. 1998). The final section "Conclusion" is a brief conclusion.

Sampling Technique and Questionnaire

Seven-page questionnaires were mailed out to two independently selected random samples of households in British Columbia in October and November 1999, with 3000 going to households in or south of Hundred Mile House and 5000 going to households north of that town. The decision to make Hundred Mile House the demarcation line between north and south was based on the relative numbers and sizes of cities above and below it. Although about 85% of the population resides in the southern part of the province, because we wanted to have useful samples from several northern towns, we drew a larger sample from the north than from the south. This was the first time northern and southern views were systematically compared in British Columbia.

The first three pages of the questionnaire listed 42 events and states of affairs that might occur in the next 100 years, and respondents were asked to indicate whether they thought "it would be good (or bad) if it happened" and then if they thought it was "probably going to happen (or not)". For example, the first item was "Canada will merge with the United States". These items were followed by a page containing 17 "things affecting people today", such as their family relations, health, jobs and so on. The extent to which people were satisfied with these things was measured on a 7-point Likert scale with response categories ranging from "very dissatisfied = 1 point", through "an even balance = 4", to "very satisfied = 7".

After these items, there was a 7-point question designed to measure the extent to which people were happy with their lives as a whole, ranging from "very unhappy = 1 point", through "an even balance = 4", to "very happy = 7".

There was then a battery of four self-reported health items designed and used extensively by the U.S. Center for Disease Control and Prevention (CDC) in all of the 50 states. This was the first time these items were used on a provincial population in Canada. An example of one of these items is "Would you say that in general your health is (a) excellent, (b) very good, (c) good, (d) fair, or (e) poor?"

These were followed by four open-ended questions asking respondents first, to describe their "greatest fear for the next few years", and then "what they most hoped for". Then we asked, "All things considered, if you could change anything about your life to improve its quality, what would you do?" Finally, we asked some questions about employment and education in the immediate future, and the questionnaire ended with two pages of demographic questions (e.g., gender, age, education).

Sample Characteristics

By the end of November, 499 (17%) useable questionnaires were returned from the south and 969 (19%) were returned from the north, which form the working data-sets for the survey. For the southern group the sampling error margin is ±4.5% points 19 times out of 20 and for the northern group it is 3.2% points.

The average age in the southern group is 51 (ranging from 18 to 93) and in the northern group it is 47 (ranging from 18 to 91). Sixty percent of the southern group and 56% of the northern group are male. The median household income for the southern group is $55,000 per year, compared to $60,000 for the northern group. Fifty-four percent of the southern group are employed full or part-time, compared to 65% of the northern group. Sixty percent of the southern group and 62% of the northern group are married. A full 30% of the southern group have a university degree, compared to 17% of the northern group.

Although we are unable to make rigorous comparisons between our samples and the northern and southern populations from which they are drawn, we can certainly say that our samples have percentages of males, married and university educated people that are a bit higher than they should be to be strictly representative according to the most recent provincial census figures. It would be possible to assign weights to our responses to get a perfect fit with census figures. However, we have no way of knowing how representative each of our respondents is of every person in the population with the same demographic profile (gender, age, education and so on). For example, maybe the 20 year old males with a university education who filled out our questionnaire are significantly different somehow from those who did not fill out our questionnaire. So multiplying our responses for such people to get a sample that is demographically more representative of the provincial population may produce a sample that is substantively more unrepresentative. Rather than risk such an anomaly, we simply note and work with unweighted samples.

Expectations and Attitudes

Table 9.1 lists the percentages of northern and southern respondents who indicated that they thought the various events and states of affairs would be good or bad if they occurred, and the percentages who thought they would actually occur in the next 100 years.

For 22 of the 42 items northerners and southerners gave responses that were identical or only one or two percentage points different; e.g.,

> 75% of northerners and southerners said it would be bad if Quebec separated from Canada,
>
> 93% of both groups said it would be good if Northern B.C. got the attention it deserves,
>
> 85% of both groups said it would be good if most people got university degrees,
>
> 96% of both groups said it would be bad if the polar ice caps melt and seaports are flooded,
>
> 94% of both groups said it would be good if the quality of their lives improved in the next 5 years.

For 3 of these 5 items, northerners and southerners agreed on the probability of the events happening, but for 2 they disagreed; i.e.,

> 45% of northerners but 61% of southerners thought Northern B.C. would get the attention it deserves,
>
> 45% of northerners but 40% of southerners thought the polar ice caps would melt and flood seaports.

The following items had the greatest levels of disagreement regarding things that might happen in the next 100 years. Percentages of people expecting that the events would happen are in parentheses.

> Ninety percent of northerners but 62% of southerners thought it would be good if there were tax breaks for northern residents (26% of northerners and 38% of southerners thought it would happen),
>
> 26% of northerners but 37% of southerners thought it would be good if religion becomes much less important (60% of northerners and 65% of southerners thought it would happen),
>
> 70% of northerners but 60% of southerners thought it would be good if capital punishment becomes reinstated in Canada (42% of northerners and 36% of southerners thought it would happen),
>
> 76% of northerners but 86% of southerners thought it would be good if provincial and federal elections began using some system of proportionate representation (56% of northerners and 61% of southerners thought it would happen),
>
> 55% of northerners but 47% of southerners thought it would be good if people lived longer than 100 years (45% of northerners and 43% of southerners thought it would happen).

If one were looking for a popular (and populist) political agenda for most British Columbians, some of its elements are discernible in Table 9.1. Fairly large majorities, north and south, think it would be bad to change our political geography by merging with the United States, separating Quebec, B.C. or aboriginal nations from the rest of the country, or breaking up the country in any way. Large

Table 9.1 Percentages of respondents indicating it would be good or bad and whether it will or will not happen

		Would it be		Will it happen?	
		Good (%)	Bad (%)	Yes (%)	No (%)
1	Canada will merge with the United States	**N = 21**	N = 79	**N = 24**	N = 76
		S = 26	S = 74	**S = 25**	S = 75
2	Quebec will separate from Canada	**N = 25**	N = 75	**N = 29**	N = 71
		S = 25	S = 75	**S = 27**	S = 73
3	Some aboriginal groups will form separate countries	**N = 14**	N = 86	**N = 24**	N = 76
		S = 15	S = 85	**S = 23**	S = 77
4	Canada will break up into several countries	**N = 7**	N = 93	**N = 14**	N = 86
		S = 9	S = 91	**S = 16**	S = 84
5	The national debt will finally be paid off	**N = 93**	N = 7	**N = 19**	N = 81
		S = 92	S = 8	**S = 22**	S = 78
6	The gap between rich and poor will widen	**N = 3**	N = 97	**N = 86**	N = 14
		S = 5	S = 95	**S = 82**	S = 18
7	Most people will live longer than 100 years	**N = 55**	N = 45	**N = 45**	N = 55
		S = 47	S = 53	**S = 43**	S = 57
8	Most people will not live in single Family detached homes	**N = 27**	N = 73	**N = 68**	N = 32
		S = 33	S = 67	**S = 73**	S = 27
9	Religion will become much less important	**N = 26**	N = 74	**N = 60**	N = 40
		S = 37	S = 63	**S = 65**	S = 35
10	Most people will have to work harder for lower pay	**N = 6**	N = 94	**N = 80**	N = 20
		S = 9	S = 91	**S = 72**	S = 28
11	Same sex couples will be more commonly accepted	**N = 45**	N = 55	**N = 86**	N = 14
		S = 52	S = 48	**S = 89**	S = 11
12	There will be fewer prejudiced people	**N = 92**	N = 8	**N = 42**	N = 58
		S = 90	S = 10	**S = 45**	S = 55
13	There will be a population shift toward the north	**N = 72**	N = 28	**N = 65**	N = 35
		S = 77	S = 23	**S = 52**	S = 48
14	All health insurance will be privatized	**N = 19**	N = 81	**N = 65**	N = 35
		S = 21	S = 79	**S = 50**	S = 50
15	Northern B.C. will get the attention it deserves	**N = 93**	N = 7	**N = 45**	N = 55
		S = 93	S = 7	**S = 61**	S = 39
16	There will be only two political parties, a united right and a united left	**N = 27**	N = 73	**N = 28**	N = 72
		S = 29	S = 71	**S = 30**	S = 70
17	There will be a provincial ministry of Northern affairs	**N = 85**	N = 15	**N = 60**	N = 40
		S = 81	S = 19	**S = 66**	S = 34
18	Global warming will increase	**N = 10**	N = 90	**N = 89**	N = 11
		S = 9	S = 91	**S = 87**	S = 13
19	Crime will increase in the North	**N = 1**	N = 99	**N = 83**	N = 17

(continued)

Table 9.1 (continued)

		Would it be		Will it happen?	
		Good (%)	Bad (%)	Yes (%)	No (%)
		S = 4	S = 96	**S = 80**	S = 20
20	Crime will increase in rural areas	**N = 2**	N = 98	**N = 81**	N = 19
		S = 5	S = 95	**S = 79**	S = 21
21	Most people will get university degrees	**N = 85**	N = 15	**N = 29**	N = 71
		S = 85	S = 15	**S = 31**	S = 69
22	An earthquake will destroy vancouver and surrounding area	**N = 6**	N = 94	**N = 45**	N = 55
		S = 5	S = 95	**S = 36**	S = 64
23	Crime will increase in most urban areas	**N = 1**	N = 99	**N = 86**	N = 14
		S = 3	S = 97	**S = 81**	S = 19
24	The mining industry in B.C. will disappear	**N = 10**	N = 90	**N = 35**	N = 65
		S = 14	S = 86	**S = 40**	S = 60
25	All natural resource industries will specialize in value-added products	**N = 86**	N = 14	**N = 73**	N = 27
		S = 85	S = 15	**S = 74**	S = 26
26	The polar ice caps will melt and many seaports will be flooded	**N = 4**	N = 96	**N = 45**	N = 55
		S = 4	S = 96	**S = 40**	S = 60
27	The quality of your own life will improve in the next 5 years	**N = 94**	N = 6	**N = 61**	N = 39
		S = 94	S = 6	**S = 61**	S = 39
28	You will find it more difficult to maintain your standard of living	**N = 6**	N = 94	**N = 66**	N = 34
		S = 8	S = 92	**S = 62**	S = 38
29	The world will witness the second coming of Jesus Christ	**N = 72**	N = 28	**N = 21**	N = 79
		S = 65	S = 35	**S = 16**	S = 84
30	There will be a catastrophic nuclear explosion somewhere in the world	**N = 2**	N = 98	**N = 75**	N = 25
		S = 3	S = 97	**S = 73**	S = 27
31	Capital punishment will be reinstated in Canada	**N = 70**	N = 30	**N = 42**	N = 58
		S = 60	S = 40	**S = 36**	S = 64
32	Abortion will be outlawed again	**N = 30**	N = 70	**N = 19**	N = 81
		S = 25	S = 75	**S = 17**	S = 83
33	There will be tax breaks for Northern residents	**N = 90**	N = 10	**N = 26**	N = 74
		S = 62	S = 38	**S = 38**	S = 62
34	B.C. will separate from the rest of Canada	**N = 20**	N = 80	**N = 8**	N = 92
		S = 21	S = 79	**S = 12**	S = 88
35	The institution of marriage will hold up in the next century	**N = 95**	N = 5	**N = 78**	N = 22
		S = 94	S = 6	**S = 80**	S = 20
36	Couples will continue to have fewer children in the next century	**N = 67**	N = 33	**N = 89**	N = 11
		S = 74	S = 26	**S = 91**	S = 9
37	The north east of B.C. will become part of Alberta	**N = 26**	N = 74	**N = 18**	N = 82
		S = 23	S = 77	**S = 16**	S = 84
38	There will be off shore oil and gas wells along the B.C. coast	**N = 63**	N = 37	**N = 74**	N = 26
		N = 59	S = 41	**S = 67**	S = 33

(continued)

Table 9.1 (continued)

		Would it be		Will it happen?	
		Good (%)	Bad (%)	Yes (%)	No (%)
39	All elections will be using some system of proportionate represent	**N = 76**	N = 24	**N = 56**	N = 44
		S = 86	S = 14	**S = 61**	S = 39
40	All aboriginal land claims will be settled	**N = 76**	N = 24	**N = 39**	N = 61
		S = 81	S = 19	**S = 34**	S = 66
41	A cure for AIDS will be found	**N = 97**	N = 3	**N = 73**	N = 27
		S = 95	S = 5	**S = 77**	S = 23
42	Gender roles will become less fixed	**N = 80**	N = 20	**N = 83**	N = 17
		S = 78	S = 22	**S = 84**	S = 16

majorities think it would be good to pay off the national debt, decrease the gap between rich and poor, create a Ministry of Northern Affairs, settle all aboriginal land claims and introduce some form of proportionate representation. Somewhat smaller majorities think it would be good to reinstate capital punishment but to continue the current legal regime regarding therapeutic abortion. Large majorities think it would be bad to have all health insurance privatized and to have only two political parties, a united left and a united right. Of course many of these issues cannot be managed at the provincial level.

Table 9.2 lists the northern and southern mean scores for the 17 satisfaction items and the one happiness item. The most striking thing about this table is the fact that 10 of the pairs of figures are exactly the same and another 5 differ by only 0.1% point for northerners and southerners. Statistically significant differences are relatively easy to get with such large sample sizes, but there are no statistically significant differences between the two groups for any of the 18 items. Since these 18 items are fairly standard measures of the quality of people's lives according to reports of their own subjective experiences, it is fair to say that the quality of life of northern and southern British Columbians is practically identical.

The most satisfying aspects of people's lives were satisfaction with their living partners (*mean* = 6.0), family relations generally (5.7 north/5.8 south), friendships and neighbourhoods (5.6). Average scores for happiness with life as a whole were fairly high (5.8), higher than the mean scores for satisfaction with life as a whole (5.6) and the overall quality of life (5.5).

Highest levels of dissatisfaction were expressed for provincial government officials (2.1), federal government officials (2.6) and local government officials (3.4/3.2).

Table 9.2 Northern and southern mean levels of satisfaction and happiness

On a 7-point scale, satisfaction with:	Northern %	Southern %
Your house, apartment or mobile home	5.5	5.6
Your neighbourhood as a place to live	5.6	5.6
Your family relations	5.7	5.8
Your living partner	6.0	6.0
Your job	5.1	5.2
How you feel about life as a whole	5.6	5.6
Your friendships	5.6	5.6
Your health	5.3	5.3
Your religion or spiritual fulfilment	5.2	5.2
Your financial security	4.4	4.5
Your recreation activities	4.8	5.0
Your self-esteem	5.3	5.4
Federal government officials	2.6	2.6
Provincial government officials	2.1	2.1
Local government officials	3.4	3.2
Your overall quality of life	5.5	5.5
Your personal safety in your neighbourhood	5.5	5.3
Your happiness with life as a whole	5.8	5.8

Health

In response to the first item from the CDC, about 82% of northerners and southerners reported that their general health was good to excellent. The second two items distinguish physical and mental health, and ask people to indicate the number of days out of the past 30 that their health was not good. The 'mean number of *good health days* in the past 30 days' for an individual is then calculated by simply summing the mean number of not good physical and mental health days and subtracting the sum from 30. Both northerners and southerners reported an average of 22.6 good health days in the past 30.

Using data from the CDC Behavioral Risk Factor Surveillance System for 1998, we were able to compare our aggregated north and south scores with scores from the 50 states plus Washington, D.C. of the USA according to gender and age. Table 9.3 shows that in every case the Americans had on average relatively more good health days in the past 30 than Canadians. Comparing our data with data for each of the states, we found very few cases in which the British Columbian figures were superior. For every state, American men and women aged 18–34 had more good health days on average than British Columbian men and women in that age group. For the 35–49 age group, with the exception of women in Utah, men and women in every state had more good health days on average than British Columbian men and women. For the 50–64 age group, with the exceptions of men in Alabama, Arizona, South Carolina and Utah and women in Alabama, Kentucky

Table 9.3 Average number of good health days in the past 30 days for Americans and British Columbians, by gender and age

Age	USA	Means	BC	Means
18–34 years	Men	25.9 (N = 17354)	Men	21.3 (N = 131)
	Women	24.0 (N = 22581)	Women	21.2 (N = 169)
35–49 years	Men	25.7 (N = 19994)	Men	23.5 (N = 271)
	Women	23.9 (N = 26751)	Women	21.9 (N = 226)
50–64 years	Men	25.1 (N = 12158)	Men	23.9 (N = 264)
	Women	23.3 (N = 16787)	Women	22.4 (N = 118)
65 years or more	Men	24.6 (N = 9443)	Men	23.2 (N = 150)
	Women	23.2 (N = 17606)	Women	21.4 (N = 82)
Totals	Men	25.5 (N = 58949)	Men	23.2 (N = 816)
	Women	23.7 (N = 83725)	Women	21.7 (N = 595)

American data covering the 50 states and Washington, D.C. of the USA were kindly provided by David Moriarty from the CDC Behavioral Risk Factor Surveillance System 1998

and Nevada, men and women in every state had more good health days on average than British Columbian men and women. For the 65 and older age group, with the exceptions of men in Alabama, Alaska, Arizona, Indiana, Massachusetts, Michigan and Minnesota and women in Alabama, Colorado, Kentucky, Michigan, Minnesota and North Carolina, men and women in every state had more good health days on average than British Columbian men and women. Recalling that people with university degrees are over-represented in our sample and that such people tend to have relatively higher incomes and better health than those without degrees, it is likely that, if anything, our sample exaggerates the healthiness of B.C. residents. Granting that, the comparisons we have just reviewed are disturbing.

We know there is some sort of cultural bias in self-reports of subjective well-being, including self-reported health, but so far nobody knows exactly how to measure or compensate for such bias (Michalos 1991a, b, 1993a, b). For example, Americans typically give fairly robust personal reports while Japanese tend to give fairly modest reports of their well-being, although the life expectancy at birth of Japanese is 80 years compared to 77 years for Americans (United Nations Development Program 1999, p. 134). Life expectancy is only one gross indicator of health status, but it is useful to illustrate our point that there is no evidence that the Japanese are generally less healthy than the Americans.

Fears, Hopes and Things to Change

For all respondents, the most frequently mentioned "greatest fears" for the next few years concerned unemployment and financial insecurity, poor health or health care, and poor government. For northerners, issues related to unemployment and financial insecurity constituted 36% of all issues mentioned, compared to 31% for southerners. Twenty percent of issues mentioned by northerners involved poor health or health care, compared to 22% for southerners. Fifteen percent of issues mentioned by northerners concerned poor government, compared to 9% for southerners.

Thirty percent of things mentioned by northerners as "most hoped for" involved employment and financial security, 20% involved good health and health care, and 13% involved good government. For southerners, issues involved good health and health care first (28%), then employment and financial security (25%) and then good government (11%).

Having determined respondents' fears and hopes, we wanted to find out what respondents would change to improve the quality of their lives, if they "could change anything". The most frequently mentioned things for northerners and southerners were the same, only the percentages of responses were a bit different. Both groups mentioned issues related to employment and financial security first (34% north, 29% south), second health (19% north, 18% south), and third educational opportunities (8% north, 7% south).

The "educational opportunities" response was especially interesting in the light of our questions about education. Forty-four percent of northerners and 40% of southerners reported that they intended to further their education. Seventy-four percent of northerners who intended to further their education planned to do it in the north, compared to only 7% of southerners. Just to clarify the preference more, we asked those who intended to further their education if they would "prefer it to be in the north although that is not presently possible". Eighty percent of northerners said they would prefer it to be in the north.

Explaining Life Satisfaction, Happiness and Overall Satisfaction with the Quality of Life from Domain Satisfaction Items

Table 9.4 provides some comparative figures resulting from regressing mean life satisfaction scores on mean scores for satisfaction with various domains of life. The simple linear model used to obtain these figures was one of the first models applied by social indicators researchers and it is still one of the most frequently used models (Michalos 1991a). Since the model merely explains overall life (global) satisfaction in terms of the (domain) satisfaction one gets from one's job, family relations and so on, it is not useful for explaining satisfaction in the generic sense. For the latter, one would require something other than satisfaction to do the explanatory work. For example, in multiple discrepancies theory (MDT) satisfaction is posited as the effect of such things as the perceived discrepancies between what one has and wants, between what one has and others have, and so on (Michalos 1985, 1991a). Nevertheless, although the simple linear model does not explain satisfaction in the generic sense, it does allow one to measure the impact of satisfaction with various domains of life on one's perceived overall satisfaction with life. We will also apply

Table 9.4 Comparison of life satisfaction regressions from 8 surveys

Sample	1979	1981	1982	1984	1985/86	1997	1997	1999
	A[a]	B	C	D	E	F	G	H
Percent of variance explained in satisfaction	57	49	53	53	49	64	65	55
Predictors								
Satisfaction with:	Standardized regression coefficients							
Health	0.11	0.18	0.17	0.12	0.11	b	0.17	0.16
Financial security	0.15	−0.01	0.24	0.11	0.16	0.09	b	07
Family relations	0.35	−0.10	0.10	0.13	0.06	0.09	0.16	b
Job	0.10	c	b	0.09	b	0.08	11	0.18
Friendships	0.20	0.08	0.07	0.17	0.08	0.07	b	0.24
Housing	−0.05	0.21	0.10	0.12	0.12	b	b	0.07
Area lived in	b	0.01	0.13	b	c	b	b	c
Recreation activity	0.08	0.08	0.05	0.12	0.13	b	b	b
Religion	c	0.13	0.07	b	b	b	b	b
Self-esteem	0.13	0.17	0.19	0.31	0.19	0.57	0.57	0.22
Transportation	0.09	0.05	0.06	b	0.05	b	c	c
Gov. services	c	0.13	0.04	c	c	b	b	c
Living partner	c	0.06	c	c	0.15	0.13	b	0.15
Education	−0.03	c	c	16	0.19	c	c	c
Fed. Gov. officials	c	c	c	c	c	c	c	0.05

$P < 0.01$
[a]A = Clerical staff (N = 312), B = Rural seniors (N = 273), C = Cochrane residents (N = 328), D = Guelph students (N = 296), E = world students (N = 5107), F = Prince George residents (N = 512), G = Jasper residents (N = 229), H = British Columbians (N = 1083)
[b]Significance level too low to enter equation
[c]Not in questionnaire

the model to explain happiness with life as a whole and satisfaction with the overall quality of life.

Briefly, the samples used in Tables 9.4 and 9.5 came from the following sources: (A) the office, clerical and technical staff of the University of Guelph (Michalos 1980), (B) rural senior citizens in Ontario (Michalos 1982), (C) residents of Cochrane, Ontario (Michalos 1983), (D) undergraduate students at the University of Guelph (Michalos 1991a), (E) undergraduates in 39 countries (Michalos 1991a), (F) residents of Prince George (Michalos and Zumbo 1999), (G) residents of Jasper, Alberta (Zumbo and Michalos 2000), (H) British Columbians.

Table 9.5 Comparison of happiness regressions from 8 surveys

Sample	1979	1981	1982	1984	1985/86	1997	1997	1999
	A[a]	B	C	D	E	F	G	H
Percent of variance explained in happiness	45	32	36	39	28	38	27	46
Predictors satisfaction with:	Standardized regression coefficients							
Health	0.12	0.12	0.18	0.17	0.09	b	b	0.08
Financial security	0.09	0.06	0.21	b	0.13	0.14	0.19	0.08
Family relations	0.38	−0.03	0.09	0.14	0.06	0.14	b	b
Job	0.03	c	0.09	0.18	b	b	b	0.16
Friendships	0.23	0.23	0.01	0.21	0.10	0.09	b	0.09
Housing	0.01	−0.01	0.10	b	0.07	b	b	b
Area lived in	b	0.01	0.05	b	c	b	b	c
Recreation activity	0.03	0.04	0.05	b	0.07	b	b	b
Religion	c	0.01	0.03	b	b	b	b	b
Self-esteem	0.07	0.09	0.14	0.26	0.13	0.27	0.25	0.32
Transportation	0.05	0.05	b	b	b	b	c	c
Gov. services	c	0.08	0.03	c	c	0.09	b	c
Living partner	c	0.30	c	c	0.18	0.22	0.22	0.13
Education	−0.03	c	c	b	0.10	c	c	c
Fed. Gov. officials	c	c	c	c	c	c	c	0.08
Personal safety	c	c	c	c	c	c	c	0.10

$P < 0.01$

[a]A = Clerical staff (N = 312), B = Rural seniors (N = 273), C = Cochrane residents (N = 328), D = Guelph students (N = 296), E = world students (N = 5036), F = Prince George residents (N = 466), G = Jasper residents (N = 210), British Columbians (N = 1061)

[b]Significance level too low to enter equation

[c]Not in questionnaire

On average, for the eight samples represented in Table 9.4, we were able to explain 56% of the variance in reported life satisfaction scores from some subset of the 15 predictor variables listed in the table. Our best success came from the Jasper sample in 1997 (column G), at 65%. For British Columbians we were able to explain 55% of the variation in life satisfaction scores. When all variables are standardized to have means of zero and standard deviations of one, the standardized regression coefficients (Betas) measure the percent of movement in the dependent variable when a predictor variable moves one full unit and every other predictor in the set is held constant. For example, under column G one finds that the Beta value for self-esteem is $\beta = 0.57$, which means that for every full standard deviation increase in satisfaction with one's own self-esteem, one's life satisfaction increases a bit over half a standard deviation. Inspection of the other figures in that column reveals that satisfaction in no other domain had as great an impact on overall life satisfaction for the 229 Jasper respondents.

It should be noted that the presence of correlation among the predictor variables affects the magnitude of the standardized regression coefficients. Therefore, it is not recommended that standardized regression coefficients be interpreted as reflecting the importance of the predictor. Thus far in this essay we are not interpreting the importance of the predictors, per se, but rather we use the standardized regression coefficients, in part, to help us make comparisons across samples. In the next section we will come back to these regression models and consider the relative importance of the predictor variables.

Reading across the row to the left from 0.57, one sees that satisfaction with one's own self-esteem was also the strongest predictor of life satisfaction for the sampled 512 Prince George residents in 1997 (column F, $\beta = 0.57$) and for the sample of 296 University of Guelph students (column D), at $\beta = 0.31$. That Guelph sample was part of the much bigger global student sample whose results are listed in column E. Inspection of that column shows that satisfaction with one's own self-esteem tied with satisfaction with one's university education as the strongest predictors of life satisfaction for the 5107 students in the global sample.

For the other four samples, satisfaction with one's self-esteem was not as powerful a predictor as (had less explanatory power than) satisfaction with one or more other domains. For the 312 sampled members of the office, clerical and technical staff of the University of Guelph (column A), satisfaction with one's family relations had the greatest explanatory power ($\beta = 0.35$). For the 273 sampled rural seniors (column B), satisfaction with their housing had the strongest predictive strength ($\beta = 0.21$); for the 328 Cochrane residents (column C), it was satisfaction with their financial security ($\beta = 0.24$); and for British Columbians, it was satisfaction with their friendships ($\beta = 0.24$). Satisfaction with one's own self-esteem was the second strongest explanatory variable for the latter group ($\beta = 0.22$). The British Columbia group was the only one for which satisfaction with friendships had the greatest impact on life satisfaction.

The figures just reviewed clearly illustrate the fact that different groups of people with different life circumstances, resources and constraints use different mixtures of ingredients to determine their life satisfaction. The explanatory model used here allowed the groups represented in Table 9.4 to draw satisfaction from roughly the same set of 15 domains. Analytically speaking, some groups used more and some used fewer of these domains to build their life satisfaction. The Jasper group used only 4 of the 12 possibilities open to them, the rural seniors group used all 12 available, while British Columbians used 8 of the 11 possibilities open to them.

Table 9.5 provides some comparative figures resulting from regressing mean happiness scores on mean scores for satisfaction with various domains of life. On average, for the eight samples represented in this exhibit, we were able to explain 36% of the variance in reported happiness with life as a whole from some subset of the 16 predictor variables listed in the table. Our best success came from our British Columbia sample, at 46%. The strongest explanatory variable for that sample was satisfaction with one's own self-esteem, which had a Beta value of $\beta = 0.32$. Thus, figuratively speaking, for every full-step increase in satisfaction with their own self-esteem, the overall happiness of these British Columbians increased 32% of a step. Put another way still, for every full-step increase in their good feelings about themselves, their overall happiness with life increased about a third of a step.

As one moves across the columns of Table 9.5, one finds that satisfaction with self-esteem was also the strongest explanatory variable for the Guelph students ($\beta = 0.26$), the Prince George sample ($\beta = 0.27$) and the Jasper sample ($\beta = 0.25$). The strongest explanatory variable for the rural seniors group was satisfaction with their friendships ($\beta = 0.23$). Satisfaction with their financial security was the strongest predictor for the Cochrane group ($\beta = 0.21$) and satisfaction with living partners for the world student sample ($\beta = 0.18$). As in the case of life satisfaction, different groups built up their overall happiness with different mixtures of ingredients and some groups drew upon more domains than others. The Jasper sample used only 3 of the 12 possibilities open to them, British Columbians used 8 of 12 and the rural seniors used all 12.

When we examined the impact of the same domain satisfaction scores on satisfaction with the overall quality of life in British Columbia, we found that there were five statistically significant predictors which collectively accounted for 56% of the variation in the global indicator scores (N = 1085). Satisfaction with one's own self-esteem was the strongest predictor ($\beta = 0.26$). Satisfaction with one's personal safety in one's own neighbourhood ($\beta = 0.20$) was second, followed by satisfaction with financial security ($\beta = 0.13$) and then a cluster of four variables including satisfaction with friendships, health, job and recreation activities ($\beta = 0.11$ for each). Next to last in relative influence came satisfaction with federal government officials ($\beta = 0.08$) and finally with family relations generally ($\beta = 0.06$).

Relative Importance of the Predictor Variables

Keeping in mind the caveat we provided in the preceding section about interpreting the relative importance of predictor variables based on the magnitude of the Beta coefficient, Thomas et al. (1998) presented a new statistical method for ordering predictor variables in a linear model in terms of their importance in the model. The Thomas, Hughes, and Zumbo method proceeds by defining importance as the relative proportion (percentage) of the resultant model R-squared that can be attributed to each predictor variable. Said another way, their method additively partitions the R-squared value so that one can attribute a certain proportion of the R-squared to each predictor variable. The computation of this new statistic is straightforward: multiply the Beta coefficient by the simple correlation of the predictor and dependent variable, and then divide this quantity by the model

Table 9.6 Variable importance for the British Columbian explanations of life satisfaction, happiness and satisfaction with the overall quality of life

	% of the R-squared attributed to the predictor
Life satisfaction (from Table 9.4)	
Satisfaction with:	
Friendships	25
Self-esteem	23
Job	16
Health	14
Living partner	10
House or apartment	5
Financial security	4
Federal gov. officials	2
Happiness (from Table 9.5)	
Satisfaction with:	
Self-esteem	41
Job	16
Living partner	10
Friendships	8
Health	7
Personal safety	7
Financial security	6
Federal gov. officials	4
Quality of life	
Satisfaction with:	
Self-esteem	29
Personal safety	16
Financial security	10
Recreation activities	9
Health	9
Friendships	9
Job	9
Family relations	4
Federal gov. officials	4

R-squared. One simply performs these computations for each predictor variable in a model.

Table 9.6 lists the results for each of the linear regression models used to explain life satisfaction, happiness and satisfaction with the overall quality of life. As an example of how to interpret these new methods, consider the explanation of British Columbians' life satisfaction reported in Table 9.4. From Table 9.6 we see that 25% of the explained variation in life satisfaction is attributable to satisfaction with friendships, 23% is attributable to satisfaction with one's own self-esteem, 16% to job satisfaction, and so on. This sort of analysis is possible because of additive properties of the Thomas-Hughes-Zumbo method. Satisfaction with friendships is clearly the most important and satisfaction with federal government officials is the least important explanatory variable in that model.

Sometimes people wonder how we or anyone else distinguishes life satisfaction from happiness and satisfaction with the overall quality of life. The answer may be found by examining the relative importance of the different sets of explanatory variables in Table 9.6. For example, notice first that for British Columbians 25% of the explained variance in *life satisfaction* is attributable to satisfaction with friendships and 23% is attributable to satisfaction with one's own self-esteem. However, only 8% of the explained variance in *happiness* is attributable to satisfaction with friendships while 41% is attributable to satisfaction with one's own self-esteem. Thus, for the British Columbians in our sample, personal happiness has much more to do with feeling good about one's self than anything else, but satisfaction with one's life as a whole is practically as much a matter of having satisfying friendships as it is feeling good about one's self. Regarding *satisfaction with the overall quality of life,* satisfaction with one's self-esteem is most important, followed by satisfaction with one's personal safety.

It is perhaps also worthwhile here to call the reader's attention to the relative unimportance of citizen dissatisfaction with provincial, local and federal government officials. In section "Expectations and Attitudes" we remarked that respondents' levels of dissatisfaction were higher for government officials than for anything else, and highest of all for provincial government officials. Nevertheless, inspection of Tables 9.4, 9.5 and 9.6 reveals that, in the context of roughly a dozen important domains of life, dissatisfaction with provincial and local government officials has no impact on life satisfaction, happiness or satisfaction with the overall quality of life. Dissatisfaction with such officials is simply totally unimportant to respondents' global assessments of their lives as a whole. On the other hand, dissatisfaction with federal government officials has some impact but it is clearly the least important explanatory variable for each of the global variables listed in Table 9.6. Although government officials at all levels tend to be public punching bags and to get more than a fair share of attention in the news media in British Columbia (and elsewhere), their impact on people's perceived well-being is negligible compared to many other things.

Conclusion

The main aims of this research were to describe some of the expectations and attitudes of British Columbians toward possible events in the first 100 years of the third millennium, and to explain their satisfaction with life as a whole, their happiness and their satisfaction with the overall quality of their lives. We reported on results of two independent surveys taken in October and November 1999, one containing 499 respondents living south of Hundred Mile House and the other containing 969 respondents living north of Hundred Mile House. About half of the expectations and attitudes of northerners and southerners were very similar to each other. Levels of satisfaction with 18 aspects of respondents' lives were practically identical for northerners and southerners. Aggregated (northern and southern) answers to self-reported health questions were shown to be inferior to the self-reported health of 142,674 Americans from the 50 states of the USA in 1998, when the samples were subdivided by age and gender. Answers to open-ended questions revealed that northerners' and southerners' greatest fears for the future concerned issues related to unemployment and financial security. Explanations of respondents' satisfaction with life as a whole, happiness and satisfaction with the overall quality of life from a limited set of 16 variables revealed that for northerners and southerners taken together, satisfaction with friendships and one's own self-esteem were most important for life satisfaction. Regarding happiness, for northerners and southerners taken together, satisfaction with their own self-esteem was most important, followed by satisfaction with their jobs. Regarding satisfaction with the overall quality of life, for northerners and southerners taken together, satisfaction with one's own self-esteem was most important, followed by satisfaction with one's personal safety.

Acknowledgements The authors would like to express their appreciation to Irene Huse, Rob van Adrichem, Peter Godfrey and John Harding for the help they gave us in the development, administration, analysis and reporting of the survey.

References

Michalos, A. C. (1980). Satisfaction and happiness. *Social Indicators Research, 8,* 385–422.

Michalos, A. C. (1982). The satisfaction and happiness of some senior citizens in rural Ontario. *Social Indicators Research, 11,* 1–30.

Michalos, A. C. (1983). Satisfaction and happiness in a rural northern resource community. *Social Indicators Research, 13,* 225–252.

Michalos, A. C. (1985). Multiple discrepancies theory (MDT). *Social Indicators Research, 16,* 347–413.

Michalos, A. C. (1991a). *Global report on student well-being, volume 1: Life satisfaction and happiness.* New York: Springer.

Michalos, A. C. (1991b). *Global report on student well-being, volume 2: Family, friends, living partner and self-esteem* New York: Springer.

Michalos, A. C. (1993a). *Global report on student well-being, volume 3: Employment, finances, housing and transportation.* New York: Springer.

Michalos, A. C. (1993b) *Global report on student well-being, volume 4: Economics, religion and morality.* New York: Springer.

Michalos, A. C., & Zumbo, B. D. (1999). Public services and the quality of life. *Social Indicators Research, 48,* 125–156.

Thomas, D. R., Hughes, E., & Zumbo, B. D. (1998). On variable importance in linear regression. *Social Indicators Research, 45,* 253–275.

United Nations Development Program. (1999). *Human development report 1999*. New York: Oxford University Press.

Zumbo, B. D., & Michalos, A. C. (2000). Quality of life in Jasper, Alberta. *Social Indicators Research, 49,* 121–145.

Chapter 10
Identifying the Horse, the Cart and Their Proper Order in Sustainable Development

Alex C. Michalos

The Fraser River Basin covers over 25% of the land area of the province of British Columbia, houses about 2.7 million people, and contributes about 80% of the province's and 10% of Canada's gross domestic product. In 1997 the Fraser Basin Council was established as a not-for-profit society with a mandate "to ensure that the decisions we make now about how we live, work and play in the Fraser Basin will protect and advance its social, economic and environmental sustainability into the future" (Fraser Basin Council 2001–2002). The first line of the Vision Statement of the Council says "We want to see the Fraser Basin as a place where *social well-being is supported by a vibrant economy and sustained by a healthy environment*" (Fraser Basin Council 2002, emphasis added).

Since 1997 I have been a member of a Fraser Basin Council Sustainability Indicators Advisory Committee, which was responsible for producing the first State of the Fraser Basin Report called *A Snapshot on Sustainability* (Fraser Basin Council 2003). When the Report was released at the Annual General Meeting in January 2003, a special conference was held in which, among other things, the British Columbia Minister of Sustainable Resource Management, Stan Hagen, made a speech saying how pleased he was to have a report on sustainable *economic* development. If he had used the phrase once, I might have missed it or at least ignored it. But he used it several times, which convinced me that he thought of the *aim* of our work on sustainable development as *economic development* rather than "social well-being supported by a vibrant economy and sustained by a healthy environment".

After spending 5 years trying to craft a useful reporting system to inform people of how well we were achieving our goals for the Fraser Basin, it was frustrating to

Michalos, A.C.: 2003. Identifying the horse, the cart and their proper order in sustainable development. Revista Italiana de Economia Demografica e Statistica, 52(1–2), pp. 151–162. © 2003 Italian Society of Economics, Demography and Statistics.

A.C. Michalos (✉)
University of Northern British Columbia, Prince George, BC, Canada
e-mail: michalos@brandonu.ca

A.C. Michalos, *Development of Quality of Life Theory and Its Instruments*,
DOI 10.1007/978-3-319-51149-8_10

hear an elected member of the provincial government totally misunderstand and misrepresent the most important goal. In fact, he had got the means and end of our exercise exactly backwards. He put the social well-being and healthy environment horse squarely behind the economic cart, assuming that our primary aim was to make people and physical resources better serve the economy rather than to make the economy better serve people and the natural environment.

Fortunately, or maybe unfortunately depending on which side you are on, around the time of the annual meeting, I was asked to give the organizers of the conference in Bari a more precise idea of what I planned to talk about related to the social and economic aspects of sustainable development. What I want to talk about is the danger of distorting a fairly progressive idea of sustainable development into the old reactionary idea that people must serve the economy instead of the economy serving people.

To begin with, it might be claimed that the original notion of sustainable development as it came out of the report of the World Commission on Environment and Development (1987) was focused on economic development. However, both the mandate of the Commission and explicit quotations in the report indicate that, unlike many other groups established by the United Nations to examine issues related to economic development, the main focus of the Brundtland Commission was elsewhere. The mandate is given on p. ix of the report.

It was an urgent call by the General Assembly of the United Nations:

- to propose long-term environmental strategies for achieving sustainable development by the year 2000 and beyond;
- to recommend ways concern for the environment may be translated into greater co-operation among developing countries and between countries at different stages of economic and social development and lead to the achievement of common and mutually supportive objectives that take account of the interrelationships between people, resources, environment and development;
- to consider ways and means by which the international community can deal more effectively with environmental concerns;
- to help define shared perceptions of long-term environmental issues and the appropriate efforts needed to deal successfully with the problems of protecting and enhancing the environment, a long-term agenda for action during the coming decades, and aspirational goals for the world community.

In the body of the report, one can find the following explicit commitment

> Sustainable development is development that meets the needs of the present without compromising the ability of future generations to meet their own needs. The satisfaction of human needs and aspirations is the major objective of development. The essential needs of vast numbers of people in developing countries - for food, clothing, shelter, jobs - are not being met, and beyond their basic needs these people have legitimate aspirations for an improved quality of life. A world in which poverty and inequity are endemic will always be prone to ecological and other crises. Sustainable development requires meeting the basic needs of all and extending to all the opportunity to satisfy their aspirations for a better life (pp. 43–44).

Clearly, then, the original notion of sustainable development had social well-being as its aim, with strong economies working within the carrying capacity of the natural environment as the means.

Apart from the original notion of sustainable development, it is important to consider the question of simple sustainability of the status quo versus progressive change to some other status that is more worthy of sustenance. For example, addressing the apparently benign aim of creating a relatively socially integrated or inclusive society, the authors of the United Nations Research Institute for Social Development (1994, p. 3) Briefing Paper on *Social Integration: Approaches and Issues* reminded us that

If not carefully thought out, a call for greater 'inclusion' in the benefits of development can be made without questioning the nature of the current process of development itself. It is intellectually easy and often politically expedient to assume that grave problems of poverty and injustice can be alleviated through 'including' people formerly 'excluded' from certain activities or benefits. Yet, in many cases, … the existing state of affairs may sometimes be not only ecologically unsustainable but also politically repressive. It is useful to remember that strongly authoritarian or totalitarian societies do in fact 'include' everyone in elaborate structures of managed participation. In such cases, the problem of improving the quality of life for most people is not one of exclusion or inclusion, but of reform.

The connection between the ideas of sustainable development and the quality of life was made explicit in the passages quoted from *Our Common Future*. When people use the phrase *quality of life*, they sometimes intend to contrast it with quantities or numbers of something. There are, then, two quite different sorts of things that one might want to refer to when using the phrase *quality of life*. In the first place, one might want to refer to sorts, types or kinds of things rather than to mere numbers of things. For example, one might want to know not merely how many people were admitted to a hospital last year and for how long, but also what sorts of people they were, male or female, young or old, rich or poor, and so on. When the term *quality* in the phrase *quality of life* is used in this sense, one may say that it and the phrase in which it occurs is intended to be primarily *descriptive*. In the second place, however, one might want to refer to the value or worth of things by using the term *quality* in the phrase *quality of life*. For example, one frequently hears of people making a trade-off between, say, a high salary on the one hand and better working or living conditions on the other. Presumably the exchange here involves monetary and some other value. That is, one exchanges the value of a certain amount of money for the value of a certain set of working or living conditions. When the term *quality* in the phrase *quality of life* is used in this sense, one may say that it and the phrase in which it occurs is intended to be primarily *evaluative*. Both senses of the phrase *quality of life* are important. It is important to be able to describe human existence in a fairly reliable and valid fashion, and it is important to be able to evaluate human existence in the same way. The philosopher Plato is still celebrated for raising the evaluative question at least 2300 years ago when he asked "What is a good life for an individual person and what is a good society?", but it is often forgotten that he also raised the descriptive question "What is the nature of an individual's or a society's life?".

The research literature concerned with the quality of life and sustainable development is enormous. To get a rough idea of how large it is, consult a website called *Compendium of SD Indicator Initiatives,* maintained by Laszlo Pinter and Mathis Wackernagel of the International Institute for Sustainable Development in Winnipeg (http://iisdl.iisd.ca/measure/compindex.asp). At the time I accessed it, there were just over 500 reports listed.

Enormous as the literature on *sustainable* development is, the body of research literature on *development* itself is even larger. Alechina (1982, p. 25) quoted an unidentified UNESCO document, presumably written before 1982 and certainly before *Our Common Future,* as follows.

> Development is **integrated**: it is an organic process involving a number of economic, social and cultural factors which overlap and constantly influence one another.
>
> Development is **endogenous**: each country carries out its development according to its own choice, and in conformity with the real values, aspirations and motivations of the population.
>
> Development is **global**: its objectives and problems are determined with relation to world problems and reflect the general nature of development…The society in which development is carried out is not isolated, but forms part of the network of relations and forces that cover the entire world, including the most economically advanced societies as well as those which, from the economic point of view, are the most deprived.

Perhaps the most interesting feature of this quotation is the absence of any reference to the environment, the earth's carrying capacity or sustainability. Things change. UNESCO (1988) contains several state-of-the-art papers on development planning.

One way to get a comprehensive measure of sustainable development that thoroughly integrates economic, environmental and social accounts is to build separate systems of environmental and social accounts, and to connect them to national systems of economic accounts. The London Group on Environmental Accounting appears to be an international ad hoc group of practitioners that began meeting in 1993 to develop a system of environmental accounts (a so-called satellite system) that would complement the United Nations's System of National Accounts (SNA). Meetings have continued periodically, with papers circulated and discussed, and a very sophisticated handbook called *System of Environmental and Economic Accounts* (SEEA) (London Group 2002) is nearing completion. Authors of the handbook emphasize early on that although "the social dimension of sustainability" is important "for a well-rounded view of sustainable development, this is not a prime focus of the SEEA" (pp. 1–2). The "prime focus" is explained briefly as follows.

> There are essentially three strands to the accounting system of the SEEA. The first is to look at physical data and marshal it according to the conventions, definitions and classifications of an economic accounting system. The second is to look at the economic accounting

> system, as it presently stands, to identify those elements which are relevant to the good management of environmental resources. The third and last is to consider how these two approaches could be united in a single system…Once the physical data are aligned with economic classifications, an obvious development is to compare the physical quantities with the matching economic flows. This is developed throughout the SEEA by means of so-called 'hybrid' accounts…*A key policy goal is to maintain or improve economic performance while simultaneously reducing or eliminating the impact on the environment. This process is sometimes referred to as 'de-coupling'* (pp. 1-5–1-6, emphasis added).

The accounts provide a means of comparing the economic contribution to the environmental burden of diverse industries by measuring, for example, the total percent of GDP or employment contributed by an industry versus that industry's

Table 10.1 Net contribution of consumption and production to GDP and to six environmental themes in the Netherlands, 1993 Percentages

	Economy	Environment				
		Greenhouse effect	Ozone-layer depletion	Acidification	Eutrophication	Solid waste
Total		100	100	100	100	100
Consumption		19	2	15	9	3
Industry		79	97	85	91	66
Capital and other sources		2	1	–	–	31
Consumption	100	100	100	100	100	100
Own transport	8	38	–	88	21	1
Other consumption	92	62	100	12	79	99
Production	100	100	100	100	100	100
Agriculture, hunting, forestry, fishing	3	15	2	47	91	7
Mining and quarrying	3	2	–	1	–	1
Manufacturing Petroleum industry	1	7	–	11	–	
Chemical industry	2	14	27	6	2	16
Metal products and machinery industry	3	2	9	1	–	2
Other manufacturing	12	12	20	7	6	25
Public utilities	2	26	–	9	1	2
Transport and storage	6	8	6	12	1	5
Other services	68	14	36	6	−1	42

Source London Group (2002)

total percent of environmental pollution. Such comparative statistics are called "environmental-economic profiles" or "eco-efficiency" profiles. Table 10.1, taken from the Netherlands, shows that the aggregated industry "agriculture, hunting, forestry and fishing" accounts for 91% of eutrophication and 47% of acidification emissions, but only 3% of GDP. If that were all the information the Dutch people had about the value of that particular "industry" to their well-being, they might be inclined to take very severe regulatory measures to reduce its environmental burden to something more similar to its economic contribution. The problem is, of course, that particular "industry" is the only one in the list that produces food, which is absolutely necessary for the survival of people and, consequently, of any other industries. The specific point is that a set of accounts that reveals an agricultural industry to be a relatively light-weight contributor to GDP and a free-riding polluter, while entirely neglecting the industry's contribution to human nourishment could be a very dangerous set of accounts. More generally, the point is that there are many more examples of this sort, showing that integrated systems of environmental and economic accounts that lack social accounts could be very dangerous for measuring human well-being. In terms of my horse and cart metaphor, the SEEA system removes the problem of deciding which should come first by simply eliminating the social well-being horse altogether!

The United States National Research Council's Committee on National Statistics's panel report by Nordhaus and Kokkelenberg (1999) covers some of the same ground as that covered in the London Group report, and members of the panel interacted and shared information with members of the London Group. The following passage from the Executive Summary of the report found on the National Academy of Science website explains the point of the exercise.

> …the NIPA's [National Income and Product Accounts] focus on market activities has raised concerns that the accounts are incomplete and misleading because they omit important nonmarket activities, such as nonmarket work, the services of the environment, and human capital. In response to these concerns about standard measures of economic activity, private scholars and governments have endeavored to broaden the national accounts in many directions. Most recently, attention has focused on extending the accounts to include natural resources and the environment. *The guiding principle in extended national accounts is to measure as much economic activity as is feasible, whether that activity takes place inside or outside the boundaries of the marketplace.* (p. 8, http://books.nap.edu/html/natures_numbers: emphasis added).

Clearly, then, an environmentally extended NIPA system is *not* a comprehensive set of indicators of sustainable development. Some extremely important things are not normally traded in the market place and cannot reasonably be measured by the yardstick of money, e.g., truth, love, hope, honour, dignity, moral virtue and justice, in fact, using what I call the Commercial Bias Argument, one might even question the wisdom of trying to get a composite measure of sustainable development whose elements have values that are positively correlated with values found in an extended NIPA.

The Commercial Bias Argument (CBA) runs as follows.

1. Suppose we regard a person's willingness to pay for a marketed good or service as a measure of its value to that person. This is a standard assumption of economists who believe that market prices reflect the real value of things bought and sold in free market economies.
2. One's willingness to pay is partly a function of one's ability to pay. If willingness to pay is indicated by actual demand, then this premise is practically guaranteed to be true, because people can not spend money that they do not have, even if they have to borrow it. Apart from actual demand, people's preferences are influenced by their life circumstances and experiences, which are always influenced by their incomes as well as other personal and social endowments.
3. There is no necessary connection between one's ability to pay and what one needs to live (e.g., extraordinary medical treatment) and what one deserves as a matter of right or fair treatment (e.g., equal treatment in law courts). Evidence from many countries, for many years clearly shows that relatively poor and weak (e.g., children, the aged and disabled) people often can not meet their basic needs and can not get fair treatment in law courts.

Cl. So, there is no necessary connection between the commercial (market) value of what one needs to live and what one deserves as a matter of right or fair treatment. That is, the market value of things one needs to live and things one deserves does not measure the real value of such things.

C2. So, there is no necessary connection between goods and services that will be favoured with market success and goods and services that may be necessary for life and may be deserved as a matter of right or fair treatment. That is, for example, things like good child care or elder care may be very poorly compensated compared to things like good soccer or baseball playing, although the real value to individual and social well-being of the former tasks is greater than that of the latter tasks.

C3. So, insofar as any composite measure of sustainable development is correlated with commercial values (e.g., Gross Domestic Product), it is bound to be biased in favour of the preferences of those with purchasing power. That is, for example, such a measure will be biased against things especially valuable to our most vulnerable populations of children, older people and disabled people.

4. Insofar as a composite measure is biased in favour of the preferences of those with purchasing power, it is inconsistent with and undermines the idea that every human being is equally valuable, and entitled to the same respect and consideration as every other. That is, it is inconsistent with and undermines the fundamental ideal of democracy.
5. A composite measure of sustainable development should not undermine democracy.

C4. Therefore, composite measures that are well-correlated with commercial values should be rejected.

I find the CBA both persuasive and very troublesome. I tried to indicate briefly after each premise and the various interim conclusions why I thought they were each true. But I am troubled by the argument for a couple reasons. First, I know there is all kinds of evidence indicating that countries with relatively higher per capita incomes are much more able to satisfy the basic human needs of their citizens and, more importantly, usually do satisfy such needs much more thoroughly than countries with relatively lower per capita incomes. There are exceptions and there are striking cases of very wealthy countries that provide relatively little help for some of their most vulnerable populations; e.g., compared to Sweden and the Netherlands, Canada and the United States provide relatively little aid for single mothers with small children. But, on the whole, countries with relatively greater resources provide more help than countries with relatively fewer resources to their most vulnerable populations. Insofar as that is the case, there would be relatively high correlations between income measures and measures of social well-being. No doubt there would also be relatively high correlations between some environmental measures (e.g., availability of clean drinking water) and income, although there would also be negative correlations between things like income and air pollution. Anyhow, the existence of such clear counter-instances to the conclusion of the CBA, suggests that there must be a mistake in the argument somewhere.

The other troublesome thing about the argument is that if its conclusion is true, then all efforts being made to make environmental and possibly social accounts consistent with our economic accounts are contributing to the further undermining of democracy. We are simply compounding the misleading messages already provided by the National Income and Product Accounts about what is really valuable to human beings.

I do not know what to do with these troublesome issues. Maybe we do not have to do anything. After all, someone might argue, if favourable economic indicators are often positively associated with favourable social and environmental indicators, then it does not matter which is regarded as our primary objective.

This is an attractive, but dangerous argument. It is attractive, because if it is a sound argument, then nobody has to change any behaviour and all interests will be served anyhow. This is really politics without tears, because the world will become a better place if everybody just keeps doing whatever they want to do.

I do not think we are so lucky. As I explained in Michalos (1989), a similar argument has been used by those who favour the commercialization of weapons of war. They say that it is ok to sell arms for profit because there are often technological spin-offs leading to economic and social benefits. Besides, some of the countries that are most successful in providing a relatively secure and high standard of living for their citizens are also the world's most successful arms merchants, e.g., the United States of America and the United Kingdom. However, using evidence assembled by Sivard (1986) and Sanger (1982), among others, it was shown that there is a clear negative correlation between a country's military expenditures and its annual growth rates of manufacturing productivity. Thus, because industrial innovation and civilian productivity tend to be retarded by the commercialization of arms, the latter ought to be resisted. Similarly, it can be argued that because improvements in social and environmental conditions tend to be retarded by focussing on economic conditions, the latter ought to be resisted. That is roughly another way of putting the central thesis of my essay.

I suppose that people whose social and environmental conditions have been undermined by economic globalization in one form or another would be sympathetic to the thesis. For example, in Michalos (1995) the evidence was reviewed showing that in a variety of ways the North American Free Trade Agreement (NAFTA) was bound to undermine the work of progressive environmentalists and trade unionists who had spent years getting legislation passed to protect the environment and workers' rights, and conserve resources. It is an agreement designed to make life better for relatively wealthy investors and to strengthen their hand when conflicts arise between their interests and those of the general public or even of particular communities. It has generally served its purposes well, as other researchers on both sides have shown, e.g., IISD/WWF (2001), Public Citizen (2001), Hufbauer et al. (2000), Graham (2000). (Of the four publications just cited, the first two are generally sympathetic to the thesis and the second two are not.)

Clearly, the people around the world who have protested against the WTO would be sympathetic to the thesis, and those who have continued to press for the expansion of the WTO rules in its various extensions to trade in services (GATS), etc. would oppose it. I can't hope to resolve these conflicts here. In fact, all 1 hope to show (in case nobody noticed) is that the battle between those who are inclined to put people in the service of economies instead of economies in the service of people is being fought within the parameters of the movement for sustainable development. So, the fact that someone or some government or organization is generally supportive of sustainable development may or may not be a good thing, all things considered. Under the banner of sustainable development, very progressive or regressive economic, social and environmental policies might be espoused. Therefore, if you see a pedlar flying the flag of sustainable development, make sure his social well-being and healthy environment horse is in front of his economic cart before you buy any of his goods.

References

Alechina, I. (1982). The contribution of the United Nations system to formulating development concepts. In *Different theories and practices of development* (pp. 9–68). Paris: UNESCO.
Fraser Basin Council. (2001–2002). *Annual Report*. Vancouver: Fraser Basin Council.
Fraser Basin Council. (2002). *Charter for sustainability*. Vancouver: Fraser Basin Council.
Fraser Basin Council. (2003). *A snapshot on sustainability*. Vancouver: Fraser Basin Council.
Graham, E. M. (2000). *Fighting the wrong enemy: Antiglobal activists and multinational enterprises*. Washington: Institute for International Economics.

Hufbauer, G. C., et al. (2000). *NAFTA and the environment: Seven years later*. Washington: Institute for International Economics.
IISD/WWF. (2001). *Private rights, public problems: A guide to NAFTA's controversial chapter on investor rights*. Winnipeg: International Institute for Sustainable Development and World Wildlife Fund.
London Group. (2002). *System of environmental and economic accounts*. SEEA. http://www4.statcan.ca/citygrp/london/publicrev/pubrev.htm.
Michalos, A. C. (1989). *Militarism and the quality of life*. Toronto: Science for Peace and Samuel Stevens.
Michalos, A. C. (1995). The case against the North American free trade agreement. In *A pragmatic approach to business ethics* (pp. 188–235). Thousand Oaks, CA: Sage Publications.
Nordhaus, W. D. & Kokkelenberg, E. C. (1999). *Nature's Numbers: Expanding the National Economic Accounts to Include the Environment*. National Academy Press: Washington D.C.
Public Citizen. (2001). *NAFTA chapter 11 investor-to-state cases: Bankrupting democracy*. Washington: Public Citizen's Global Trade Watch.
Sanger, C. (1982). *Safe and sound: Disarmament and development in the eighties*. Ottawa: Deneau Pub.
Sivard, R. L. (1986). *World military and social expenditures 1986*. Washington: World Priorities.
UNESCO. (1988). *Innovative approaches to development planning*. Paris: UNESCO.
United Nations Research Institute for Social Development. (1994).
World Commission on Environment and Development. (1987). *Our common future*. New York: Oxford University Press.

Chapter 11
Connecting Communities with Community Indicators

Alex C. Michalos

Introduction

The question I would like to begin answering in this essay is this. How can one connect communities of diverse sizes by means of a system of statistical indicators in the interests of building solidarity and embracing diversity? I say "begin answering" because I have only been able to see some salient aspects of a beginning. A complete and logically tidy vision is not yet clear.

The general structure and approach to answering the question before us is that used by the team of researchers building the Canadian Index of Wellbeing System (CIWS). The main sponsor of the CIWS work is the Atkinson Charitable Foundation. Since the team is fairly large (a few dozen people), we do not have complete agreement about everything, but we generally aim for consensus as our work progresses.

Besides following the structure and approach of the CIWS, my remarks are significantly informed by discussions with the governing Board and participants at meetings of the Community Indicators Consortium and the newly formed National Neighbourhood Network in Canada. There are levels of theoretical and practical expertise, and of enthusiasm and energy in the CIWS, CIC and NNN groups that are quite remarkable. Indeed, adding the new initiatives of the OECD to these grass roots organisations and those of the International Society for Quality of Life Studies promises a very bright future for work in the general field of quality of life, well-being and progress measurement.

Michalos, A.C.: 2008. Connecting communities with community indicators. In O.E.C.D. Statistics, Knowledge and Policy 2007: Measuring and Fostering the Progress of Societies, (pp. 133–146). Paris: O.E.C.D. © OECD 2008.

A.C. Michalos (✉)
University of Northern British Columbia, Prince George, BC, Canada
e-mail: michalos@brandonu.ca

A.C. Michalos, *Development of Quality of Life Theory and Its Instruments*,
DOI 10.1007/978-3-319-51149-8_11

Because our time is limited, I will make several assumptions immediately.

First, as explained in detail elsewhere (e.g., Michalos 2003, 2005), it is assumed that a good life or a life that is qualitatively good may be measured in quantitative terms with statistical time series data, broadly referred to as social, economic and environmental indicators.

Second, it is assumed that the progress referred to in the title of this conference is progress toward precisely such a life.

Third, the communities referred to in our research question are primarily place-based, i.e., communities of place, and secondarily communities of interest. Although there are frequently interactions among these two kinds of communities, it seems more likely that people sharing the same space would have common interests than that people having common interests would share the same space. The people assembled at this conference to discuss issues of common interests illustrate my point precisely, since we come from all parts of the globe. What is perhaps extraordinary about our meeting here is the fact that our particular common interest concerns issues related to connecting the earth's great variety of place-based communities by identifying additional common interests.

Fourth, it may be useful to distinguish what we might call *fundamental definitions* of 'community' from *derived definitions.* Fundamental definitions would have individuals (people) as their constituents, while derived definitions would have groups (collectivities) as their constituents. A fundamental definition of a 'place-based community' would be a network of people sharing some common place or space (e.g., the city of Prince George, the Carney Hill Neighbourhood in Prince George, the province of British Columbia, or Canada), while a fundamental definition of an 'interest-based community' would be a network of people sharing some common interests (e.g., dentists, city mayors, sociologists, book publishers). A derived definition of a 'place-based 3 community' would be a network of place-based communities (e.g., the network of municipalities of British Columbia, the network of Canadian provinces, the network of countries in the European Union or the United Nations), while a derived definition of an 'interest-based community' would be a network of interest-based communities (e.g., the Canadian Labour Congress or the Social Sciences and Humanities Federation of Canada).

Fifth, following Aristotle (1999) in the fourth century BCE, I think that a good life for an individual or community is a function of the actual conditions of that life and what an individual or community makes of those conditions. What a person or community makes of those conditions is in turn a function of how the conditions are perceived, what is thought and felt about those conditions, what is done and, finally, what consequences follow from all these things. People's perceptions, thoughts, feelings and actions, then, have an impact on their own and others' living conditions, as illustrated in Fig. 11.1.

Sixth, the basic components of a good life from the time of Aristotle to today, across all cultures, are familiar to most people. In the ancient philosopher's terms, they included goods of the body (e.g., good physical health, strength, vitality, bodily pleasures), goods of the mind (e.g., wisdom, moral virtue and mental pleasures) and external goods (e.g., wealth, security, good friends, loved ones,

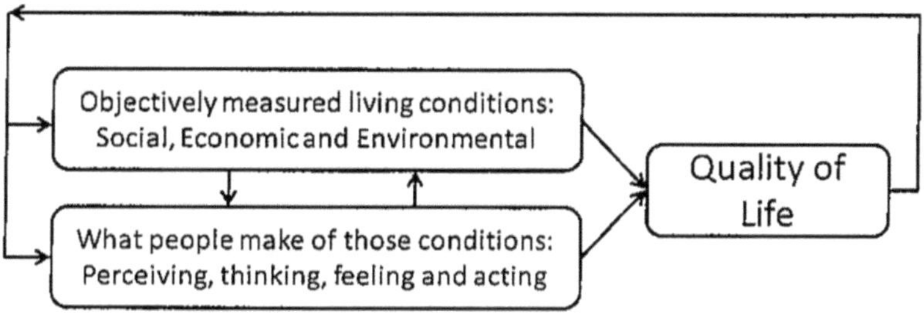

Fig. 11.1 General quality of life model

beautiful built and natural environments, and good communities). People whose lives are characterised by such features have generally been regarded as happy, enjoying *eudaimonia* or "living well and doing well" in Aristotle's phrase, or briefly in contemporary terms, enjoying well-being.

Seventh, and finally, at least since the report of the Brundtland Commission (1987), the idea of a good quality of life has been essentially connected to that of sustainable development.

> "Sustainable development", we are told in the Report, "is development that meets the needs of the present without compromising the ability of future generations to meet their own needs…The satisfaction of human needs and aspirations is the major objective of development. The essential needs of vast numbers of people in developing countries – for food, clothing, shelter, jobs – are not being met, and beyond their basic needs these people have legitimate aspirations for an improved quality of life…Sustainable development requires meeting the basic needs of all and extending to all the opportunity to satisfy their aspirations for a better life" (pp. 43–44).

Acceptability Criteria and Critical Issues

Over some years of work on indicators of a good life, I have gradually produced lists of Acceptability Criteria and Critical Issues that must be addressed by anyone interested in constructing such indicators. Briefly, acceptable indicators and/or indexes should be:

Acceptability Criteria

1. Relevant to the concerns of our main target audiences
2. Easy to understand
3. Reliable and valid
4. Politically unbiased
5. Easy to obtain and periodically update
6. Comparable across jurisdictions and groups
7. Objective or subjective, or both

8. Positive or negative, or both
9. A constituent or determinant of well-being, or both
10. Attributable to individuals or groups of animate or inanimate objects, or all of these
11. Obtained through an open, transparent and consultative review process
12. Going to contribute to a coherent and comprehensive view of a good life or human well-being

Acceptability Criteria are not usually specified with great precision (e.g., see Hagerty 2001), but they provide useful guidelines for discussions and negotiations over particular indicators and indexes. Some judgment is required in their application in order to prevent the achievement of some goals at the expense of others, e.g., measures that are easy to obtain and update must not be allowed to arrest the development of new measures that might have greater validity and make a greater contribution to a comprehensive view of well-being.

Additional complications arise when one considers the array of Critical Issues that have to be settled in order to assemble a set of indicators or indexes satisfying the final criterion in the list, i.e., contributing to a coherent and comprehensive set. Explicitly or implicitly, every indicator or index must be specified by addressing the 21 issues listed below. The issues are not categorised or presented in any particular order of priority or importance because no single principle or set of principles seems sufficient to provide a single rank order of the total set. Some are clearly logically prior to others in the sense that answers to some must be obtained before others, e.g., one cannot assess causal relations (#17) or benefits and costs (#9) without knowing what sorts of things (#5) have been selected for measurement or evaluation. Other ordering principles would lead to different orders, e.g., one might suppose that the most important question in the lot is who gets to assess the adequacy of answers to all other questions (#20), or perhaps, who is entitled to any consideration at all (#4). As well, it is unlikely that the issues in this list are mutually exclusive in pairs and collectively exhaustive. Nevertheless, for all their limitations, in order to identify and measure *a life, way of life or quality of life worthy of pursuit*, an individual or community must make decisions concerning the following issues.

Critical Issues

1. Individual well-being, group well-being or both: e.g., per capita incomes are inferred attributes applying to individuals, while unemployment rates are inferred attributes applying to groups.
2. Spatial coordinates: e.g., the best size to understand air pollution may be different from the best size to understand crime.
3. Temporal coordinates: e.g., the optimal duration to understand resource depletion may be different from the optimal duration to understand the impact of sanitation changes.
4. Population composition: e.g., analyses by language, sex, age, education, ethnic background, income, etc. may reveal or conceal different things.

5. Domains of life composition: e.g., different domains like health, job, family life, housing, etc. give different views and suggest different agendas for action.
6. Objective versus subjective indicators: e.g., relatively subjective appraisals of housing and neighbourhoods by actual dwellers may be very different from relatively objective appraisals by "experts".
7. Positive versus negative indicators: negative indicators seem to be easier to craft for some domains, which may create a biased assessment, e.g., in the health domain measures of morbidity and mortality may crowd out positive measures of well-being.
8. Input versus output indicators: e.g., expenditures on teachers and school facilities may give a very different view of the quality of an education system from that based on student performance on standardised tests, and both may be very different from assessing whether the populace at large is becoming more literate, knowledgeable, educated and wise.
9. Benefits and costs: different measures of value or worth yield different overall evaluations as well as different evaluations for different people, e.g., the market value of child care is far below the personal, social or human value of having children well cared for.
10. Recipient populations: Who should be included as a recipient for particular benefits and costs?
11. Measurement scales: e.g., different measures of well-being provide different views of people's well-being and relate differently to other measures.
12. Research personnel: e.g., different stakeholders often have very different views about what is important to monitor and how to evaluate whatever is monitored.
13. Report readers: e.g., different target audiences need different reporting media and/or formats.
14. Aggregation function: e.g., once indicators are selected, they must be combined or aggregated somehow in order to get a coherent story or view.
15. Distributions: e.g., because average figures can conceal extraordinary and perhaps unacceptable variation, choices must be made about appropriate representations of distributions.
16. Distance impacts: e.g., people living in one place may access facilities (hospitals, schools, theatres, museums, libraries) in many other places at varying distances from their place of residence.
17. Causal relations: Prior to intervention, one must know what causes what (interaction effects), which requires relatively mainstream scientific research, which may not be available yet. At a minimum, correlations among variables should be explored with a view to discovering possible evidence of dependence or independence, redundancy and double-counting.
18. Discount rates: How much should one discount costs and benefits delivered some time in the future compared to those delivered today?
19. Confidence levels: What levels of confidence should one require to accept any particular claim or measure?

20. Auditors: Who should decide if any assessments are adequate or appropriate?
21. Auditing criteria: What criteria should be used to assess the adequacy of auditors' assessments, the adequacy of the procedures used for audits and even the adequacy of the answers to questions raised with the previous 20 issues?

The last question reveals the threat of either an infinite regress, a circular argument or an arbitrary end to analysis. Clearly, none of these options is very attractive, but it is in the very nature of foundational work that such a point must be reached. In any event, supposing that one had only two alternatives for each of the 21 Critical Issues (an absurdly conservative supposition), at least 2 097 152 different sets of indicators might be constructed. If nothing else, this suggests the size of the working space for indicator and index development.

Multi-level Nesting of Indicators

Given the particular question of this essay, our attention should be directed to the critical issues of individual versus group well-being (#1), spatial coordinates (#2), distance impacts (#16) and causal relations (#17). Assuming that we are seeking indicators in the form of statistical time series to connect diverse kinds of communities, Fig. 11.2 illustrates an array of 8 kinds of entities that are usually nested within larger entities. The entities in the figure are not exhaustive of all those that

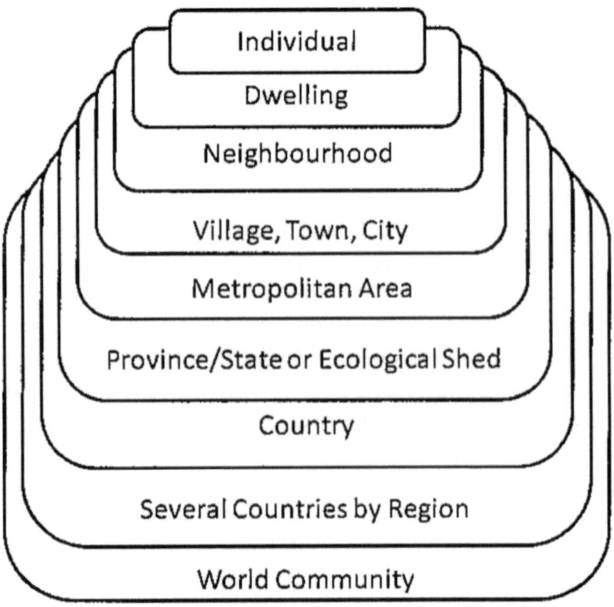

Fig. 11.2 Multi-level nesting of indicators

might have been included and, since they are nested, they are not mutually exclusive. People often talk about places of work or places of worship, and statistical agencies routinely collect data on "establishments" of various kinds. Such places might be given an appropriate slot in a more robust figure. Apart from the smallest nest in the figure, that of individuals, all the other nests are place-based communities with diverse geographical, cultural and other component features.

As the figure clearly shows, individuals are multi-nested entities. Because each type of nest has some distinctive features and requirements for its own existence, multi-nested individuals typically have multiple roles to play throughout their own existence. Different nests produce different rights, privileges and obligations. For example, we are family members (fathers, mothers, sons, cousins), friends, neighbours, residents of some city, province and country. As fathers, for example, we have special obligations to our wives and children, as neighbours we have somewhat less distinct obligations, as residents of cities and so on, still other kinds of obligations as well as rights and privileges.

It seems to me that the most fundamental problem faced by people with an interest in community indicators is to precisely identify the particular nest or set of nests that they are thinking of when they think of community indicators, and then to clearly identify its or their essential features by working through the list of Critical Issues. Identification of the nest or nests is essential because of the diverse roles, rights, privileges and obligations that are attached to individuals and groups in the nests. It is impossible to begin taking stock of a community's strengths and weaknesses, opportunities and challenges, obligations and rights without community identification. Until there is common consent regarding community identification, there is no way to know who is or should be responsible or accountable for what, and no way to begin constructing a strategic plan for change or development. For example, homelessness will be addressed in different ways if it is regarded as a personal problem of some individuals, a problem of some neighbourhoods, some cities, provinces or the country as a whole. If people living in certain areas of a city do not perceive those areas to be neighbourhoods and do not think of the problem of homelessness as a neighbourhood problem, it will be impossible to address the problem at a neighbourhood level. Similar remarks apply to each of the kinds of nests named in Fig. 11.2. At the broadest level, the so-called international or world community often fails to act (e.g., to reduce global warming, the spread of AIDS or genocide) because the community and its interests are so vaguely defined. If these colossal problems are neglected for lack of a sufficient definition of a 'global community', it is difficult to be optimistic about the chances of global action for common measures of progress toward an economically, socially and environmentally sustainable future. Nevertheless, it is necessary to try to build a consensus for the development of such measures because, after all, we all inhabit a single planet with a limited capacity for growth and waste disposal.

In Fig. 11.2, individuals are the smallest units of analysis. They are not places, certainly not in any geographical sense. Social scientists might suppose these "units" are individual human beings, but biologists of various sorts might imagine individuals of other animal or plant species and other kinds of scientists might have still other paradigm cases of individuals. Regarding human beings, individual-level indicators for any place-based community would include things like simple census counts of total numbers of individuals, men, women, people of a certain age, born in a certain place educated to certain level, with an income of a certain amount and a Body Mass Index of a certain size. The place-based community might be as small as a single household or a remote village or a neighbourhood within a city, or as large as a province, a whole country or set of countries.

It is important to emphasise that even though social scientists might collect individual-level information about people (e.g., Body Mass) without collecting any information about the place(s) occupied by those people, human beings are not disembodied spirits. So, they are always occupying some place(s) and the missing information would frequently, if not always, be relevant to the measures obtained. This happens all the time, for example, when psychologists gather information from students in diverse places. Depending on the issues being investigated, being in one rather than another, or in one school or university rather than another, or in a particular family, neighbourhood and so on might be relevant, whether or not any such Place-based information is collected. If such variables are just missing from the survey research instruments used, then it is impossible to test for place-based effects or interaction effects, or to undertake any kind of multi-level modeling involving place. Researchers' explanatory equations are then bound to be misspecified, as it so often happens, and their purported causal analyses are bound to be faulty.

Individual-level indicators are routinely aggregated in uncontroversial ways to form group-level indicators. For example, we might calculate the percentages of men and women in a certain place-based community, and find that 52% of the individuals women and 48% are men. Since only individuals can be characterised as men or women while only groups can be characterised as having a certain percent of men or women, it is clear that the properties of being a man or women are distinctive of individuals while the properties of being a certain percent of men or women are distinctive of groups. There was a time when social scientists hotly debated the question of whether all social scientific data could be reduced to individual-level data or not, with those on the individualist side insisting on the possibility of reduction and those on the holist side insisting on its impossibility. We need not address this question here, but I have always been on the holist side (Michalos 1978).

Dwellings occupy the second level of Fig. 11.2, typically "our places" for most people and most often family places. The tasks of taking account of people without dwellings (homeless people), in the simple sense of counting them as part of the official population and in the more profound sense of accounting for their very livelihood, usually do not fall on statistical agencies. Such tasks are routinely left to public or private welfare service agencies.

One might suppose that the aggregation of individuals into families is a relatively simple matter, but it is not. For example, for some years Statistics Canada had two definitions of a family. A *census family* was either a husband or wife couple, including common-law couples, with or without children, or a lone-parent with a child sharing a dwelling, while an *economic family* was any group of people, including all census families, sharing a dwelling and related by blood, marriage, common-law or adoption. Thus, the idea of an economic family was broader than that of a census family and both kinds of families were essentially place-based communities of people, the places being the particular dwelling units occupied by those people. More recently, 'census families' have dropped out of usage, and we now have 'economic families' and 'unattached individuals'. For the purposes of their study of family violence, Poff and Michalos (1991) had to construct an even broader notion of family which they called a *socio-psychological family.* They defined such families as "economic or census families, or groups of individuals with self-avowed, personally and socially constructed, relatively intimate relationships without sexual or temporal boundaries" (p. 155). Socio-psychological families must also occupy some place, which may differ from that of particular economic families.

If one went no further down the pyramid of nested entities in Fig. 11.2, one would still have to address the issues concerning the interactions and causal relations among individuals and groups occupying particular dwelling units. After all, individuals with different genetic and learned capabilities and attributes act and react in different ways in groups with different capabilities and attributes. So, what resources and constraints are present or absent, and what it might be necessary to provide or remove in the interests of improving the quality of the lives of individuals and groups can only be determined by individual and group-level research, with some notion of family or at least occupants of a single dwelling providing the group-level unit of analysis. Thus, if one went no farther down the pyramid of nested entities, it is obvious that the chances of appropriately measuring and understanding only the socio-psychological dynamics affecting the individuals and families would be very small unless one engaged the expertise of multidisciplinary and trans-disciplinary teams of researchers. Nevertheless, because the basic building blocks of human communities are human beings, one can be sure that the Aristotelian core of internal and external goods will merit attention, be capable of measurement, periodic monitoring and some deliberate manipulation in the interests of improving the quality of life.

The term 'neighbourhood' in the third nest of Fig. 11.2 is intended to do double duty, designating a set of contiguous streets and/or blocks with residents whose children often share a single public school as well as a set of contiguous rural properties. While the former idea and situation is probably familiar to more people because most people live in relatively urban areas, people living in sparsely populated rural and remote areas also think of themselves as having neighbours. That is, residents of urban and rural or remote areas all have neighbours sharing a common place, only those in urban areas might be just around the comer, across the street or upstairs while those in rural and remote areas might be several acres or even hundreds or thousands of acres away. That is why when we speak of neighbourhoods as place-based centres of community activities, we must be sensitive to the fact that the geography of the places occupied by some communities can be the most important feature of those communities, the greatest asset or liability for mobilising community action.

It is worth mentioning that there is no more agreement over definitions of 'urban' and 'rural' than there is over 'community' and 'neighbourhood'. Statistics Canada's concept of rurality is a function of population density and distance from an urban centre. So, for example, "one's measure of rurality would change, depending upon whether one was considering access to a monthly ballet performance or access to a curling rink or access to a sizable number of organic restaurants to market your organic farm products" (Bollman 2007, p. 7). Since there is very little information about the size of most people's living space, how far they are willing to and actually do travel to access shops of various kinds (groceries, clothes, household appliances, automobile services), leisure activities (theatres, restaurants, arenas, golf courses, parks, ballparks, museums), health care (clinics, hospitals, medical specialists and general practitioners), education and information (public and private trade and other kinds of schools, universities, libraries), it is very hazardous to assess the quality of people's lives by simply counting kinds of facilities and services available within a relatively well-defined political jurisdiction (e.g., within a particular town or city). For example, when I moved from the city of Guelph, Ontario to Prince George, British Columbia, both cities had populations of 70–80 thousand people, a university, hospital and symphony. However, Guelph is about a 1 h drive from downtown Toronto and the Hamilton-Niagara region, giving Guelph residents access to practically all the facilities and services of these two larger communities, while the closest relatively large city to Prince George is Edmonton, Alberta, at least a 7 h drive away. Residents of Toronto can escape the city congestion and enjoy the theatres and more leisurely paced lives of the small towns of Stratford or Niagara on the Lake, Ontario by simply driving a couple hours west. Clearly, the so-called 'spillover problem' that researchers encounter when they try to assess neighbourhood facilities and services is a problem for researchers assessing the facilities and services of communities of all sizes in most places. Even in a relatively small city like Prince George, road maintenance is sometimes primarily the responsibility of the municipal government and sometimes the provincial government, depending on which road. A local survey respondent asked to approve or disapprove of the government's performance on road maintenance would seldom know which government is praise-worthy or blame-worthy.

The fourth nest in Fig. 11.2 is set aside for villages, towns and cities, settlement areas which seem to have no universally agreed upon definitions. This is also true of metropolitan areas, our fifth nest. Although the diversity and complexity of facilities, services, institutions and organisations tends to increase with the populations of such settlement areas, there are no new Critical Issues so far as quality of life, well-being or progress measurement are concerned. I would not under-estimate the significance of the additional diversity and complexity introduced by great increases in population or population density in particular places. However, the changes that occur with such increases seem to me to be differences of degree rather than differences of kind. Villages, towns, cities and metropolitan areas are communities of communities insofar as each of the larger settlement areas contains smaller settlement areas. Each of the larger places contains smaller places, with diverse kinds of interactions and causal relations among the individuals and groups in the diverse places.

I mentioned the Community Indicators Consortium earlier and there will be a presentation at this conference focused specifically on the work of this group. However, Fig. 11.3 has been included to briefly provide an overview of the sort of information, knowledge and wisdom generated at the most recent meeting of the group in Jacksonville, Florida in March 2007. Participants in the meetings of this group are primarily interested in the development of indicators and indexes, tools of measurement, advocacy and change for communities of the fourth and fifth levels of Fig. 11.2. Hopefully, this essay will make it easier to see connections between these two levels and all the others.

It might be thought that differences of kind would appear at the sixth nest, involving relatively large political jurisdictions like provinces or states, or ecological water sheds or air sheds. But such a view does not seem warranted. The province of British Columbia, for example, has two large river basins, for the Columbia and Fraser Rivers. The largest of the two, the Fraser River runs approximately 1 400 km from Mount Robson in the Rocky Mountains to the Pacific Ocean at the Straight of Georgia. About 2.8 million people live in the basin, which is two-thirds of the province's population. According to the most recent "state of the basin" report of the Fraser Basin Council (2007, p. 2), "The Fraser Basin is a special place". The Basin supports

> ...six salmon species, including steelhead, and 65 other species of fish...British Columbia's most productive waterfowl breeding area, home to hundreds of species of birds and mammals as well as reptiles, amphibians and insects. From Prince George to Williams Lake to Kamloops, and throughout the most populated stretches of the Fraser Valley and Greater Vancouver, communities depend on the Basin to support a range of economic activity–from natural resource industries, to agriculture to businesses of all types. This is the land where we live, work and play. Our well-being is so closely tied to the Fraser Basin that its future is our own.

Such is the diversity and complexity of the Basin, that to make a reasonable assessment of the "state of the Basin", the total area covered has been divided into 5 regions with a common set of indicators applied to each region. Prince George is the largest city in the most northern region of the Basin, a region that enjoys the best water quality and the worst air quality of all 5 regions. Regardless of the fact that the Basin occupies much more space and has a considerably greater variety of natural species than, say, the metropolitan area of Toronto, measuring the quality of life in the Basin does not seem to introduce new Critical Issues. One would expect greater variability in the air and water quality across the length of the Basin than across the length of the metropolitan Toronto area, but not necessarily different kinds of indicators of air and water quality. Sampling techniques and quality standards that would apply to air and water in the Basin would apply in the metropolitan area. Measures of family violence, mortality and morbidity, educational attainment, employment, income and so on would be as relevant to the people

Aim to build a culture of evidence-based policy making
Be as inclusive as possible and find the best talent
Inclusiveness is more important than speed
Expect mistakes, be patient, be very patient
The process is at least as important as the product
Let media and friends know how much they are appreciated
Agency responsible for reports needs recognised integrity
City level reports can influence state/provincial, federal gov.
QOL reports provide vision and allow goal setting
Benchmarking is important
Results-based accountability is important
QOL is connected to place and to heritage
Facts and perceptions are important
Different communities have different champions
Produce shorter and longer versions of reports
Use diverse media and means to communicate messages
Pictures are better than numbers
Provide user training sessions for diverse potential users
Identify key change agents for diverse kinds of changes
Allow elected and appointed officials to do their jobs
Undertake evaluations to find what works or does not work
Recognise that communities are not homogeneous
Don't try to do know everything or do everything
Focus on something, identify critical variables for action
From Bishop Tutu: Mobilise, mobilise, mobilise
From trade unions: analyse, organise, educate, agitate

Fig. 11.3 Some results from the CIC Jacksonville meeting: lessons learned, March 2007

in the smaller communities and neighbourhoods within communities within the "special place" known as the Fraser Basin as in the place known as metropolitan Toronto.

For a huge country like Canada, diversity and complexity significantly increase as one moves to the seventh level or nest, the whole country. Unlike the States of the United States of America, Canadian provinces have constitutionally guaranteed jurisdictional rights to the natural resources found in the provinces, e.g., the oil and gas of Alberta is primarily a provincial resource and source of tax revenue. Apart from constitutional provisions, the geography of the country creates its own divisions. For example, to address the issue of a sustainable fishing industry in Canada, one must consider problems of the Pacific herring and salmon on the coast and inside of British Columbia as well as problems of the cod fish across the continent to the coasts of Newfoundland and Labrador. Forestry is vitally important to the economy of British Columbia but not to Manitoba. Air pollution is a significant problem in Toronto, but not a problem in Nova Scotia.

The community of communities that is Canada is not only vertically laced with many levels of nested communities, but horizontally laced with distinct geographic features that individually and collectively make distinct as well as causally interacting contributions to what we call 'the Canadian Mosaic'. A comprehensive assessment of the progress of the Canadian community over time must somehow take account of this great diversity and complexity, and so far we have not developed a vocabulary, much less a general theory to allow us to make such an assessment (Michalos 1997; Michalos et al. 2007).

Additional complications arise at the eighth level, the level concerning international relations, whether they are bi-lateral (e.g., Canada-United States Free Trade Agreement), tri-lateral (e.g., North American Free Trade Agreement) or multi-lateral (e.g., World Trade Organization). Such agreements create new opportunities and constraints on a country's capacity to act in the interests of national progress, and additional problems in measuring and accounting for progress (Michalos in press). Then, of course, such problems are multiplied again when one moves to the global level, the nest of all nests. In a recent issue of *Prospect* magazine, Cooper (2007, p. 24) wrote,

"In the 21st century, the new forms of communication have brought us a new world and we need a new constitutional form too. The big question is how to organise this world in which politics and identity are national, but we can survive and prosper only if we act internationally. It is fíne to talk about "the international community," but who is it and how can it function?

As already suggested, the form and functions of the international community are yet to be defined (constructed), but conferences like this one are helpful. Hopefully, so are observations on the multi-leveled forms and functions of communities of necessarily diverse and smaller sizes.

References

Aristotle. (1999). *Nicomachean ethics* (2nd ed., T. Irwin, Trans.). Indianapolis: Hackett Publishing Company.

Bollman, R. D. (2007). *Factors driving Canada's rural economy*. Agriculture and Rural Working Paper Series, Cat. No. 21-601-MIE-No.083, Statistics Canada, Ottawa.

Brundtland Commission. (1987). *Our common future*. New York: World Commission on Environment and Development, Oxford University Press.

Cooper, R. (2007). Untitled, *Prospect,* March, p. 24.

Fraser Basin Council. (2007). *2006 State of the Fraser Basin Report: Sustainability Snapshot, Inspiring Action 3, Vancouver.*

Hagerty, M. R. (2001). Quality of life indexes for national policy: Review and agenda for research. *Social Indicators Research, 55*(1), 1–96.

Michalos, A. C. (1978). *Foundations of decision-making*. Ottawa: Canadian Library of Philosophy.

Michalos, A. C. (1997). Combining social, economic and environmental indicators to measure sustainable human wellbeing. *Social Indicators Research, 40*, 221–255 (reprinted in Michalos, 2003).

Michalos, A. C. (2003). *Essays on the quality of life*. Dordrecht: Kluwer Academic Publishers.

Michalos, A. C. (Ed.). (2005). *Citation classics from social indicators research.* Dordrecht: Springer.

Michalos, A. C. (in press). *Trade barriers to the public good: The NAFTA and AIT cases concerning MMT.* Montreal: McGill-Queen's University Press.

Michalos, A. C., Sharpe, A., & Muharjarine, N. (2007). *An approach to a Canadian index of wellbeing.* Working Paper prepared for the Atkinson Charitable Foundation, Toronto.

Poff, D. C., & Michalos, A. C. (1991). *Family violence: A literature review.* Halifax: Institute for the Study of Women, Mount Saint Vincent University.

Chapter 12
Stability and Sensitivity in Perceived Quality of Life Measures: Some Panel Results

Alex C. Michalos and P. Maurine Kahlke

Introduction

In what later became a citation classic from *Social Indicators Research* (Michalos 2005), Tom Atkinson (1982) published results from a panel study involving "a representative sample of 2,162 Canadians interviewed in 1977 and again in 1979". Apart from some results dealing with a subset *(N* = 285) of the national sample used in Campbell et al. (1976), this was the first published report "on the stability of QOL [quality of life] measures over time". The particular measures employed included a single-item life satisfaction measure with 11 response categories running from 1 = completely dissatisfied to 11 = completely satisfied, similar to those used in Great Britain and in the European Community; an 11-step (0–10) self-anchoring ladder scale adapted from Cantril (1965); the Gallup 3-step ("very happy, fairly happy, or not too happy") happiness scale and single-item domain satisfaction scales for five domains; job, finances, housing, health and marriage/romance. A General Quality of Life Index was formed by combining responses for the life satisfaction, happiness and Cantril scales, and a Domain Satisfaction Index was formed by combining domain satisfaction scores. In order to assess levels of change in people's lives from the first to the second survey, respondents were asked in the second wave if their current status was the same, better or worse, for life in general and for specific domains. They were also asked which of 16 significant life events

Michalos, A.C., & Kahlke, P.M.: 2010a. Stability and sensitivity in perceived quality of life measures: some panel results, Social Indicators Research, 98(3), pp. 403–434.

A.C. Michalos (✉)
University of Northern British Columbia, Prince George, BC, Canada
e-mail: michalos@brandonu.ca

P.M. Kahlke
9005 College Drive, Coldstream, BC V1B 2P7, Canada

A.C. Michalos, *Development of Quality of Life Theory and Its Instruments*,
DOI 10.1007/978-3-319-51149-8_12

they had experienced in that period, e.g., divorce/separation, serious injury, new job or house.

His most important conclusions were summarized as follows.

> Opinions have been expressed in some quarters that subjective measures such as satisfaction are poor social indicators because they were so conditioned by expectations and restricted awareness as to be insensitive to changing circumstances. It is also argued that expectations and aspirations adjust very quickly to new situations and that satisfaction and other measures revert to their original levels immediately. This position would have led to predictions that (a) very few individuals would indicate any change in their situation, and/or (b) virtually no adjustment in subjective indicators would occur when changes did occur.
>
> Our findings contradict both hypotheses in that significant numbers of respondents perceive changes in their lives and those changes were reflected, for better or worse, in their satisfaction levels. The fact that these changes took place over a two year period indicates that, while adaptation probably does occur, it is not instantaneous and will be detected by an indicator series which utilizes fairly frequent measurements (Atkinson 1982, pp. 128–129).

Because the questionnaire included respondents' perceived changes (subjective indicators) and numbers of specific life events experienced (objective indicators), Atkinson was able to compare levels of association between each of these measures and QOL measures. Among other things, he found that

> The hypothesis that the No Change group would have more stable QOL scores than those reporting change is supported when the perceptual indicator of change is used as the independent variable but not when the event measures are involved… [As well] Relationships between self-reported change and satisfaction levels are always higher than between events and changes in satisfaction (Atkinson 1982, pp. 122, 126).

About a decade after the Atkinson article appeared, Headey and Wearing (1992) published results of their Australian/Victorian Quality of Life Panel Study that monitored the lives of "…a representative sample of 942 people in Australia's most densely populated State, Victoria". Panel members were interviewed in five waves for 1981, 1983, 1985, 1987 and 1989, with the "central question posed" being "What causes *change* in people's levels of well-being?". Given the 5 waves of data and a diverse array of particular measures, these authors were able to develop and test some very sophisticated models to explain changes in respondents' reported wellbeing. Their main preference was for something they called "a dynamic equilibrium model". In a sequel to this paper we will address the causal question, the model of Headey and Wearing, some others and especially Multiple Discrepancies Theory (MDT; Michalos 1985). In this paper our focus is on measuring stability and sensitivity to change following Atkinson's work. We are concerned here to show *that* appropriate changes in variable values and correlations did or did not occur, leaving the question of *why* to the sequel.

Headey and Wearing had a list of 93 kinds of life events that respondents might experience, including all the discrete, relatively objective events used by Atkinson (e.g., respondent got married, lost a close family member through death, got a new job) and a variety of continuing or possibly repetitive occurrences (e.g., respondent had arguments with children, increased the number of family outings, took courses that "seemed pointless"). For each event, respondents were asked if it occurred in the past 2 years, when, if it was continuing, if not then when it ended and its level of satisfaction or distress on a 10-point scale (Headey and Wearing 1992, pp. 30–31, 193–208). The dependent variable that was tracked over time with the occurrence of various life events was called the "life satisfaction (2) index". It was an average score based on two singleitem, 10-point measures, one of life satisfaction and another of life fulfillment. The correlation of the values of this index for 1981–1983 was $r = 0.64$ and for 1981–1989 it was $r = 0.43$. On the basis of several analyses using their "dynamic equilibrium model" the authors concluded that "life events in fact have a significant impact over and above personality", that "favourable events seem to have at least as much impact on well-being as adverse events" in the expected directions and that, therefore, whatever adaptation there is to new circumstances is not so rapid as to put people on "a hedonic treadmill" (pp. 138–143).

In another citation classic from *Social Indicators Research,* Veenhoven (1994) summarized overtime correlations of a variety of happiness-related variables in 26 longitudinal studies. (Atkinson's study was not one of the 26.) The variables were all employed as dependent and included Bradburn's Affect Balance Scale, some single-item measures of happiness, life satisfaction, contentment with life, appreciation of life and cheerfulness. The time-spans involved ranged from 4 months to 40 years, although the latter were based on interviewer assessments rather than self-reports of happiness. In a nutshell, he concluded that those studies plus others reviewed in the article showed that "happiness is no trait…[because]…happiness is not temporally stable…is not situationally consistent…and not entirely an internal matter" (Veenhoven 1994, pp. 145–146). Considering the 26 studies as a whole, he wrote,

> It appears that the stability of happiness is a short-term matter. The highest correlations concern mainly time lags of several months; overtime correlations are around +0.60. Over the years the correlations drop considerably. After five years overtime-correlation is almost halved and varies around +0.30. Over periods of ten to fifteen years the correlation shrinks back to about +0.15. Extrapolation of this trend predicts complete disappearance of all overtime-correlation after twenty years (p. 109).

Taking into consideration measurement errors, he thought that "the true stability of happiness is probably somewhat higher than the correlations suggest…about +0.77 after 1 year, about +0.50 after 5 years, and about +0.40 after 10 years" (p. 110).

Given the mixed bag of happiness-related measures used in the 26 studies, these are fairly bold estimates. Only two of the 26 studies provided somewhat comparable data for our purposes. Using a single-item measure of happiness, Eels (1985) reported a 2-year correlation of $r = 0.41$ for an adult sample of $N = 1{,}188$ in Nebraska, and using a single-item, 10 step life satisfaction measure, Landua (1992) reported a 2-year correlation of $r = 0.46$ for an adult German sample of $N = 7{,}091$. More to the point, based on results from 7 longitudinal studies (2 from the set of 26 plus 5 new ones), he found that the values of some sort of happiness-related dependent variables did decrease for people who became unemployed, had a spouse die, got divorced or had a net balance of negative versus positive events in their lives between surveys taken in time-spans of from 6 months to 11 years (pp. 121–124).

Ehrhardt et al. (2000) studied changes and stability in values of a 0–10-point single-item scale of life satisfaction over the 11 year period from 1984 to 1994 using the German Socio-Economic Panel. Respondents were interviewed annually, beginning with an $N = 9{,}000$ and including $N = 5{,}483$ people who responded to the life satisfaction question in each survey. For present purposes the following results should be noted.

> Year-to-year correlation started at +0.45 and increased gradually to +0.54. The correlation between the first and later reports declined through the years, the correlation between the 1st and the 11th report was only +0.29…life-changes explained 30% of the variance…These results mark a considerable mobility along the life-satisfaction ladder in a modern society: over a lifetime less than 30% of the original rank order in life-satisfaction will be left. That outcome is at odds with common theories of class and personality (Ehrhardt et al. 2000, p. 177).

The correlation between the first and third year values of their dependent variable was $r = 0.38$.

So far as we know, Richard E. Lucas and colleagues have made the most extensive use of the German Socio-Economic Panel in explorations of stability and change over time, using a 0–10-point single-item scale of happiness. Lucas et al. (2003) traced the impact of "marital transitions" on values of this variable over 15 years with an $N = 1{,}761$ respondents who "began the study unmarried, became married at some point during the study, and stayed married until the most recent wave of data (or until they were unreachable)". (Over 24,000 individuals participated in the surveys.) Their general "take-home message" follows.

> Brickman and Campbell (1971) were correct that adaptation to events does occur. People initially react strongly to both good and bad events, but then their emotional reactions dampen. Headey and Wearing (1989) were also correct that people return to a positive rather than to a neutral baseline, and this baseline is probably influenced by one's personality. Our study adds to the understanding of adaptation to marital transitions by following individuals for many years before and after events have occurred. Our results show that (a) selection effects appear to make happy people more likely to get and stay married, and these selection effects are at least partially responsible for the widely documented association between marital status and SWB [Subjective Wellbeing]; (b) on average, people adapt quickly and completely to marriage, and they adapt more slowly to widowhood (though even in this case, adaptation is close to complete after about 8 years); (c) there are substantial individual differences in the extent to which people adapt; and (d) the extent to which people adapt is strongly related to the degree to which they react to the initial event - those individuals who reacted strongly were still far from baseline levels years after the event…Thus, life circumstances are necessary for our understanding of long-term SWB; all happiness is not due to temperament" Lucas, Clark, Georgellis and Diener 2002003, p. 538).

In another study using the German Panel over the same 15 year period, Lucas et al. (2004) showed that

> In accordance with set-point theories, individuals reacted strongly to unemployment and then shifted back toward their baseline levels of life satisfaction. However, on average, individuals did not completely return to their former levels of satisfaction, even after they became reemployed. Furthermore, contrary to expectations from adaptation theories, people who had experienced unemployment in the past did not react any less negatively to a new bout of unemployment than did people who had not been previously unemployed. These

> results suggest that although life satisfaction is moderately stable over time, life events can have a strong influence on long-term levels of subjective well-being (Lucas et al. 2004, p. 8).

Using the German Panel to track changes over 18 years, Lucas (2005) showed that

> …there is considerable variability in the extent to which people react and adapt to major life events…just as people vary in their average levels of happiness, people vary in the degree to which their happiness changes following life events. Many people actually experience an increase in satisfaction following their divorce, whereas many others experience a greater drop in satisfaction…This study adds to a small but growing body of research showing that adaptation is not always quick and complete…Reactions vary for different events and even for different individuals who experience the same event…some people may never adapt to some life events, at least not without intervention. The challenge for future research will be to identify which events cause lasting changes and why (Lucas 2005, pp. 948–949; see also the summary paper by Diener et al. 2006 and Chap. 6 of Diener et al. 2009)

Reflecting on all these longitudinal studies, then, it is fair to say that at least for some single-item measures of life satisfaction, there is compelling evidence that variable values change with some significant changes and/or perceived changes in people's life circumstances, i.e., these life satisfaction measures are appropriately sensitive to changes in life circumstances over considerable lengths of time. In the present article, we provide some evidence from 3 relatively small panels tracked over 3 years showing that among 27 frequently used quality of life variables and indexes there is considerable variety in their sensitivity to changes in life circumstances measured in different ways. Efforts put into exploring the sensitivity of a few single-item, life satisfaction measures must be extended to these frequently used other variables and indexes.

The structure of this paper is as follows. In the next section we describe our questionnaires and sampling technique. Following that, there is a section "Sample Characteristics" describing our sample characteristics. Descriptive statistics and test-retest correlations of our substantive variables are presented in the fourth section. The longest section "Bivariate Relationships" describes a variety of bivariate relationships, tracking changes in the values of our variables and correlations among them over time and with different measures of changing conditions. Following this section, there is a conclusion.

Questionnaires and Sampling Technique

Two questionnaires were used in our study. The first questionnaire was 5 pages long. It began with 33 items asking respondents to assess their levels of satisfaction with 30 aspects or domains of life (e.g., housing, job, family relations, air quality) and with their life as a whole, their overall standard of living and the overall quality of their life. The scale used had 7 response categories running from 1 = very dissatisfied, 2 or 3 = dissatisfied, 4 = even balance of satisfaction and dissatisfaction, 5 or 6 = satisfied, to 7 = very satisfied. These items were followed by a happiness item also containing 7 response categories running from 1 = very unhappy to 7 = very happy. A self-reported general health item came next, with 5 response categories running from 1 = poor to 5 = excellent. There were then 7 items designed to test some of the basic hypotheses of Multiple Discrepancies Theory (MDT, Michalos 1985), e.g., Considering your life as a whole, how does it measure up to your general aspirations or what you want out of life?, How does it measure up to the best in your previous experience? Eleven items were included to allow us to construct the Satisfaction With Life Scale (SWLS) from Diener et al. (1985) and the Contentment with Life Assessment Scale (CLAS) from Lavallee et al. (2007). Finally, there were 6 demographic items, e.g., gender, age, highest level of education completed.

The second questionnaire had all of the items in the first one plus items borrowed from Atkinson (1982) designed to measure changes in respondents' life circumstances since the previous survey. First there was an item asking "Since the last survey, would you say that your life has (1) become better, (2) become worse or (3) stayed pretty much the same?". Following that, there was a list of 16 questions about events that may or may not have occurred in the lives of respondents since the last survey, e.g., Did you get married?, Become separated or divorced?, Did you have a close friend die? For each event, respondents were asked to indicate whether it occurred or not; if so, in what month and year, and whether it made their life (1) better, (2) worse or (3) had little or no effect. An event was only counted if it occurred within the last year of the survey and counted as negative or positive as indicated in the complete list of events given in the Appendix.

Two random samples of households were taken from the whole province of British Columbia and one was taken from the city of Prince George. One British Columbia sample (BF) and the Prince George sample (PG) were taken in February 2005, and a second British Columbia sample (BM) was taken in May 2005. These initial surveys contained a separate sheet asking respondents if they would be willing to complete the same questionnaire plus a page of new items two more times in the future, one in February 2006 and a final one in February 2007. Respondents who agreed to complete two more questionnaires became the initial members of one of 3 panels, but only those who actually completed questionnaires at three points of time were retained in panels.

Sample Characteristics

A total of 462 people distributed across three different panels (BF, PG, BM) completed questionnaires at three points in time. Members of panels BF and PG completed questionnaires at two 12-month intervals (February 2005, 2006, 2007) and members of panel BM completed questionnaires at one 9-month interval (May 2005–February 2006) and one 12-month interval (February 2006–February 2007). For all analyses, we treated panel BM the same as the other two.

Table 12.1 summarizes some demographic features of the total sample and each of the three panels. Two hundred and forty-five (53.0%) of the total sample were females and the mean age for the sample was 54. One hundred and sixty-eight (38.0%) of the total sample completed university, 171 (40.0%) were employed full-time and 268 (60.0%) were married.

Panel BF was the largest with *N* = 192 or 41.6% of the total sample, panel BM was second with N = 151 (32.7%) and panel PG was smallest with N = 119 (25.7%). The largest panel (BF) had the smallest percentage of females (50.5%) and full-time employed respondents (34.2%), and the highest mean age of respondents (55). The middle-sized panel (BM) had the largest percentage of females (57.0%) and respondents who had completed university (43.7%), the smallest percentage of married respondents (54.5%) and the lowest mean age of respondents (52). The smallest panel (PG) had the largest percentage of full-time employed (48.7%) and

Table 12.1 Demographics for panel survey 2005 to Feb./May 06 to Feb. 07 (in PanelTable_2007_Summary_Demographics.doc)

Variable	3 Panels	BC (BF)	BC (BM)	PG
Sample size	462	192	151	119
%	100	41.6	32.7	25.7
Male *N*	217	95	65	57
%	47	49.5	43.0	47.9
Female *N*	245	97	86	62
%	53	50.5	57.0	52.1
Mean age	54	55	52	54
Age range	21–97	21–97	22–86	26–88
21–34 years old *N*	59	23	25	11
%	13	12.2	16.8	9.4
35–64 years old *N*	286	116	92	78
%	63	61.4	61.7	66.7
65 years and older *N*	110	50	32	28
%	24	26.5	21.5	23.9
Completed trade/college *N*	97	42	26	29
%	22	23.2	18.3	25.9
Completed university *N*	168	72	62	34
%	38	39.8	43.7	30.4
Employed full-time *N*	171	63	52	56
%	40	34.2	35.6	48.7
Self-employed *N*	53	21	22	10
%	12	11.4	15.1	8.7
Married *N*	268	112	79	77
%	60	60.5	54.5	64.7
Live-in/common-law *N*	39	22	11	6
%	8	11.9	7.6	5.0

married respondents (64.7%), and the smallest percentage of respondents who had completed university (30.4%). The panels are not representative of the province or the city.

Descriptive Statistics and Test-Retest Correlations

Table 12.2 lists the 27 substantive variables of primary concern in this essay with their mean scores of three waves for each panel, their mean scores and standard deviations for the total sample, and the Ns available for the total score calculations. Each variable was standardized to have seven response categories and each one was put into one of five clusters, with subtotal means and standard deviations recorded for each cluster.

There are seven overall life assessment variables, including four single-item measures (satisfaction with life as a whole and with the overall quality of life, happiness and general health) and three indexes (SWLS, CLAS and SWB). SWB is a 4-item index of Subjective Wellbeing calculated by combining scores on four single-item measures (satisfaction with life as a whole, with the overall quality of life and one's standard of living, and happiness). Following these two clusters, there is a cluster of seven single-item discrepancy measures for the gap between what respondents have and want (self-wants), others of the same sex and age have (self-others), deserve (self-deserve), need (self-need), expected 3 years ago to have (self-progress), expect to have in 5 years (self-future), and the best they ever had (self-best). Then, there is a cluster of ten domain satisfaction items for home, neighbourhood, family relations, living partner, job, friendships, religion/spirituality, financial security, recreation activities and self-esteem. Finally, there are three domain satisfaction indexes for physical/mental health, environment and government. The measure for health is the mean of the physical and mental health satisfaction items, the measure for the environment is the mean of the air, land and drinking water satisfaction items and the measure for the government is the mean of the federal, provincial and local government satisfaction items.

Examining the table beginning with the total sample score column in the lower right- hand corner, one finds that the mean score (5.19) for all 27 items is clearly on the positive side of the 7-point scale, with a standard deviation of 1.16. Looking at the mean scores for the five clusters, one finds that the cluster of single-item overall life assessment measures has the highest mean (5.56) and that the cluster of three domain satisfaction indexes has the lowest mean (4.68). The latter is low as a result of the very low government satisfaction score (3.65). All of the measures in the first three clusters involve some kind of an overall life assessment, while those of the last two clusters involve assessments of distinct domains of life. While the mean score of the three overall life assessment clusters (5.10) is lower than that of the mean score of the two domain satisfaction clusters (5.28), it is the mean scores of the cluster of single-item discrepancy measures (4.87) and the overall life assessment indexes (5.01) that drags the mean score of the three overall life assessment clusters

Table 12.2 Panel survey 2005 to Feb./May 06 to Feb. 07 (in PanelTable_2007_SummaryTot_3Waves_Std)

	3-Waves BC (BF) mean	3-Waves BC (BM) mean	3-Waves PG mean	3-Waves for all 3 panels		
				Mean	*N*	SD
Life as a whole	5.69	5.67	5.58	5.65	462	1.10
Happiness	5.86	5.85	5.82	5.85	462	1.22
Overall quality of life	5.78	5.74	5.59	5.72	462	1.04
General health (Std.)	5.04	5.04	4.89	5.00	461	1.24
Subtotal mean	5.59	5.58	5.47	5.56	462	1.15
SWLS (Std.)	5.00	4.87	4.77	4.90	461	1.25
CLAS (Std.)	4.49	4.41	4.41	4.44	461	1.26
SWB (Std.)	5.76	5.71	5.61	5.70	462	1.01
Subtotal mean	5.08	5.00	4.93	5.01	461	1.17
Self-want	5.55	5.41	5.40	5.46	462	0.98
Self-other	5.33	5.26	5.09	5.25	462	1.10
Self-deserve	4.84	4.57	4.71	4.72	461	1.08
Self-need	5.00	4.85	4.82	4.90	462	1.16
Self-progress	4.64	4.57	4.52	4.59	462	1.17
Self-future	4.80	4.82	4.63	4.76	462	0.98
Self-best	4.44	4.55	4.26	4.43	462	1.26
Subtotal mean	4.94	4.86	4.78	4.87	462	1.10
3-Group subtotal mean	5.16	5.09	5.01	5.10	462	1.14
Home	5.83	5.71	5.67	5.75	462	1.19
Neighbourhood	5.89	5.90	5.59	5.81	462	1.14
Family relations	5.78	5.76	5.80	5.78	461	1.06
Living partner	5.88	5.87	5.95	5.90	400	1.31
Job	5.17	5.31	5.11	5.20	408	1.33
Friendships	5.68	5.69	5.48	5.63	462	1.13
Religion/spirituality	5.18	5.26	5.18	5.21	458	1.19
Financial security	5.02	4.86	4.78	4.91	462	1.49
Recreation activities	4.97	5.01	4.81	4.94	462	1.32
Self-esteem	5.53	5.52	5.53	5.53	462	1.18
Subtotal mean	5.49	5.49	5.39	5.47	450	1.23
Physical/mental health	5.31	5.39	5.27	5.32	462	1.13
Environmental sat.	5.20	5.38	4.47	5.07	462	1.17
Governmental sat.	3.70	3.64	3.59	3.65	462	1.16
Subtotal mean	4.74	4.80	4.44	4.68	462	1.15

(continued)

Table 12.2 (continued)

	3-Waves BC (BF) mean	3-Waves BC (BM) mean	3-Waves PG mean	3-Waves for all 3 panels		
				Mean	*N*	SD
13-Domain subtotal	5.32	5.33	5.17	5.28	453	1.22
Total mean	5.24	5.21	5.09	5.19	458	1.16

down. On average, the four single-item overall life assessment scores are higher than the ten single-item domain satisfaction scores. As well, on average, there is less variability (1.15) in the four single-item overall life assessment scores than in the singleitem domain satisfaction scores (1.23). Among single-item domain satisfaction scores for the total sample, on average, living partner scores are highest (5.90) and financial security scores are lowest (4.91).

Although none of the panels is representative of the populations from which they were drawn, the two provincial panels are relatively similar compared to the city sample. The mean scores of the total set of 27 variables and of each of the five clusters for the PG panel are lower than those of the corresponding mean scores for the BF and BM panels. In fact, mean scores of 21 of the 27 variables are lower for the PG panel than for the other two panels. On average, among the ten single-item domain satisfaction scores for the three panels, neighbourhoods have the highest scores for the BF and BM panels, while living partner has the highest score for PG. Government satisfaction scores are the lowest of all 27 variables in all three panels.

Table 12.3 lists the 27 substantive variables with their average test-retest correlations for two 1-year intervals and a test-retest correlation for one 2-year interval, for each panel and for the total sample, and the average Ns available and their ranges for the total score calculations. All correlations are significant at $P < 0.05$ or better. The 27 variables are again grouped into five clusters with average values calculated for each cluster.

Beginning with the total sample score column in the lower right-hand corner, one finds that the average year-to-year correlation ($r = 0.63$) for all 27 variables is slightly higher than the 2-year correlation ($r = 0.61$). This is also true for each of the average scores for the five clusters. However, it is not true for all 27 variables. There are 7 (25.9%) cases in which the 2-year correlation is higher than the average year-to-year correlation, i.e., happiness, SWB, self-deserve, job, friendships, health and self-esteem. Besides the fairly high average correlations for the total set of variables in both columns, it is worth noticing that while the range runs from $r = 0.41$ to $r = 0.80$, there are only six cases out of 54 (11.1%) in which the correlations are in the 0.40 s. Three of these six cases occur with single-item discrepancy measures, including two with the self-future variable.

Examining the column of average year-to-year correlations and the column of 2-year correlations for the five clusters, one finds that the cluster of three overall life assessment indexes has the highest mean in both columns, $r = 0.77$ and $r = 0.76$, respectively. Since multi-item measures tend to have less random error than

Table 12.3 Correlations for panel survey 2005 to Feb./May 06 to Feb. 07 (in PanelTable_2007_SummaryCorrelationsTot_3Waves)

Variable names	BC (BF)		BC (BM)		Prince George		All 3 panels		
	Average		Average		Average		Average	2-year	N
	05–06 & 06–07	2-year 05–07	05–06 & 06–07	2-year 05–07	05–06 & 06–07	2-year 05–07			Range (average)
Life as a whole	0.65	0.71	0.74	0.62	0.61	0.63	0.67	0.65	116–187 (150)
Happiness	0.57	0.69	0.72	0.64	0.55	0.59	0.61	0.64	117–187 (151)
Overall quality of life	0.55	0.53	0.71	0.68	0.62	0.57	0.63	0.59	119–189 (153)
General health	0.66	0.51	0.73	0.56	0.66	0.75	0.68	0.61	75–132 (104)
Subtotal average	0.61	0.61	0.73	0.63	0.61	0.64	0.65	0.62	75–189 (140)
SWLS	0.79	0.73	0.85	0.79	0.77	0.74	0.80	0.75	115–180 (146)
CLAS	0.76	0.78	0.76	0.79	0.75	0.69	0.76	0.75	110–177 (142)
SWB	0.73	0.78	0.81	0.76	0.72	0.76	0.75	0.77	114–179 (145)
Subtotal average	0.76	0.76	0.81	0.78	0.75	0.73	0.77	0.76	110–180 (144)
Self-want	0.63	0.56	0.67	0.73	0.68	0.68	0.66	0.66	117–187 (151)
Self-other	0.67	0.63	0.75	0.66	0.64	0.67	0.69	0.65	118–188 (152)
Self-deserve	0.56	0.54	0.60	0.68	0.44	0.64	0.53	0.62	117–187 (151)
Self-need	0.64	0.61	0.62	0.58	0.58	0.62	0.61	0.60	117–188 (151)
Self-progress	0.56	0.39	0.58	0.57	0.56	0.41	0.57	0.46	118–189 (152)
Self-future	0.47	0.50	0.52	0.45	0.48	0.27	0.49	0.41	119–188 (151)
Self-best	0.55	0.53	0.59	0.52	0.62	0.62	0.59	0.56	119–190 (152)
Subtotal average	0.58	0.54	0.62	0.60	0.57	0.56	0.59	0.57	117–190 (151)
3-Group subtotal avg.	0.63	0.61	0.69	0.65	0.62	0.62	0.65	0.62	75–190 (145)
Home	0.61	0.58	0.67	0.70	0.64	0.62	0.64	0.63	118–192 (153)
Neighbourhood	0.57	0.43	0.63	0.62	0.67	0.65	0.62	0.57	119–192 (154)
Family relations	0.59	0.54	0.58	0.49	0.41	0.37	0.53	0.47	116–189 (151)
Living partner	0.62	0.59	0.73	0.64	0.59	0.41	0.65	0.55	88–138 (112)
Job	0.50	0.54	0.49	0.60	0.39	0.29	0.46	0.48	89–132 (111)
Friendships	0.69	0.66	0.63	0.71	0.54	0.58	0.62	0.65	116–189 (152)

(continued)

Table 12.3 (continued)

Variable names	BC (BF)		BC (BM)		Prince George		All 3 panels		
	Average		Average		Average		Average	2-year	N
	05–06 & 06–07	2-year 05–07	05–06 & 06–07	2-year 05–07	05–06 & 06–07	2-year 05–07			Range (average)
Religion/spirituality	0.61	0.55	0.63	0.61	0.49	0.38	0.58	0.51	102–173 (138)
Financial security	0.76	0.73	0.75	0.66	0.69	0.60	0.73	0.66	117–188 (151)
Recreation activities	0.65	0.61	0.66	0.59	0.62	0.56	0.64	0.59	119–188 (152)
Self-esteem	0.72	0.74	0.71	0.70	0.63	0.71	0.69	0.72	117–190 (152)
Subtotal average	0.63	0.60	0.65	0.63	0.57	0.52	0.62	0.58	88–192 (143)
Physical/mental health	0.57	0.61	0.69	0.71	0.56	0.65	0.61	0.66	119–191 (154)
Environmental sat.	0.71	0.71	0.71	0.66	0.66	0.68	0.69	0.68	119–192 (154)
Governmental sat.	0.62	0.61	0.51	0.52	0.59	0.37	0.57	0.50	118–190 (152)
Subtotal average	0.63	0.64	0.64	0.63	0.60	0.57	0.62	0.61	88–192 (153)
13-Domain subtotal	0.63	0.61	0.65	0.63	0.58	0.53	0.62	0.59	88–192 (145)
Total average	0.63	0.61	0.67	0.64	0.60	0.57	0.63	0.61	75–192 (145)

All correlations significant at $P < 0.05$ or better

single-item measures, one might have expected the average correlations for the two clusters of indexes should have been higher than the averages for the other three clusters. In fact, closer examination of the two columns reveals that the correlations for each overall life assessment index are higher than those for any other measure. The range of correlation values for the three overall life assessment indexes is also narrower and higher than that for any other cluster, running from $r = 0.75$ to $r = 0.80$. However, examination of the scores for the domain satisfaction indexes are not particularly extra-ordinary compared to many of the single-item scores in those two columns.

The patterns of higher average year-to-year correlations and 2-year correlations for the means of the five clusters for each of the three panels are the same as for the total sample, with four exceptions. The subtotal average year-to-year correlations and 2-year correlations for the mean of the four single-item overall life assessment measures and the mean of the three overall life assessment indexes are equal in the BF panel, the subtotal average year-to-year correlation is lower than the 2-year correlation for the mean of the four single-item overall life assessment measures in the PG panel and the three domain satisfaction indexes in the BF panel. Close examination of the two columns for each of the three panels reveals that the correlations for each overall life assessment index are higher than those for any other measure, with five exceptions in 162 cases (3.1%). The exceptions are the 2-year correlations for satisfaction with general health and self-esteem in the PG panel, the average year-to-year correlation for satisfaction with financial security in the BF panel, and the 2-year correlations for satisfaction with financial security and self-esteem in the BF panel.

Bivariate Relationships

Table 12.4 is a correlation matrix for the 27 substantive variables for the total sample ($N \geq 372$). Respondents' mean scores for the three waves for all three panels (Table 12.2) were used for the calculations. All correlations are significant at $P < 0.01$ except for three that are significant at $P < 0.05$. As one would expect, SWB has the highest correlations

with three of its component parts (satisfaction with life as a whole ($r = 0.92$) and with the overall quality of life ($r = 0.94$), and happiness ($r = 0.90$)). Of the four single-item overall life assessment variables, general health has the lowest correlations with the other three, running from $r = 0.44$ to $r = 0.52$, and indicating again that respondents recognize a difference between assessments of their health and of their life as a whole. This recognition is carried over to the correlations among the three overall life assessment indexes and general health, which run from $r = 0.44$ to $r = 0.51$.

On average, the single-item discrepancy measures correlate at $r = 0.59$ with the singleitem life satisfaction measure, $r = 0.63$ with the overall quality of life satisfaction measure, $r = 0.62$ with happiness and $r = 0.37$ with general health, $r = 0.67$

Table 12.4 Panel Survey 2005 to Feb./May 06 to Feb. 07 correlations with $N > 372$, $P < 0.01$ except for 3 entries with *, where $P < 0.05$ (in PanelTable_2007_CorrelationsTot_3Waves_Std.doc)

Variable	1	2	3	4	5	6	7	8	9	10	11	12	13	14	15	16	17	18	19	20	21	22	23	24	25	26
1. Life as a whole	1.0																									
2. Happiness	0.82	1.0																								
3. Overall QOL	0.85	0.80	1.0																							
4. General health	0.44	0.49	0.52	1.0																						
5. SWLS	0.76	0.79	0.77	0.47	1.0																					
6. CLAS	0.75	0.74	0.73	0.44	0.85	1.0																				
7. SWB	0.92	0.90	0.94	0.51	0.83	0.79	1.0																			
8. Self-want	0.77	0.79	0.79	0.45	0.84	0.78	0.85	1.0																		
9. Self-other	0.63	0.66	0.72	0.40	0.72	0.62	0.75	0.75	1.0																	
10. Self-deserve	0.57	0.59	0.60	0.29	0.64	0.61	0.65	0.67	0.66	1.0																
11. Self-need	0.61	0.63	0.66	0.36	0.69	0.63	0.72	0.72	0.70	0.79	1.0															
12. SelfProgress	0.59	0.61	0.60	0.33	0.64	0.60	0.65	0.63	0.60	0.59	0.62	1.0														
13. Self-future	0.34	0.40	0.42	0.30	0.47	0.34	0.42	0.42	0.44	0.31	0.41	0.49	1.0													
14. Self-best	0.59	0.64	0.61	0.44	0.68	0.66	0.66	0.64	0.56	0.53	0.55	0.73	0.57	1.0												
15. Home	0.62	0.53	0.63	0.19	0.54	0.55	0.66	0.58	0.52	0.50	0.50	0.40	0.16	0.35	1.0											
16. Neighbourhood	0.47	0.40	0.51	0.25	0.39	0.38	0.51	0.42	0.40	0.34	0.35	0.32	0.16	0.27	0.56	1.0										
17. Family	0.64	0.51	0.59	0.24	0.48	0.49	0.60	0.49	0.40	0.37	0.38	0.36	0.21	0.35	0.43	0.40	1.0									
18. Living partner	0.60	0.52	0.49	0.23	0.46	0.48	0.55	0.44	0.35	0.38	0.38	0.35	0.13*	0.41	0.41	0.28	0.54	1.0								
19. Job	0.71	0.55	0.61	0.29	0.58	0.59	0.65	0.57	0.52	0.46	0.44	0.44	0.30	0.46	0.43	0.40	0.51	0.48	1.0							
20. Friendships	0.68	0.59	0.66	0.35	0.52	0.52	0.67	0.57	0.43	0.39	0.42	0.38	0.26	0.42	0.49	0.42	0.60	0.43	0.50	1.0						
21. Health	0.73	0.68	0.73	0.71	0.59	0.62	0.74	0.61	0.52	0.44	0.46	0.46	0.29	0.52	0.38	0.37	0.50	0.43	0.51	0.63	1.0					
22. Religion	0.61	0.55	0.57	0.34	0.49	0.54	0.60	0.45	0.39	0.37	0.42	0.41	0.27	0.41	0.40	0.40	0.44	0.39	0.45	0.56	0.62	1.0				
23. Financial sec.	0.56	0.49	0.64	0.29	0.55	0.57	0.68	0.64	0.67	0.56	0.62	0.47	0.24	0.40	0.56	0.39	0.35	0.36	0.47	0.39	0.46	0.38	1.0			
24. Recreation	0.61	0.58	0.66	0.50	0.55	0.62	0.66	0.61	0.51	0.43	0.45	0.41	0.22	0.43	0.44	0.30	0.38	0.37	0.45	0.60	0.67	0.52	0.53	1.0		
25. Self-esteem	0.73	0.67	0.72	0.43	0.60	0.64	0.73	0.63	0.53	0.45	0.46	0.43	0.29	0.46	0.44	0.39	0.52	0.45	0.56	0.61	0.73	0.59	0.46	0.59	1.0	
26. Environ. sat.	0.36	0.28	0.42	0.25	0.29	0.33	0.39	0.33	0.28	0.27	0.28	0.29	0.11*	0.28	0.33	0.43	0.32	0.24	0.30	0.26	0.37	0.34	0.36	0.33	0.32	1.0
27. Govern. sat.	0.32	0.29	0.39	0.20	0.31	0.36	0.38	0.34	0.32	0.29	0.32	0.27	0.11*	0.22	0.31	0.32	0.24	0.14	0.28	0.17	0.30	0.26	0.39	0.29	0.26	0.37

with SWLS, $r = 0.61$ with CLAS and $r = 0.67$ with SWB. The correlations among the average of the 13 domain satisfaction scores and the 7 overall life assessment scores are $r = 0.59$ for the single-item life satisfaction measure, $r = 0.59$ for the overall quality of life satisfaction measure, $r = 0.51$ for happiness and $r = 0.33$ for general health, $r = 0.49$ for SWLS, $r = 0.51$ for CLAS and $r = 0.60$ for SWB. It is worthwhile to notice that with the exception of the single-item life satisfaction measure, on average the single-item discrepancy measures had stronger associations than the domain satisfaction measures with the overall life assessment measures.

A basic assumption of those using measures of the sort listed in our tables is that these measures are sensitive to changing life circumstances. As Diener et al. (2009, pp. 93, 97) emphasized, "if no gold-standard measure exists" to match against another's performance, one way to validate the latter is to "compare the results that we get from the new measure to our expectations for how the measure should behave based on our theories of the underlying construct, as well as with other established measures...well-being measures will be most valuable when they behave in ways that often match our intuition...". While most of the measures considered here are not new, the validating strategy those authors suggest is still appropriate. Strictly speaking, as those authors also explained (p. 84), the strategy involves testing two things at the same time, namely, the assumption that individual's views about life as a whole or some domain of life actually changes with some change or other in their life circumstances and the further assumption that our measures are sensitive enough to capture changes in their views. Here we have generally proceeded as if the first assumption is true and only the second is being tested.

Table 12.5 contains results addressing the question of whether or not respondents who perceived changes in their overall life circumstances for the better or worse since the last survey would have variable mean scores increasing or decreasing more than respondents who did not perceive such changes. (This summary table and the following 5 (Tables 12.6, 12.7, 12.8, 12.9 and 12.10) are based on 115 pages of detailed tables covering the three waves of data for the three panels, which are available on request.) We separated the cases in which perceived changes were for the better from those in which perceived changes were for the worse in order to see if on average the two sorts of changes had different impacts compared to no-change cases.

Beginning in the lower right-hand corner of the last column of Table 12.5, one finds that on average there is pretty good support for the basic assumption. Mean scores are higher in the change groups than in the no-change groups for 71.3% (231/324) of the cases compared. The percentage of cases favourable to our basic assumption is higher when perceived changes are for the worse (77.8%) than when they are for the better (64.8%). For respondents in our samples, on average negative changes in life circumstances have a greater impact than positive changes, at least over a 12-month period. This is true for four of the five clusters as well as for the total set of measures. For the three domain satisfaction indexes, on average positive changes have a greater impact than negative changes.

Table 12.5 Summary of 3 waves for 3 panels, numbers and percents of cases in which variable mean scores in 2006 and 2007 are higher or lower given perceived changes in overall life circumstances for the better or worse since 2005 and 2006, respectively, than they are given no perceived changes

Variable names	Mean scores are higher given changes for the better		Mean scores are lower given for the worse		Total	Percent
	Yes	No	Yes	No	Yes	Yes
Life satisfaction	3	3	5	1	8	66.7
Happiness	5	1	6	0	11	91.7
QOL satisfaction	4	2	6	0	10	83.3
General health	5	1	4	2	9	75.0
Subtotal % yes	17/24 = 70.8		21/24 = 87.5		38/48 = 79.2	
SWLS	6	0	6	0	12	100.0
CLAS	5	1	6	0	11	91.7
SWB	3	3	6	0	9	75.0
Subtotal % yes	14/18 = 77.8		18/18 = 100.0		32/36 = 88.9	
Self/wants	5	1	6	0	11	91.7
Self/others	4	2	3	3	7	58.3
Self/deserves	4	2	6	0	10	83.3
Self/needs	4	2	4	2	8	66.7
Self/progress	6	0	6	0	12	100.0
Self/future	4	2	4	2	8	66.7
Self/best	4	2	5	1	9	75.0
Subtotal % yes	31/42 = 73.8		34/42 = 81.0		65/84 = 77.4	
3-group subtotal	62/84 = 73.8		73/84 = 86.9		135/168 = 80.4	
House satisfaction	3	3	4	2	7	58.3
Neighborhood sat.	4	2	6	0	10	83.3

(continued)

Table 12.5 (continued)

Variable names	Mean scores are higher given changes for the better		Mean scores are lower given for the worse		Total	Percent
	Yes	No	Yes	No	Yes	Yes
Family sat.	3	3	4	2	7	58.3
Partner sat.	3	3	4	2	7	58.3
Job sat.	3	3	5	1	8	66.7
Friendships sat.	1	5	4	2	5	41.7
Religion sat.	3	3	5	1	8	66.7
Financial sec. sat.	4	2	3	3	7	58.3
Recreation sat.	2	4	5	1	7	58.3
Self-esteem sat.	4	2	5	1	9	75.0
Subtotal % yes	30/60 = 50.0		45/60 = 75.0		75/120 = 62.5	
Health sat.	5	1	5	1	10	83.3
Environment sat.	3	3	1	5	4	33.0
Government sat.	5	1	2	4	7	58.3
Subtotal % yes	13/18 = 72.2		8/18 = 44.4		21/36 = 58.3	
13-Domain subtot.	43/78 = 55.1		53/78 = 67.9		96/156 = 61.5	
Total percent yes	105/162 = 64.8		126/162 = 77.8		231/324 = 71.3	

Table 12.6 Summary of 3 waves for 3 panels, numbers and percents of cases in which variable test-retest correlations 2005–2006 and 2006–2007 are higher given no perceived changes in overall life circumstances for the better or worse since 2005 and 2006, respectively, than they are given perceived changes

Variable names	Correlations are higher given no changes than given changes for better		Correlations are higher given no changes than given changes for worse		Total	Percent
	Yes	No	Yes	No	Yes	Yes
Life satisfaction	3	3	1	2	4	44.4
Happiness	4	1	1	2	5	62.5
QOL satisfaction	3	3	2	2	5	50.0
General health	5	1	0	3	5	55.6
Subtotal % yes	15/23 = 65.2		4/13 = 30.8		19/36 = 52.8	
SWLS	5	1	5	1	10	83.3
CLAS	3	3	5	1	8	66.7
SWB	5	1	3	2	8	72.7
Subtotal % yes	13/18 = 72.2		13/17 = 76.5		26/35 = 74.3	
Self/wants	6	0	1	3	7	70.0
Self/others	2	4	1	4	3	27.3
Self/deserves	5	1	2	1	7	77.8
Self/needs	4	2	0	3	4	44.4
Self/progress	5	0	0	3	5	62.5
Self/future	2	2	0	3	2	28.6
Self/best	4	2	0	4	4	40.0
Subtotal % yes	28/39 = 71.8		4/25 = 16.0		32/64 = 50.0	
3-Group subtotal	56/80 = 70.0		21/55 = 38.2		77/135 = 57.0	
House satisfaction	3	3	05		3	27.3
Neighborhood sat.	3	3	03		3	33.3
Family sat.	4	1	03		4	50.0
Partner sat.	3	3	03		3	33.3
Job sat.	3	1	00		3	75.0
Friendships sat.	2	4	0	3	2	22.2
Religion sat.	4	1	0	2	4	57.1
Financial sec. sat.	5	1	3	2	8	72.7
Recreation sat.	3	2	1	4	4	40.0
Self-esteem sat.	4	2	3	2	7	63.6
Subtotal % yes	34/55 = 61.8		7/34 = 20.6		41/89 = 46.1	
Health sat.	3	2	1	3	4	44.4
Environment sat.	4	2	2	2	6	60.0
Government sat.	3	3	2	4	5	41.7
Subtotal % yes	10/17 = 58.8		5/14 = 35.7		15/31 = 48.4	
13-Domain sub.	44/72 = 61.1		12/48 = 25.0		56/120 = 46.7	
Total percent yes	100/152 = 65.8		33/103 = 32.0		133/255 = 52.2	

Table 12.7 Summary of 3 waves for 3 panels, numbers and percents of cases in which variable mean scores in 2006 and 2007 are higher or lower given a net balance of selected positive or negative events since 2005 and 2006, respectively, than they are given an equal number of positive and negative events

Variable names	Mean scores are higher given a net balance of +1 positive events		Mean scores are higher given a net balance of +2 positive events		Mean scores are higher given a net balance of +3 or +4 pos. events		Totals for all net positive balance	
	Yes	No	Yes	No	Yes	No	Yes	No
Life satisfaction	4	2	3	3	2	4	9	9
Happiness	3	3	3	3	2	4	8	10
QOL satisfaction	2	4	3	3	3	3	8	10
General health	3	3	3	3	1	5	7	11
Subtotal % yes	12/24 = 50.0		12/24 = 50.0		8/24 = 33.3		32/72 = 44.4	
SWLS	4	2	4	2	4	2	12	6
CLAS	5	1	3	3	6	0	14	4
SWB	3	3	3	3	4	2	10	8
Subtotal % yes	12/18 = 66.7		10/18 = 55.6		14/18 = 77.8		36/54 = 66.7	
Self/wants	3	3	3	3	2	4	8	10
Self/others	6	0	3	3	5	1	14	4
Self/deserves	2	4	2	4	5	1	9	9
Self/needs	4	2	3	3	2	4	9	9
Self/progress	4	2	3	3	3	3	10	8
Self/future	5	1	6	0	4	2	15	3
Self/best	4	2	4	2	4	1	12	5
Subtotal % yes	28/42 = 66.7		24/42 = 57.1		25/41 = 61.0		77/125 = 61.6	
3-Group subtotal	52/84 = 61.9		46/84 = 54.8		47/83 = 56.6		145/251 = 57.8	
House satisfaction	4	2	4	2	2	4	10	8
Neighborhood sat.	3	3	3	3	2	4	8	10

(continued)

Table 12.7 (continued)

Variable names	Mean scores are higher given a net balance of +1 positive events		Mean scores are higher given a net balance of +2 positive events		Mean scores are higher given a net balance of +3 or +4 pos. events		Totals for all net positive balance	
	Yes	No	Yes	No	Yes	No	Yes	No
Family sat.	3	3	2	4	2	4	7	11
Partner sat.	2	4	2	4	4	2	8	10
Job sat.	3	3	5	1	5	1	13	5
Friendships sat.	1	5	3	3	3	3	7	11
Religion sat.	1	5	2	4	3	3	6	12
Financial sec. sat.	3	3	3	3	6	0	12	6
Recreation sat.	3	3	2	4	4	2	9	9
Self-esteem sat.	3	3	2	4	4	2	9	9
Subtotal % yes	26/60 = 43.3		28/60 = 46.7		35/60 = 58.3		89/180 = 49.4	
Health sat.	4	2	1	5	4	2	9	9
Environment sat.	5	1	1	5	3	3	9	9
Government sat.	4	2	4	2	3	3	11	7
Subtotal % yes	13/18 = 72.2		6/18 = 33.3		10/18 = 55.6		29/54 = 53.7	
13-Domain sub.	39/78 = 50.0		34/78 = 43.6		45/78 = 57.7		118/234 = 50.4	
Total percent yes	91/162 = 56.2		80/162 = 49.4		92/161 = 57.1		263/485 = 54.2	
Variable names	Mean scores are lower given a net balance of −1 negative events		Mean scores are lower given a net balance of −2 or −3 negative events		Totals for all net negative balance		Total yes for all net positive or negative balance	
	Yes	No	Yes	No	Yes	No	Yes	% Yes
Life satisfaction	4	2	3	3	7	5	16	53.3
Happiness	2	4	4	2	6	6	14	46.7

(continued)

Table 12.7 (continued)

Variable names	Mean scores are lower given a net balance of −1 negative events		Mean scores are lower given a net balance of −2 or −3 negative events		Totals for all net negative balance		Total yes for all net positive or negative balance	
	Yes	No	Yes	No	Yes	No	Yes	% Yes
QOL satisfaction	4	2	2	4	6	6	14	46.7
General health	2	4	3	3	5	7	12	40.0
Subtotal % yes	12/24 = 50.0		12/24 = 50.0		24/48 = 50.0		56/120 = 46.7	
SWLS	3	3	4	2	7	5	19	63.3
CLAS	4	2	5	1	9	3	23	76.7
SWB	3	3	3	3	6	6	16	53.3
Subtotal % yes	10/18 = 55.6		12/18 = 66.7		22/36 = 61.1		58/90 = 64.4	
Self/wants	4	2	4	2	8	4	16	53.3
Self/others	2	4	2	4	4	8	18	60.0
Self/deserves	3	3	4	1	7	4	16	55.2
Self/needs	2	4	2	3	4	7	13	44.8
Self/progress	2	4	3	2	5	6	15	51.7
Self/future	2	4	1	5	3	9	18	60.0
Self/best	3	3	5	1	8	4	20	69.0
Subtotal % yes	18/42 = 42.9		21/39 = 53.8		39/81 = 48.1		116/206 = 56.3	
3-Group subtotal	40/84 = 47.6		45/81 = 55.6		85/165 = 51.5		230/416 = 55.3	
House satisfaction	2	4	4	2	6	6	16	53.3
Neighborhood sat.	2	4	3	3	5	7	13	43.3
Family sat.	2	4	1	5	3	9	10	33.3

(continued)

Table 12.7 (continued)

Variable names	Mean scores are lower given a net balance of −1 negative events		Mean scores are lower given a net balance of −2 or −3 negative events		Totals for all net negative balance		Total yes for all net positive or negative balance	
	Yes	No	Yes	No	Yes	No	Yes	% Yes
Partner sat.	4	2	3	3	7	5	15	50.0
Job sat.	3	3	2	4	5	7	18	60.0
Friendships sat.	3	3	2	4	5	7	12	40.0
Religion sat.	2	4	1	5	3	9	9	30.0
Financial sec. sat.	3	3	0	6	3	9	15	50.0
Recreation sat.	2	4	5	1	7	5	16	53.3
Self-esteem sat.	3	3	3	3	6	6	15	50.0
Subtotal % yes	26/60 = 43.3		24/60 = 40.0		50/120 = 41.7		139/300 = 46.3	
Health sat.	3	3	6	0	9	3	18	60.0
Environment sat.	2	4	2	4	4	8	13	43.3
Government sat.	2	4	3	3	5	7	16	53.3
Subtotal % yes	7/18 = 38.9		11/18 = 61.1		18/36 = 50.0		47/90 = 52.2	
13-Domain sub.	33/78 = 42.3		35/78 = 44.9		68/156 = 43.6		186/390 = 47.7	
Total percent yes	73/162 = 45.1		80/159 = 50.3		153/321 = 47.7		416/806 = 51.6	

Table 12.8 Summary of 3 waves for 3 panels, numbers and percents of cases in which variable test-retest correlations 2005–2006 and 2006–07 are higher given an equal number of selected positive and negative events since 2005 and 2006, respectively, than they are given a net positive or negative balance of events

Variable names	Correlations are higher given an even versus a net balance of +1 positive events		Correlations are higher given an even versus a net balance of +2 positive events		Correlations are higher given an even versus a net balance of +3 or +4 pos. events		Totals for all net positive balance	
	Yes	No	Yes	No	Yes	No	Yes	No
Life satisfaction	3	1	0	3	0	3	3	7
Happiness	4	1	0	3	0	2	4	6
QOL satisfaction	0	5	0	2	0	1	0	8
General health	3	1	0	1	0	1	3	3
Subtotal % yes	10/18 = 55.6		0/9 = 00.0		0/7 = 00.0		10/34 = 29.4	
SWLS	3	3	1	3	0	2	4	8
CLAS	2	4	1	3	0	3	310	
SWB	1	5	0	4	0	2	111	
Subtotal % yes	6/18 = 33.3		2/12 = 16.7		0/7 = 00.0		8/37 = 21.6	
Self/wants	0	2	0	2	0	2	0	6
Self/others	1	4	1	2	0	1	2	7
Self/deserves	1	5	0	1	0	0	1	6
Self/needs	1	4	0	3	0	1	1	8
Self/progress	2	3	0	4	0	1	2	8
Self/future	1	4	0	2	0	3	1	9
Self/best	3	3	0	2	0	2	3	7
Subtotal % yes	9/34 = 26.5		1/17 = 5.9		0/10 = 00.0		10/61 = 16.4	
3-Group subtotal	25/70 = 35.7		3/38 = 7.9		0/24 = 00.0		28/132 = 21.2	
House satisfaction	5	0	1	1	0	2	6	3
Neighborhood sat.	2	3	0	3	0	0	2	6

(continued)

Table 12.8 (continued)

Variable names	Correlations are higher given an even versus a net balance of +1 positive events		Correlations are higher given an even versus a net balance of +2 positive events		Correlations are higher given an even versus a net balance of +3 or +4 pos. events		Totals for all net positive balance	
	Yes	No	Yes	No	Yes	No	Yes	No
Family sat.	2	2	0	2	0	1	2	5
Partner sat.	1	5	0	3	0	0	1	8
Job sat.	0	3	0	1	0	0	0	4
Friendships sat.	2	2	1	1	0	3	3	6
Religion sat.	1	4	0	2	0	1	1	7
Financial sec. sat.	3	2	1	2	1	0	5	4
Recreation sat.	2	3	1	1	0	3	3	7
Self-esteem sat.	2	4	0	2	0	2	2	8
Subtotal % yes	20/48 = 41.7		4/22 = 18.2		1/13 = 7.7		25/83 = 30.1	
Health sat.	0	5	0	2	0	1	0	8
Environment sat.	2	4	2	2	0	1	4	7
Government sat.	1	4	0	1	0	3	1	8
Subtotal % yes	3/16 = 18.8		2/7 = 28.6		0/5 = 0.0		5/28 = 17.9	
13-Domain sub.	23/64 = 35.9		6/29 = 20.7		1/18 = 5.6		30/111 = 27.0	
Total percent yes	48/134 = 35.8		9/67 = 13.4		1/42 = 2.4		58/243 = 23.9	
Variable names	Correlations are higher given an even versus a net balance of −1 negative events		Correlations are higher given an even versus a net balance of −2 or −3 negative events		Totals for all net negative balance		Total yes for all net positive or negative balance	
	Yes	No	Yes	No	Yes	No	Yes	% Yes
Life satisfaction	0	5	1	1	1	6	4	23.5
Happiness	2	4	0	4	2	8	6	30.0

(continued)

Table 12.8 (continued)

Variable names	Correlations are higher given an even versus a net balance of −1 negative events		Correlations are higher given an even versus a net balance of −2 or −3 negative events		Totals for all net negative balance		Total yes for all net positive or negative balance	
	Yes	No	Yes	No	Yes	No	Yes	% Yes
QOL satisfaction	0	5	1	2	1	7	1	6.3
General health	1	4	0	2	1	6	4	30.8
Subtotal % yes	3/21 = 14.3		2/11 = 18.2		5/32 = 15.6		15/66 = 22.7	
SWLS	1	5	1	4	2	9	6	26.1
CLAS	2	4	1	2	3	6	6	27.3
SWB	1	5	1	3	2	8	3	13.6
Subtotal % yes	4/18 = 22.2		3/12 = 25.0		7/30 = 23.3		15/67 = 22.4	
Self/wants	1	5	0	2	1	7	1	7.1
Self/others	0	6	0	3	0	9	2	11.1
Self/deserves	1	5	0	0	1	5	2	15.4
Self/needs	2	4	1	0	3	4	4	25.0
Self/progress	1	4	1	0	2	4	4	25.0
Self/future	1	4	0	1	1	5	2	12.5
Self/best	2	4	0	1	2	5	5	29.4
Subtotal % yes	8/40 = 20.0		2/9 = 22.2		10/49 = 20.4		20/110 = 18.2	
3-Group subtotal	15/79 = 19.0		7/32 = 21.9		22/111 = 19.8		50/243 = 20.6	
House satisfaction	2	3	0	2	2	5	8	50.0
Neighborhood sat.	2	2	0	3	2	5	4	26.7
Family sat.	0	4	0	1	0	5	2	16.7
Partner sat.	1	4	0	3	1	7	2	11.8

(continued)

Table 12.8 (continued)

Variable names	Correlations are higher given an even versus a net balance of −1 negative events		Correlations are higher given an even versus a net balance of −2 or −3 negative events		Totals for all net negative balance		Total yes for all net positive or negative balance	
	Yes	No	Yes	No	Yes	No	Yes	% Yes
Job sat.	2	3	0	0	2	3	2	22.2
Friendships sat.	1	4	0	2	1	6	4	25.0
Religion sat.	2	3	0	1	2	4	3	21.4
Financial sec. sat.	3	3	2	1	5	4	10	55.6
Recreation sat.	2	4	1	1	3	5	6	33.3
Self-esteem sat.	4	2	1	1	5	3	7	38.9
Subtotal % yes	19/51 = 37.3		4/19 = 21.1		23/70 = 32.9		48/153 = 31.4	
Health sat.	2	2	0	3	2	5	2	13.3
Environment sat.	0	5	0	1	0	6	4	23.5
Government sat.	2	4	0	1	2	5	3	18.8
Subtotal % yes	4/15 = 26.7		0/5 = 0.0		4/20 = 20.0		9/48 = 18.8	
13-Domain sub.	23/66 = 34.8		4/24 = 16.7		27/90 = 30.0		57/201 = 28.4	
Total percent yes	38/145 = 26.2		11/56 = 19.6		49/201 = 24.4		107/444 = 24.1	

Table 12.9 Summary of final column results from Tables 12.5, 12.6, 12.7 and 12.8, percentages of cases in which assumptions of year-by-year variable mean score changes and variable correlation changes were consistent with changes in perceived life circumstances or changes in the net balance of life events

Variable names	Percent of cases with variable scores consistent with perceived changes	Percent of cases with variable scores consistent with life events changes	Average of percents of cases with scores consistent with assumptions
Life satisfaction	55.6	38.4	47.0
Happiness	77.1	38.4	57.7
QOL satisfaction	66.7	26.5	46.6
General health	65.3	35.4	50.4
Subtotal mean	66.2	34.7	50.4
SWLS	91.7	44.7	68.2
CLAS	79.2	52.0	65.6
SWB	73.9	33.5	53.7
Subtotal mean	81.6	43.4	62.5
Self/wants	80.9	30.2	55.6
Self/others	42.8	35.6	39.2
Self/deserves	80.6	35.3	57.9
Self/needs	55.6	34.9	45.2
Self/progress	81.3	38.4	59.8
Self/future	47.7	36.3	42.0
Self/best	57.5	49.2	53.4
Subtotal mean	63.8	37.1	50.5
3-Group mean	68.3	37.8	53.0
House sat.	42.8	51.7	47.2
Neighbd sat.	58.3	35.0	46.7
Family sat.	54.2	25.0	39.6
Partner sat.	45.8	30.9	38.4
Job sat.	70.9	41.1	56.0
Friendships sat.	32.0	22.5	32.2
Religion sat.	61.9	25.7	43.8
Financial sec. sat.	65.5	52.8	59.2
Recreation sat.	49.2	43.3	46.2

(continued)

Table 12.9 (continued)

Variable names	Percent of cases with variable scores consistent with perceived changes	Percent of cases with variable scores consistent with life events changes	Average of percents of cases with scores consistent with assumptions
Self-esteem sat	69.3	44.5	56.9
Subtotal mean	55.0	37.3	46.6
Health sat.	63.9	36.7	50.3
Environment sat.	46.5	33.4	40.0
Government sat.	50.0	36.1	43.1
Subtotal mean	53.5	35.4	44.5
13-Domain sub	54.6	36.8	46.1
Total mean	61.7	37.3	49.7

Examining the subtotal percentage figures for the five clusters, one finds that the cluster of three overall life assessment indexes has the highest value (88.9%) and the cluster of three domain satisfaction indexes has the lowest value (58.3%). In fact, the cluster of 13 domain satisfaction variables has a lower value (61.5%) than the 3-group subtotal including all three clusters pertaining to some sort of overall life assessment (80.4%) as well as to each of the three clusters in that group; i.e., the clusters of four single-item overall life assessment variables (79.2%), three indexes (88.9%) and seven single-item discrepancy measures (77.4%). What's more, this low status of the two domain satisfaction clusters compared to the other three clusters in the two kinds of change situations is the same as that in the total change column, with one exception. On average, given change for the better, the three domain satisfaction indexes have a higher success rate (72.2%) than the four single-item overall life assessment variables (70.8%). While the exact values of these clusters were not expected, we did expect to find more support for our basic assumption from the overall life assessment variables than from the domain satisfaction variables because the perceived changes respondents were asked about concerned their life in general (i.e., life as a whole), not any specific domain of life. It is quite possible for one to perceive that one's life got better or worse, on the whole or all things considered, over the past year, although some aspects or domains of life got worse or did not change at all. In fact, it is also possible to perceive that some particular domain got better or worse on the whole even though some domain-relevant event occurred that had an opposite impact, e.g., one might judge that on the whole relations with one's friends improved over the past year although a close friend passed away.

Table 12.10 Summary of 3 waves for 3 panels, numbers and percents of cases in which variable test-retest correlations 2005–2006 and 2006–2007 are higher given no events since 2005 and 2006, respectively, than they are given some positive and/or negative events

Variable names	Correlations are higher given no events versus one event		Correlations are higher given no event versus two events		Correlations are higher given no event versus three or more events		Totals for all	
	Yes	No	Yes	No	Yes	No	Yes	No
Life satisfaction	2	4	1	4	2	3	3	7
Happiness	1	4	3	2	1	3	4	6
QOL satisfaction	2	4	2	4	1	3	0	8
General health	2	4	2	3	0	2	3	3
Subtotal % yes	7/23 = 30.4		8/21 = 38.1		4/15 = 26.7		19/59 = 32.2	
SWLS	2	4	3	3	2	3	4	8
CLAS	2	4	4	2	2	3	3	10
SWB	1	5	3	3	0	4	1	11
Subtotal % yes	5/18 = 27.8		10/18 = 55.6		4/14 = 28.6		19/50 = 38.0	
Self/wants	3	3	3	2	2	1	0	6
Self/others	1	5	2	3	0	5	2	7
Self/deserves	1	5	0	3	0	3	1	6
Self/needs	2	4	1	5	1	4	1	8
Self/progress	2	2	1	4	3	1	2	8
Self/future	2	4	1	2	0	4	1	9
Self/best	2	3	1	4	0	2	3	7
Subtotal % yes	13/39 = 33.3		9/32 = 28.1		6/26 = 23.1		28/97 = 28.9	
3-Group subtotal	25/80 = 31.3		27/71 = 38.0		14/55 = 25.5		66/206 = 32.0	
House satisfaction	4	2	3	3	2	2	6	3

(continued)

Table 12.10 (continued)

Variable names	Correlations are higher given no events versus one event		Correlations are higher given no event versus two events		Correlations are higher given no event versus three or more events		Totals for all	
	Yes	No	Yes	No	Yes	No	Yes	No
Neighborhood sat.	4	2	1	3	2	2	2	6
Family sat.	1	3	0	4	1	3	2	5
Partner sat.	0	5	1	4	0	5	1	8
Job sat.	1	4	0	2	1	1	0	4
Friendships sat.	3	3	2	2	1	4	3	6
Religion sat.	3	2	1	1	3	2	1	7
Financial sec. sat.	4	2	5	1	4	0	5	4
Recreation sat.	4	2	3	1	3	0	3	7
Self-esteem sat.	3	2	1	4	2	2	2	8
Subtotal % yes	27/54 = 50.0		17/42 = 40.5		19/40 = 47.5		63/136 = 46.3	
Health sat.	4	2	2	4	2	2	0	8
Environment sat.	2	4	2	3	1	4	4	7
Government sat.	1	4	2	3	1	3	1	8
Subtotal % yes	7/17 = 41.2		6/16 = 37.5		4/13 = 30.8		17/46 = 37.0	
13-Domain sub.	34/71 = 47.9		23/58 = 39.7		23/53 = 43.4		80/182 = 44.0	
Total percent yes	59/151 = 39.1		50/129 = 38.8		37/108 = 34.3		146/388 = 37.6	

The variety of percentage values among the 27 variables is remarkable, ranging from 33.0 to 100.0%. The sample size for each variable is of course small, but that would not imply success or failure of our basic assumption. For our most successful cluster, the success rates run from 100.0% for SWLS, to 91.7% for CLAS and 75.0% for SWB. For the cluster of single-item overall life assessment measures, the happiness variable has the greatest success (91.7%), followed by satisfaction with the overall quality of life (83.3%), general health (75.0%) and life satisfaction (66.7%). Since some sort of single-item life satisfaction measure is probably the most frequently used overall life assessment scale in the literature, these results should provoke some concern and second thoughts about the wisdom of having so many eggs in one basket. For the cluster of discrepancy measures, the range is from 58.3% for self-others to 100.0% for self-progress. In previous studies with MDT (e.g., Michalos 1991a, b, 1993a, b), the self-others measure was usually one of the two strongest predictors in the set of seven discrepancy measures, self-wants being the other one. So, it is encouraging to see the self-wants variable with a high success rate of 91.7% but not encouraging to see the relatively low success rate of the self-others variable. For the cluster of three domain satisfaction indexes, it is perhaps not surprising to find the health satisfaction measure with a relatively high success rate of 83.3% because it usually has fairly strong associations with overall life assessments, but it is unclear why the single-item neighbourhood satisfaction measure would be equally successful to the health satisfaction index.

The assumption leading to the exploration of results displayed in Table 12.5 has a variant leading to the exploration of results displayed in Table 12.6. Insofar as our measures are sensitive to changing life circumstances, variable test-retest correlations for 2005–2006 and 2006–2007 should be higher given no perceived changes in overall life circumstances for the better or worse since 2005 and 2006, respectively, than they are given perceived changes. As before, we separated the cases in which perceived changes were for the better from those in which perceived changes were for the worse in order to see if on average the two sorts of changes had different impacts compared to no-change cases. The only correlations counted were those significant at least at $P < 0.05$.

Beginning in the lower right-hand corner of the last column of Table 12.6, one finds that on average there is just barely support for our assumption. Mean scores are higher in the no-change groups than in the change groups for 52.2% (133/255) of the cases compared. Contrary to results found in Table 12.5, the percentage of cases favourable to our assumption is higher when perceived changes are for the better (65.8%) than when they are for the worse (32.0%). For respondents in our samples, on average given no perceived changes in life circumstances, the year-by-year test-retest correlations for our variables tend to be higher than the test-retest correlations given perceived changes for the better but not given perceived changes for the worse. This is true for four of the five clusters as well as for the total set of measures. The overall life assessment index cluster is the exception. For this cluster, on average 76.5% of cases are favourable to our assumption when perceived changes are for the worse, and 72.2% of cases are favourable when perceived changes are for the better.

Examining the subtotal average percentage figures for the five clusters in the total sample, one finds that (like Table 12.5) the cluster of three overall life assessment indexes has the highest value (74.3%) and the cluster of ten single-item domain satisfaction variables has the lowest value (46.1%). In fact, the cluster of ten single-item domain satisfaction variables has a lower average value than the 3-group subtotal including all three clusters pertaining to some sort of overall life assessment (57.0%) as well as to each of the three clusters in that group; i.e., the clusters of four single-item overall life assessment variables (52.8%), three indexes (74.3%) and seven single-item discrepancy measures (50.0%). This low status of the ten single-item domain satisfaction cluster compared to the other four clusters in the two kinds of change situations is the same as that in the total change column, with one exception. On average, in the changes-for-worse column, the seven single-item discrepancy measures had correlations favourable to our assumption for only 16.0% of cases. On average, the three domain satisfaction indexes scored marginally better (48.4%) than the ten single-item domain satisfaction measures.

The variety of percentage values among the 27 variables in the total sample column is again remarkable, ranging from 22.2 to 83.3%. For our most successful cluster, the success rates run from 83.3% for SWLS, to 72.7% for SWB and 66.7% for CLAS. For the cluster of single-item overall life assessment measures, the happiness variable again has the greatest success (62.5%), followed by general health (55.6%), satisfaction with the overall quality of life (50.0%), and life satisfaction (44.4%). As we remarked concerning results in Table 12.5, these results should provoke some concern about the wisdom of relying heavily on a single-item measure of life satisfaction. For the cluster of discrepancy measures, the range is from 27.3% for self-others to 77.8% for self-deserves. From the point of view of MDT, it is not particularly encouraging to see the self-wants variable with a success rate of 70.0% and encouraging to see the relatively higher success rate of the self-deserves variable. For the cluster of three domain satisfaction indexes, it is surprising to find the health satisfaction measure with a relatively low success rate of 44.4% and a lower success rate than the single-item general health variable (55.6%). It is also surprising and unclear why the job satisfaction (75.0%) and financial security satisfaction (72.7%) measures would be so much more successful than the other eight variables in the ten item cluster.

Tables 12.7 and 12.8 were constructed like Tables 12.5 and 12.6, by counting cases favourable or not to the basic assumption that our 27 measures are sensitive to changing life circumstances. The main difference between the earlier tables and these is that to create these tables we counted the net balance of reported positive and negative events in respondents lives instead of perceived changes for the better or worse in respondents' overall life circumstances. Following the patterns of Tables 12.5, 12.6 and 12.7 concerns changes in variable mean scores and Table 12.8 concerns changes in variable test-retest correlations.

Table 12.7 contains results addressing the question of whether or not respondents who experienced a net balance of positive or negative life events since the last survey would have variable mean scores increasing or decreasing more than respondents who experienced an equal number of positive and negative events.

Assuming that the chances of producing a variable mean score change would increase as the year-by-year net balance increased either positively from +1 to +2 to +3 or +4 or negatively from −1 to −2 or −3, we counted positive changes for three kinds of cases and negative changes for two kinds of cases. There were not enough cases with four negative events to get complete symmetry, and even for positive events there were often relatively few cases of four events.

Beginning in the lower right-hand corner of the last column of Table 12.7, one finds that on average there is just barely support for our basic assumption. Mean scores are appropriately higher or lower in the net-positive-or-negative-balance-of-events groups ('net-change groups' for short) than in the equal-balance-of-positive-and-negative-events groups ('no-net-change groups' for short) for 51.6% (416/806) of the cases compared. Contrary to results concerning perceived changes in Table 12.5, the percentage of cases favourable to our basic assumption is higher when there is a net balance of positive events (54.2%) than when there is a net balance of negative events (47.7%). The progressive increases in variable mean scores that we anticipated to follow net increases in the balance of positive events was somewhat achieved. Mean scores are higher given a net balance of +1 positive events in 56.2% of cases, higher given a net balance of +2 positive events in only 49.4% of cases and highest given a net balance of +3 or +4 positive events in 57.1% of cases. For negative events, anticipated results hardly followed. Mean scores are lower given a net balance of −1 negative event in only 45.1% of cases, and lower given a net balance of −2 or −3 negative events in 50.3% of cases.

Examining the subtotal average percentage figures for the five clusters in the total sample column, one again finds that the cluster of three overall life assessment indexes has the highest value (64.4%). The cluster of ten single-item domain satisfaction variables has the lowest value (46.3%). As expected the 3-group subtotal average including all three clusters pertaining to some sort of overall life assessment was higher (55.3%) than the average for the cluster of 13 domain satisfaction scores (47.7%), for the 10 single-item scores (46.3%) and the 3 domain satisfaction indexes (52.2%). On average, the seven single-item discrepancy measures performed relatively well at 56.3%.

Turning to the column summarizing results for cases with a net balance of positive events, we find nearly the same pattern as in the total sample results column. On average, the three overall life assessment indexes have the greatest success (66.7%), the four single-item overall life assessment measures have the least success (44.4%), the seven discrepancy measures come in second (61.6%), the three domain satisfaction indexes third (53.7%) and the ten single-item domain satisfaction measures fourth (49.4%). This pattern is altered in the column summarizing results for cases with a net balance of negative events. While the three overall life assessment indexes still perform best (61.1%), the ten single-item domain satisfaction measures perform worst (41.7%), with the four single-item overall life assessment measures and the three domain satisfaction indexes coming second (50.0%) and the seven discrepancy measures third (48.1%).

The anticipated progressive changes in mean scores for the positive and negative net-change versus no-net change groups were not achieved in most clusters.

Considering the subtotal average scores for the positive net-change groups first, one finds that as one moves from the +1 column to the +2 column, for three clusters there is less rather than more success, i.e., for the three overall life assessment indexes, seven discrepancy measures and three domain satisfaction indexes. For the four single-item overall life assessment variables there is no change and for the ten single-item domain satisfaction measures there is the anticipated increase in scores. As one moves from the +2 column to the +3 or +4 column, one finds the anticipated progressive changes in four of the five clusters, with the cluster of four single-item overall life assessment variables out of line. Our assumption of progressive changes was supported for three clusters in the negative net-changes groups. As one moves from the −1 column to the −2 or −3 column, on average our assumption is supported for the cluster of three overall life assessment indexes, three domain satisfaction indexes and seven discrepancy measures, but not for the four single-item overall life assessment measures or the ten single-item domain satisfaction measures.

Returning to the total sample column, there is relatively less variety than we have seen before in the percentage values among the 27 variables, ranging from 30.0 to 76.7%. Most success for our assumption was achieved by CLAS, at 76.7%, and least success was achieved by the satisfaction with religion or spiritual fulfillment variable (30.0%).

Table 12.8 contains results addressing the question of whether or not variable test-retest correlations would be higher for respondents who experienced an equal number of positive and negative events since the last survey than for respondents who experienced a net balance of positive or negative life events. Again assuming that the chances of producing a variable test-retest correlation change would increase as the year-by-year net balance increased either positively from +1 to +2 to +3 or +4 or negatively from −1 to −2 or −3 versus the no-net change situation, we counted positive changes for three kinds of cases and negative changes for two kinds of cases. As before, one should view the results in this table with caution because of the small sample sizes for each variable.

Beginning in the lower right-hand corner of the last column of Table 12.8, one finds that on average there is very little support for our basic assumption. Test-retest correlations are higher in the no-net-change groups than in the net-change groups for only 24.1% (107/444) of the cases compared. The percentage of cases favourable to our basic assumption is practically the same whether there is a net balance of negative events (24.4%) or a net balance of positive events (23.9%). Considering only positive net-change groups versus no-net-change groups, changes in correlations are exactly opposite to expectations. Test-retest correlations are higher for the no-net-change groups versus groups with a net balance of +1 positive event in 35.8% of cases, higher for the no-net-change groups versus groups with a net balance of +2 positive events in only 13.4% of cases and higher for the no-net-change groups versus groups with a net balance of +3 or +4 positive events in 2.4% of cases. Considering only negative net-change groups versus no-net-change groups, results are equally disappointing. Test-retest correlations are higher for the no-net-change groups versus groups with a net balance of −1 negative events in only 26.2% of cases, and higher for the no-net-change groups versus groups with a net balance of −2 or −3 negative events in 19.6% of cases.

Examining the subtotal average percentage figures for the five clusters in the total sample column, surprisingly one finds that the cluster of ten single-item domain satisfaction variables has the highest success ratio (31.4%) and the cluster of seven discrepancy measures has the lowest success ratio (18.2%). The average success ratio for the four single-item overall life assessment variables (22.7%) is practically the same as that of the three overall life assessment indexes (22.4%). The three domain satisfaction indexes have the second lowest success rate (18.8%).

Turning to the column summarizing results for cases with a net balance of positive events, we find the same pattern as that in the total sample column. On average the ten single-item domain satisfaction variables have the greatest success (30.1%), the seven discrepancy measures have the least success (16.4%), the four single-item overall life assessment measures come in second (29.4%), the three overall life assessment indexes third (21.6%) and the three domain satisfaction indexes fourth (17.9%). The pattern in the column summarizing results for cases with a net balance of negative events is different from the pattern in the total sample and positive net balance columns. While the ten domain satisfaction measures still perform best (32.9%), the four single-item overall life assessment measures perform worst (15.6%), with the three overall life assessment indexes coming second (23.3%), the seven discrepancy measures third (20.4%) and the three domain satisfaction indexes fourth (20.0%).

The anticipated progressive changes for the positive and negative net-change versus no-net change groups were not achieved in most clusters. Considering the subtotal scores for the positive net-change groups first, one finds that as one moves from the +1 column to the +2 column and from that column to the +3 or +4 column there is less rather than more success for each cluster except that of the 3 domain satisfaction indexes. However, our assumption of progressive changes was supported for 3 clusters in the negative net-changes groups. As one moves from the −1 column to the −2 or −3 column, our assumption is supported for the cluster of four single-item overall life assessment measures, the cluster of three overall life assessment indexes and seven discrepancy measures, but not for the two clusters of domain satisfaction measures.

Returning to the total sample column, there is again considerable variety in the percentage values among the 27 variables, ranging from 6.3 to 55.6%. Most success for our assumption was achieved by the financial security satisfaction (55.6%) and housing satisfaction variables (50.0%), and least success was achieved by the satisfaction with one's overall quality of life (6.3%).

Given the great variety of results in Tables 12.5, 12.6, 12.7 and 12.8, it is worthwhile to provide a summary table. Table 12.9 was constructed by calculating the average percentage figures from the final column results of Tables 12.5 and 12.6 for perceived changes and Tables 12.7 and 12.8 for net balances of life events, then taking the average of these two mean scores to form the final column of Table 12.9. Our basic question has been this: On average, are the 27 frequently used quality-of-life measures sensitive to (1) respondents' reported year-by-year perceived changes in their life circumstances for the better or worse and (2) calculated changes in the net balance of their reported positive and negative life events? Besides answering this most basic question for the 27 measures collectively, we have addressed the question from the point of view of average scores for five different clusters of measures in the total set and of each measure taken individually.

Beginning with the last figure in the lower right-hand column of Table 12.9, one finds that on average, the 27 measures were appropriately sensitive to year-by-year changes in respondents' life circumstances in 49.7% of the cases examined. In other words, measuring year-by-year changes in respondents' life circumstances by reports of their own perceptions and experienced life events, on average the values of the 27 variables changed in ways that were consistent with respondents' reported changes in about half of the cases examined. Clearly, a success rate struggling to equal a random chance rate is not a spectacular achievement for the total set of 27 measures. However, if one examines the bottom line of the other two columns in the table, one finds a substantial difference between the results in the perceived changes and net balance of life events changes columns. The former has a success rate of 61.7% while the latter has a rate of only 37.3%.

Considering only the final column of results, one finds that on average, measures in the three overall life assessment clusters had a higher success rate (53.0%) than measures in the domain satisfaction clusters (46.1%). In fact, on average measures for each of the three former clusters was higher than that of the latter cluster. The three overall life assessment indexes had the highest average (62.5%), followed by the seven discrepancy measures (50.5%) and then the four single-item overall life assessment measures (50.4%). Within the three overall life assessment index cluster, SWLS had the highest success rate (68.2%). Within the discrepancy cluster, self-progress was highest (59.8%) and for the single-item overall life assessment cluster it was happiness (57.7%). For the ten single-item domain satisfaction cluster, satisfaction with one's financial security (59.2%) and self-esteem (56.9%) were highest. For the three domain satisfaction index cluster, satisfaction with one's health was highest (50.3%).

Considering the column of worst results (column two), one finds again that on average, measures in the three overall life assessment clusters had a higher success rate (37.8%) than measures in the domain satisfaction clusters (36.8%). The three overall life assessment indexes again had the highest average (43.4%), followed by the ten single-item domain satisfaction measures (37.3%) and then the seven discrepancy measures (37.1%). The three domain satisfaction indexes came in fourth (35.4%) and the four single-item overall life assessment measures average came in last (34.7%). Within the three overall life assessment index cluster, CLAS had the highest success rate (52.0%). Within the discrepancy cluster, self-best was highest (49.2%) and for the four single-item overall life assessment cluster, happiness was tied with life satisfaction (38.4%). For the ten single-item domain satisfaction cluster, satisfaction with one's financial security (52.8%) had the best score, followed by housing satisfaction (51.7%). The latter figure was the only one in the first two columns of the table in which a value of a variable in the second column (51.7%) was greater than its corresponding value in the first column (42.8%).

Considering finally the column of best results (column one), one finds again that on average, measures in the three overall life assessment clusters had a higher success rate (68.3%) than measures in the domain satisfaction clusters (54.6%). The three overall life assessment indexes again had the highest average (81.6%), followed by the four single-item overall life assessment measures (66.2%). Then, the seven discrepancy measures came in third (63.8%), the ten domain satisfaction measures came fourth (55.0%) and finally, the three domain satisfaction indexes (53.5%). Within the three overall life assessment index cluster, SWLS had the highest success rate (91.7%). Within the four single-item overall life assessment cluster, happiness had the highest rate (77.1%). For the discrepancy cluster, self-progress was highest (81.3%), for the cluster of ten domain satisfaction measures, job satisfaction was highest (70.9%), followed by self-esteem satisfaction (69.3%). Within the three domain satisfaction indexes cluster, health satisfaction was highest (63.9%).

Conclusion

Recall that Atkinson's most important conclusions directly challenged the hypotheses that satisfaction measures "are poor social indicators because they were so conditioned by expectations and restricted awareness as to be insensitive to changing circumstances" and that "expectations and aspirations adjust very quickly to new situations and that satisfaction and other measures revert to their original levels immediately". Predictions following these hypotheses were contradicted by his results "in that significant numbers of respondents perceive changes in their lives and those changes were reflected, for better or worse, in their satisfaction levels". The changes he tracked "took place over a two year period" and he thought they showed that "while adaptation probably does occur, it is not instantaneous and will be detected by an indicator series which utilizes fairly frequent measurements". Using two different measures of changing life circumstances, he found that "The hypothesis that the No Change group would have more stable QOL scores than those reporting change is supported when the perceptual indicator of change is used as the independent variable but not when the event measures are involved".

We have some similar and some dissimilar results. Since about 46% of our respondents reported changes in their life circumstances using each of the two different measures of change, it is fair to say that we also found "significant numbers of respondents perceive changes in their lives". Considering nearly three times as many relevant variables as Atkinson (i.e., 27 compared to 10) and 1 year change periods, we also found that they behaved more often than not (61.7%) as expected using "the perceptual indicator of change" but less often than not (37.3%) as expected using "event measures".

We did not find as he did that single-item domain satisfaction measures performed better than overall life assessment measures. As reported in Table 12.9, using both kinds of measures of change, on average the ten single-item domain satisfaction measures had a 46.6% success rate, compared to 53.0% for the 14 overall life assessment measures. Using "the perceptual indicator of change", on average the ten single-item domain satisfaction measures had a 55.0% success rate, compared to 68.3% for the 14 life assessment measures. It should also be noticed that within the cluster of all domain satisfaction measures, on average the three indexes did not perform better than the ten single-item measures, i.e., 53.5% compared to 55.0%, respectively. Generally speaking, then, considering the relative performance of overall life assessment measures versus domain satisfaction measures, our results are consistent with those summarized by Diener et al. (2009, pp. 72–73). They found "no systematic differences" among such measures and reported that "Overall, the content of well-being measures has surprisingly little influence on the reliability of well-being measures".

Regarding single-item overall life assessment measures, Atkinson's worst performer was the Gallup 3-step happiness measure. He suspected that "the item's problems stem from the use of a three-point response scale". As indicated in Table 12.9, our 7-step happiness measure had the highest success rate of the four single-item overall life assessment measures using both measures of change (57.7%) and perceived changes measure (77.1%). The 2-year test-retest correlation for his 3-step happiness measure was $r = 0.39$ (p. 120, Table 12.2), while our 7-step happiness measure scored $r = 0.64$ (Table 12.3). His 11-step life satisfaction scale had a 2-year test-retest correlation of $r = 0.41$, while our 7-step scale scored $r = 0.65$. Concerning response categories, Diener et al. (2009, p. 74) claimed that "the evidence suggests that, at least in the range from 2 to 11 response categories, the more response categories produce higher reliability…We strongly urge researchers to use scales with more response options and to phase out measures with three or four response categories that are still in use".

Atkinson's General QOL Index had a 2-year test-retest correlation of $r = 0.53$, while the average of our three overall life assessment indexes was $r = 0.76$. In fact, each of our three indexes displayed greater stability than Atkinson's General QOL Index, with SWB having the highest 2-year test-retest correlation of $r = 0.77$, followed by SWLS and CLAS at $r = 0.75$ each. Most importantly, considering the general stability of our three indexes regardless of changing life circumstances (Table 12.3) and the average superior sensitivity of these indexes to perceived changes in life circumstances (81.6%; Table 12.9), a fairly strong case has been made for preferring any of these indexes to any single-item overall life assessment measure. It is, therefore, worth emphasizing that any general survey of the perceived quality of life and especially the World Values Survey and the Gallup World Poll would be strengthened if they included any of these indexes. Since Michalos and Kahlke (2008) showed that our single-item measure of satisfaction with the overall quality of life was more sensitive to arts-related activities than any of the three overall life assessment indexes, we still believe that the wisest course to follow in any assessment of perceived quality of life is to use more than one measure for one's dependent variable. One of the strongest messages we have had from over 40 years of quality of life research is that different measures are more or less sensitive to different features of people's lives (Michalos 2005), and the best way to avoid oversimplification in our assessments is to use more rather than fewer measures. In Michalos (2008) additional arguments were presented against the use of any single life satisfaction measure as a criterion variable for overall quality of life studies. Of course, if one must choose between having a single life satisfaction (index or single-item) measure and none at all in such studies, one should opt for such a measure. However, the use of any such single measure as a criterion variable for assigning importance weights to aspects or domains of life should be resisted or undertaken with great caution.

Considering the average stability of our seven discrepancy measures regardless of changing life circumstances ($r = 0.59$ and $r = 0.57$ for one- and 2-year test-retest correlations, respectively; Table 12.3) and their average sensitivity to perceived changes in life circumstances (63.8%; Table 12.9), these measures should be used with caution. Since they are essential components of MDT, we are aware of the significance of this finding for that theory. While the success rates of measures of self/wants (80.9%), self/deserves (80.6%) and self/progress (81.3%) are fairly acceptable, those of the other 4, especially self/others (42.8%), are problematic. The reliability and usefulness of these four variables could prove to be a fatal blow to the theory as currently crafted. Results of our causal analyses in the next paper will help us decide what role, if any, these variables should continue to have in MDT.

Finally, in one of our email exchanges with Lucas, he suggested that "when looking at stability coefficients, it might be worth comparing people with more events (regardless of valence) to those with fewer events". Table 12.10 summarizes the results of our exploration of this suggestion. Beginning with the last figure in the lower right-hand column of Table 12.10, one finds that on average for the stability coefficients of the 27 variables under consideration, the hypotheses that correlations are higher given no events versus one, two and three or more events are supported in only 37.6% of the cases examined. Reviewing the sub-total average figures for the five main clusters, one finds that the ten single-item domain satisfaction measures performed most consistently with the hypotheses (46.3%), but still more often than not failed to support them. The three overall life assessment indexes performed no better than average (38.0%). Comparing the bottom lines of the other three columns, one would expect to find increasing support for the basic hypothesis, i.e., more events produces smaller stability coefficients. In fact, we find decreasing support, from 39.1% (0 events vs. 1) to 38.8% (0 vs. 2) to 34.3% (0 vs. 3 or more). Examining all the subtotals in the three columns, there are no cases of a steady increase across all three columns in support of the basic hypotheses. There are, however, two cases in which there are increases consistent with the hypotheses, namely, for the four single-items and the three indexes of overall life assessment clusters as one moves from 0 versus 1 to 0 versus 2 events. All things considered, we find little support for the hypothesis that, regardless of valence, respondent experiences of more versus fewer salient life events produces lower stability coefficients.

Acknowledgement We would like to express our thanks to the Social Sciences and Humanities Research Council for funding this research through the Gold Medal for Achievement in Research 2004. As well, we would like to thank John Helliwell and Richard Lucas for suggestions that improved the paper, and Joyce Henley, Office Manager of ISRE and all the anonymous respondents who shared their time and thoughts with us to make this report possible.

Appendix: List of Life Events

1. Did you get married? p*
2. Become separated or divorced? n
3. Did you (your wife) have a child? p
4. Did you start a close romantic relationship? p
5. Did you have a romantic relationship break up? n
6. Did you lose a close family member through death? n
7. Did you have a close friend die? n
8. Did you suffer a serious injury or illness? n
9. Did you form a new very close friendship? p
10. Did you lose touch with a very close friend? n
11. Did you get a new job? p
12. Did you get a job promotion? p
13. Did you have an outstanding honour or achievement? p
14. Did you change your place of residence? p
15. Did you have a large increase in your or your family's income? p
16. Did you have a large decrease in your or your family's income? n
    *p = positive event, n = negative event

References

Atkinson, T. (1982). The stability and validity of quality of life measures. *Social Indicators Research, 10*(2), 113–132.

Brickman, P., & Campbell, D. T. (1971). Hedonic relativism and planning the good society. In M. H. Appley (Ed.), *Adaptation-level theory* (pp. 287–305). New York: Academic Press.

Campbell, A., Converse, P. E., & Rodgers, W. L. (1976). *The quality of american life: Perceptions, evaluations, satisfactions*. New York: Russell Sage Foundation.

Cantril, H. (1965). *The patterns of human concerns*. New Brunswick: Rutgers University Press.

Diener, E., Emmons, R. A., Larsen, R. J., & Griffin, S. (1985). The satisfaction with life scale. *Journal of Personality Assessment, 49*(1), 71–75.

Diener, E., Lucas, R. E., Schimmack, U., & Helliwell, J. F. (2009). *Well-being for public policy*. Onxford: Oxford University Press.

Diener, E., Lucas, R. E., & Scollon, C. N. (2006). Beyond the hedonic treadmill. *American Psychologist, 61*(4), 305–314.

Eels, L. W. (1985). *The effect of role change on physical health, mental health and general life-satisfaction: A panel analysis [dissertation]*. Lincoln: University of Nebraska.

Ehrhardt, J. J., Saris, W. E., & Veenhoven, R. (2000). Stability of life-satisfaction over time: Analysis of change in ranks in a national population. *Journal of Happiness Studies, 1*(2), 177–205.

Headey, B., & Wearing, A. J. (1989). Personality, life events and subjective well-being: Towards a dynamic equilibrium model. *Journal of Personality and Social Psychology, 57,* 731–739.

Headey, B., & Wearing, A. J. (1992). *Understanding happiness: A theory of subjective well-being.* Melbourne: Longman Cheshire.

Landua, D. (1992). Satisfaction changes. *Social Indicators Research, 26*(3), 221–241.

Lavallee, L. F., Hatch, P. M., Michalos, A. C., & McKinley, T. (2007). Development of the contentment with life assessment scale (CLAS): Using daily life experiences to verify levels of self-reported life satisfaction. *Social Indicators Research, 83*(2), 201–244.

Lucas, R. E. (2005). Time does not heal all wounds: A longitudinal study of reaction and adaptation to divorce. *Psychological Science, 16*(12), 945–950.

Lucas, R. E., Clark, A. E., Georgellis, Y., & Diener, E. (2003). Reexamining adaptation and the set point model of happiness: Reactions to changes in marital status. *Journal of Personality and Social Psychology, 84*(3), 527–539.

Lucas, R. E., Clark, A. E., Georgellis, Y., & Diener, E. (2004). Unemployment alters the set point for life satisfaction. *Psychological Science, 15*(1), 8–13.

Michalos, A. C. (1985). Multiple discrepancies theory (MDT). *Social Indicators Research, 13,* 347–413.

Michalos, A. C. (1991a). *Global report on student well-being, vol. 1: Life satisfaction and happiness.* New York: Springer.

Michalos, A. C. (1991b). *Global report on student well-being, vol. 2: Family, friends, living partner and self-esteem.* New York: Springer.

Michalos, A. C. (1993a). *Global report on student well-being, vol. 3: Employment, finances, housing and transportation.* New York: Springer.

Michalos, A. C. (1993b). *Global report on student well-being, vol. 4: Religion, education, recreation and health.* New York: Springer.

Michalos, A. C. (Ed.). (2005). *Citation classics from social indicators research: The most cited articles edited and introduced by Alex C. Michalos.* Dordrecht: Springer.

Michalos, A. C. (2008). Education, happiness and wellbeing. *Social Indicators Research, 87*(3), 347–366.

Michalos, A. C., & Kahlke, P. M. (2008). Impact of arts-related activities on the perceived quality of life. *Social Indicators Research, 89*(2), 193–258.

Veenhoven, R. (1994). Is happiness a trait? *Social Indicators Research, 32*(2), 101–160.

Chapter 13
Arts and the Perceived Quality of Life in British Columbia

Alex C. Michalos and P. Maurine Kahlke

Introduction

In Michalos and Kahlke (2008) we reported the results of a 2006 survey of 1,027 adults in five communities of British Columbia (Comox Valley, Kamloops, Nanaimo, Port Moody and Prince George). The aim of that survey was to measure the impact of arts-related activities on the perceived quality of respondents' lives. The sample was not drawn in any way that it could be regarded as representative of the whole provincial population. However, our plan was to undertake an independent survey in 2007 that would be representative of the whole province. This paper is a report of the results of that province-wide survey. Specifically, then, the aims of this investigation are (1) to measure the impact of arts-related activities on the perceived quality of life of a representative sample of British Columbians aged 18 years or more, and (2) to compare the findings of this study with those of the earlier study.

As in Michalos (2005b) and Michalos and Kahlke (2008), the term 'arts' is used here in a very broad sense to include such things as music, dance, theatre, painting, sculpture, pottery, literature (novels, short stories, poetry), photography, quilting, gardening, flower arranging, textile and fabric art. Although we regard 'culture' as a term with a broader connotation than 'arts' and many people seem to treat the two

Michalos, A.C., & Kahlke, P.M.: 2010b. Arts and the perceived quality of life in British Columbia. Social Indicators Research, 96, pp. 1–39.

A.C. Michalos (✉)
University of Northern British Columbia, Prince George, BC, Canada
e-mail: michalos@brandonu.ca

P.M. Kahlke
Institute for Social Research and Evaluation (ISRE), University of Northern British Columbia, 3333 University Way, Prince George, BC V2N 4Z9, Canada
e-mail: hatchp@unbc.ca

A.C. Michalos, *Development of Quality of Life Theory and Its Instruments*,
DOI 10.1007/978-3-319-51149-8_13

terms as synonyms, such distinctions should not create any confusion here because we will give a complete list of everything we consider to be an arts-related activity for the purposes of this study. Again following the strategy of the two earlier studies, we are not attempting any distinction between high/fine and low/popular art or culture.

The structure and analyses in this essay follow closely those of Michalos and Kahlke (2008). In the next section "Sampling Technique and Questionnaire" we describe our sampling technique and questionnaire, and in the section after that section "Sample Characteristics" we summarize the characteristics of the sample. The descriptive statistics resulting from the substantive items in the questionnaire are reviewed in section "Descriptive Statistics". In section "Bivariate Relationships" the results of a variety of bivariate analyses are presented, and variables shown to have statistically significant bivariate associations are used in multivariate analyses in section "Multivariate Relationships". The concluding section "Conclusion" provides an overview of our results compared to results from the earlier study.

Sampling Technique and Questionnaire

The 13-page questionnaire used in the survey undertaken for this investigation was a revised version of one used for the five-community survey described in Michalos and Kahlke (2008). In May 2007, 5,000 questionnaires were mailed out to a random sample of households across the whole province of British Columbia. The first three pages of the questionnaire listed 66 activities that are related in one way or another to the arts, e.g., listening to music, teaching painting or drawing, singing in a group, attending live theatre performances. Because people participate in different artistic activities in very different time periods, from daily (e.g., listening to music) to a few times per year (e.g., attending live theatre performances), to properly estimate the amount of time committed to such activities, two different questions were included. For activities involving frequent participation, respondents were asked to estimate the average amount of time per week that they spent on them, in hours. If they never engaged in some particular activity, they were asked to write 0 for *hours per week*. For activities involving infrequent participation, respondents were asked to estimate the number of times per year that they participated in them. If they never engaged in some particular activity, they were asked to write 0 for *times per year*. For those activities in which they participated, they were asked to rate the average level of satisfaction obtained on a 7-point scale running from 1 = very dissatisfied, 2 or 3 = dissatisfied, 4 = even balance of satisfaction and dissatisfaction, 5 or 6 = satisfied, to 7 = very satisfied. The Appendix attached to this paper has a complete list of all the activities sorted and ordered by (1) the numbers of people participating in each, (2) the average number of hours per week people engaged in each and (3) the average number of times per year that people engaged in each. Copies of the questionnaire and detailed responses to all items are available from the corresponding author on request.

Following the frequency-of-participation items, there was a page of questions designed to get more information about the arts-related activity (out of the 66) that respondents perceived as "most important". For examples, there were questions about levels of satisfaction with their access to the activity, with the price of engagement and with the usual venue, and questions about where they first learned about the activity, e.g., in school, watching television, listening to a friend, and how old they were at the time.

The next two pages listed 45 statements culled from the literature describing people's beliefs and feelings about the arts, usually phrased in personal terms, e.g., My artistic activities help me preserve my cultural heritage, I engage in artistic activities to express my spirituality, I enjoy art for its own sake. Sometimes the phrasing was impersonal, e.g., Artistic activity strengthens a community, Good art needs no justification beyond itself. Respondents were given a 5-point Likert scale and asked to indicate for each item their level of agreement or disagreement, with strongly disagree = 1 and strongly agree = 5.

There were then two pages of standard questions about respondents' health and quality of life. These included questions about life as a whole and about specific domains and aspects of life, e.g., family relations, friendships, sense of meaning in life. Seven overall assessments of life were used as dependent variables in this study: (1) self-reported general health using a 5-point scale from poor to excellent, (2) satisfaction with life as a whole using a 7-point scale from very dissatisfied to very satisfied, (3) satisfaction with the overall quality of life using a 7-point scale from very dissatisfied to very satisfied, (4) happiness with life as a whole using a 7-point scale from very unhappy to very happy, (5) satisfaction with life as a whole using a 5-item index drawn from Diener et al. (1985), (6) contentment with life using a 5-item index drawn from Lavallee et al. (2007) and (7) subjective wellbeing using a 4-item index (Michalos et al. 2005). All measures of satisfaction with particular domains or aspects of life were formatted as 7-point scales running from very dissatisfied to very satisfied and these measures have been used around the world for over 30 years (Michalos 2005a).

Following these standard questions, there were two pages of questions designed to test some of the basic hypotheses of Multiple Discrepancies Theory (MDT, Michalos 1985), e.g., Considering your life as a whole, how does it measure up to your general aspirations or what you want out of life?, How does it measure up to the best in your previous experience? This is only the second survey allowing some testing of MDT in the context of a wide variety of information about arts-related activities and the perceived quality of life.

Finally, there were 2 pages of demographic questions about, e.g., age, sex, marital status, income and education.

Sample Characteristics

A total of 708 (14.2%) useable questionnaires were returned, which form the working data-set for the survey. Table 13.1 summarizes the main features of the respondent sample.

Table 13.1 Sample demographics, unweighted and weighted numbers and % and census (Statistics Canada, *2006 census data*) values, numbers and %

Characteristic	Unweighted		Weighted		Census values	
	N	%	*N*	%	*N*	%
Gender						
Female	455	65.7	457	65.9	1,745,320	51.4
Male	238	34.3	236	34.1	1,649,585	48.6
Total	693	100.0	693	100.0	3,394,905	100.0
Age						
20–34	86	12.4	167	24.2	762,435	24.4
35–44	140	20.3	137	19.9	622,615	19.9
45–54	165	23.9	146	21.1	661,485	21.2
55–64	167	24.2	113	16.4	502,645	16.2
65 and over	133	19.2	127	18.4	572,420	18.3
Total	691	100.0	690	100.0	3,121,600	100.0
Education—highest level						
Secondary—incomplete	32	4.7	110	16.0	502,270	16.1
Secondary—complete	165	24.0	189	27.5	858,115	27.5
Diploma, certificate etc.	165	24.0	205	29.7	924,820	29.6
Some university	100	14.5	40	5.8	182,695	5.9
University degree	226	32.8	144	21.0	653,700	20.9
Total	688	100.0	688	100.0	3,121,600	100.0
Employment status						
Unemployed	11	1.6	11	1.6	115,000	3.7
Employed	416	60.4	408	59.6	1,973,335	63.2
Not in the labour force	262	38.0	266	38.8	1,033,285	33.1
Total	689	100.0	685	100.0	3,121,620	100.0
Marital status						
Now married	406	58.2	395	56.6	1,728,875	54.7
Live-in partner	72	10.3	70	10.0	276,130	8.8
Single—never married	72	10.3	95	13.6	653,715	20.7
Divorced	73	10.5	68	9.8	212,535	6.7
Separated	19	2.7	20	2.9	92,705	2.9
Widowed	56	8.0	50	7.1	196,365	6.2
Total	698	100.0	698	100.0	3,160,325	100.0

The first substantive column of the table lists statistics for the unweighted sample, the second lists those statistics weighted by age and education according to the census of 2006 and the final column lists the 2006 census values for comparative purposes. All of our analyses are based on the weighted sample.

For the weighted sample, of those respondents who revealed their gender ($N = 693$), nearly two-thirds (65.9%) were female. Of 690 respondents answering the age question, 44.1% were aged 20–44 and 34.8% were 55 or older, ranging from 18 to 96. Twenty-one percent of 688 respondents held a university degree and another 29.7% held a diploma or certificate from a trade, technical, business or community college. Sixty percent of 685 respondents answering the question were employed full-time and 56.6% of 698 respondents were married, with another 10.0% having a live-in partner.

Comparing the figures for the weighted sample with those of the 2006 census, one finds that the age and education values are practically the same, the weighted sample has 3% points fewer of employed people, 2% points more of married people and 15% points more of females than the census. Since some studies have found women to be generally more supportive than men of the arts (Decima 2002, p. 50; DiMaggio and Pettitt 1999, p. 34), the over-representation of women in our sample may create a bias in favour of arts-related activities. In fact, split-file analyses (not shown here) by gender revealed very few differences. If the weighted sample has a bias in favour of arts-related activities, it is a bias shared fairly equally among respondents regardless of their gender, i.e., it is a bias resulting from self-selection of respondents. Gender had no significant impact on any dependent variables in our multiple regression analyses (section "Multivariate Relationships"). In any event, with the exception of gender, our weighted sample is fairly representative of the total population of British Columbia.

Descriptive Statistics

Table 13.2 lists the top 10 arts-related activities by numbers and percent of participants, with average *hours per week* participation and mean levels of satisfaction. The activity with the highest percentage of participants was listening to music, followed by reading novels, short stories, plays or poetry. Eighty-four percent (593) reported listening to music an average of 14.0 h per week with a mean level of satisfaction of 6.0. Fifty-eight percent (412) reported reading novels, etc. an average of 7.4 h per week with a mean level of satisfaction of 6.1. The third and fourth activities with the highest percentages of participants were watching films on dvd or video and singing alone, respectively. Forty-one percent (293) of respondents reported watching films on dvd or video on average 5.4 h per week with a mean level of satisfaction of 5.6. Thirty-seven percent (260) of respondents reported singing alone on average 4.3 h per week with a mean level of satisfaction of 5.7. The activity with the fifth highest percentage of participants was reading to others. Thirty-one percent (216) reported reading to others an average of 3.5 h per week with a mean level of satisfaction of 6.0. Comparing the figures in the first five rows of Table 13.2 with their counterparts in Table 2 of Michalos and Kahlke (2008), one finds the same activities ordered in the same way, practically the same average levels of satisfaction, and a bit more disparity among percentages and hours per week of participation.

Table 13.3 lists the top 10 arts-related activities by numbers and percent of participants, with average *times per year* participation and mean levels of

Table 13.2 Top 10 arts-related activities by number and percent of participants, with average number of *hours per week* participation and mean levels of satisfaction

Activities	N	%	Hours per week	Mean sat.
Listening to music	593	83.8	14.0	6.0
Reading novels, etc.	412	58.2	7.4	6.1
Watching films, dvd	293	41.4	5.4	5.6
Singing alone	260	36.7	4.3	5.7
Reading to others	216	30.5	3.5	6.0
Telling stories	141	19.9	3.0	5.9
Gourmet cooking	124	17.5	4.6	6.2
Painting or drawing	120	17.0	5.0	5.9
Singing in a group	100	14.1	2.8	6.1
Watching TV art shows	92	13.0	3.7	5.6

Table 13.3 Top 10 arts-related activities by number and percent of participants, with average number of *times per year* participation and mean levels of satisfaction

Activities	N	%	Times per year	Mean sat.
Go to movies	409	57.7	6.2	5.6
Go to concerts	384	54.2	3.5	6.0
Go to community festivals	353	49.9	2.9	5.6
Go to historic sites	348	49.2	3.0	5.9
Go to art museums	345	48.7	3.4	5.7
Go to other museums	295	41.6	2.3	5.7
Go to public library	295	41.7	8.2	5.6
Go to amateur theatre	264	37.3	2.4	5.8
Go to prof. theatre	254	35.8	2.7	6.2
Decorating a home	212	29.9	5.9	5.8

satisfaction. The activity with the highest percentage of participants was going to films (cinema, movie theatres). Fifty-eight percent (409) reported going to films an average of 6.2 times per year with a mean level of satisfaction of 5.6. The activity with the second highest percentage of participants was going to concerts. Fifty-four percent (384) reported going to concerts an average of 3.5 times per year, with a mean level of satisfaction of 6.0. The activity with the third highest percentage of participants was attending community festivals. Fifty percent (353) of respondents reported attending community festivals an average of 2.9 times per year, with a mean level of satisfaction of 5.6. The activities with the fourth and fifth highest percentages of participants were going to historic, heritage sites and going to art museums and galleries, and the figures were similar. Forty-nine percent (348) reported going to historic, heritage sites an average of 3.0 times per year, with a mean level of satisfaction of 5.9, while 49% (345) reported going to art museums and galleries an average of 3.4 times per year, with a mean level of satisfaction of 5.7.

Table 13.4 Percent of respondents indicating first thoughts about the meaning of 'arts' or 'artistic activity', respondents' most important arts-related activity, place of and age at first encounter with the activity, and mean levels of satisfaction with aspects of that activity

Item	Activity, place, age, % and sat.
First thoughts %	Painting, drawing 37.9%
Most important %	Music 35.8%
Place where first learned about it %	School 55.4%
Mean age when first learned about it	12 years
Mean level of satisfaction with	
Access to activity itself (*N*)	5.4 (599)
Access to information re activity (*N*)	5.3 (616)
Place where activity occurs (*N*)	5.2 (463)
Access to the activity facility (*N*)	5.0 (558)
Price ($) for participating (*N*)	4.8 (479)
City government support for activity (*N*)	4.1 (501)
Provincial government support (*N*)	3.8 (481)
Federal government support (*N*)	3.5 (474)
Other support for the activity (*N*)	4.4 (455)

Comparing the figures in the first five rows of Table 13.3 with their counterparts in Table 3 of Michalos and Kahlke (2008), one again finds the same activities ordered in the same way, practically the same average levels of satisfaction, and a bit more disparity among percentages and times per year of participation.

Table 13.4 lists the percent of respondents indicating the first thing they think of when they hear the word 'arts' or the phrase 'artistic activity' and respondents' most important arts-related activity, with mean levels of satisfaction with nine aspects of that activity. The most frequently mentioned activity that respondents think of when they hear the word 'arts' or the phrase 'artistic activity' is painting and/or drawing. Thirty-eight percent of the sample gave that response. The most frequently mentioned "most important" arts-related activity is music in some form. Thirty-six percent gave that response. The most frequently mentioned place where respondents first learned about their most important arts-related activity is in school. Fifty-five percent gave that response. The mean age at which respondents first learned about their most important arts-related activity was 12.0 years. Mean satisfaction levels reported for respondents' access to information about their most important arts-related activity (5.3), access to the activity itself (5.4), access to the place where the activity occurs (5.0) and about the place itself (5.2) were all on the positive side of the 7-point satisfaction scale. For the remaining five items in the list, three items had mean satisfaction levels in the middle range and two were on the negative side. Mean satisfaction levels reported for the price ($) paid for participating in respondents' most important arts-related activity, for city government support and support from other sources for the activity were 4.8, 4.1 and 4.4, respectively. For the amount of provincial government support and federal government support, the mean satisfaction levels were 3.8 and 3.5, respectively.

Comparing the items in Table 13.4 with their counterparts in Table 4 of Michalos and Kahlke (2008), one again finds the same two activities ordered in the same way, the same age and place of first encounter, and practically the same average levels of satisfaction for all items.

Twenty-three of the 45 statements in our questionnaire about beliefs and feelings about arts-related activities were used to construct four indexes of beliefs and feelings that might motivate people to engage in arts-related activities. Since correlation coefficients cannot identify the direction of causality between significantly related variables, it is possible that significant correlations arise because the experience with arts-related activities leads to certain beliefs and feelings about the activities. Most likely, the causal arrows run in both directions although we are using the general label of 'motivational indexes' for the four. Table 13.5 lists each of the four indexes by name, gives the statements included in each, the percent of respondents agreeing or strongly agreeing with each statement, the item-total correlation of each statement with the index and Cronbach's Alpha Coefficient of Reliability. Each index is formed by simply summing the values of the variables included in it. Besides the four arts-related indexes, Table 13.5 also lists the same information for three overall life assessment indexes.

Table 13.5a describes the *Index of Arts as Self-Health Enhancers,* which has six items and an Alpha Coefficient of $\alpha = 0.87$. A good representative item is 'My artistic activities contribute to my emotional wellbeing', which has an item-total correlation of $r = 0.80$. Eighty-eight percent of respondents agreed or strongly agreed with this statement.

Table 13.5b describes the *Index of Arts as Self-Developing Activities,* which has six items and an $\alpha = 0.86$. A good representative item is 'My artistic activities contribute to my self esteem', which has an item-total correlation of $r = 0.71$. Seventy-five percent of respondents agreed or strongly agreed with this statement.

Table 13.5c describes the *Index of Arts as Community Builders,* which has six items and an $\alpha = 0.82$. A good representative item is 'Artistic activity strengthens a community', which has an item-total correlation of $r = 0.61$. Seventy-eight percent of respondents agreed or strongly agreed with this statement.

Table 13.5d describes the *Index of Arts and Arts-Related Activities as Ends in Themselves,* which has five items and an $\alpha = 0.71$. A good representative item is 'I enjoy art for its own sake', which has an item-total correlation of $r = 0.64$. Eighty-eight percent of respondents agreed or strongly agreed with this statement.

Table 13.5e describes the *Satisfaction With Life Scale* (SWLS) developed by Diener et al. (1985), which has five items and an $\alpha = 0.90$. A good representative item is 'I am satisfied with my life', which has an item-total correlation of $r = 0.83$. Forty-nine percent of respondents agreed or strongly agreed with this statement.

Table 13.5f describes the *Contentment with Life Assessment Scale* (CLAS) developed by Lavallee et al. (2007), which has five items and an $\alpha = 0.87$. A good representative item is 'I am very content with my life', which has an item-total correlation of $r = 0.76$. Forty-eight percent of respondents agreed or strongly agreed with this statement.

Table 13.5 Indexes of beliefs and feelings that might motivate arts-related activity, whole group, satisfaction with life scale (SWLS), contentment with life assessment scale (CLAS) and subjective wellbeing (SWB)

	% Agreeing or strongly agreeing	Item-total correlation
a. Index of arts as self-health enhancers, N = 648, α = 0.87[a]		
Description: my artistic activities…		
Have a positive effect on my life	90.8	0.58
Help me to relax	89.8	0.70
Help relieve stress	86.0	0.72
Contribute to my emotional wellbeing	88.0	0.80
Help me to stay healthy	66.8	0.55
Contribute to my overall wellbeing	78.8	0.70
b. Index of arts as self-developing activities, N = 642, α = 0.86[b]		
Description: my artistic activities…		
Give me self-confidence	76.1	0.64
Help me to learn about myself	73.8	0.65
Help me to reveal my thoughts, feelings or physical skills to others	72.3	0.64
Contribute to my self-esteem	74.5	0.71
Help me develop my social skills	59.9	0.53
Help me express my personal identity	67.4	0.69
c. Index of arts as community builders, N = 637, α = 0.82[c]		
Item		
My artistic activities help me to learn about other people	74.6	0.55
My artistic activities help me to accept differences among people	71.4	0.55
My artistic activities help me feel connected to this community	49.0	0.53
Artists help build community solidarity	70.2	0.59
Artistic activity strengthens a community	77.7	0.61
Artistic activity in a community increases its social capital	62.9	0.62
d. Index of arts and arts-related activities as ends in themselves, N = 639, α = 0.71[d]		
Item		
The appreciation of art is an art-lover's reward	66.2	0.39
Good art needs no justification beyond itself	72.5	0.51
I enjoy art for its own sake	88.3	0.64
Without art, life would be very dull	84.1	0.42
I engage in artistic activities for the sake of the activities themselves	68.2	0.38

(continued)

Table 13.5 (continued)

	% Agreeing or strongly agreeing	Item-total correlation
e. Satisfaction with life scale (SWLS), N = 667, α = 0.90[e]		
Item		
In most ways my life is close to my ideal	35.3	0.78
The conditions of my life are excellent	42.3	0.79
I am satisfied with my life	49.1	0.83
So far I have gotten the important things I want out of life	52.6	0.78
If I could live my life over, I would change nothing	34.5	0.60
f. Contentment with life assessment scale (CLAS), N = 661, α = 0.87[f]		
Item		
Nothing is currently lacking in my life	32.5	0.71
I am living my life to the fullest	32.8	0.79
I am very content with my life	48.1	0.76
When I examine my life as a whole, I feel that I am not meeting my aspirations (reverse coded)	29.2	0.60
I feel dissatisfied because I'm not doing everything that I want to be doing in my life (reverse coded)	28.3	0.64
	% Very or somewhat sat.	Item-total correlation
g. Subjective wellbeing (SWB), N = 675, α = 0.87[g]		
Item		
How satisfied are you with		
Your life as a whole	67.2	0.76
Your overall standard of living	64.7	0.63
Your overall quality of life	65.8	0.80
	% Very or somewhat hap.	Item-total correlation
How happy would you say you are?	76.4	0.68

[a]Scale mean = 24.6, standard deviation = 3.7
[b]Scale mean = 22.8, standard deviation = 4.1
[c]Scale mean = 22.5, standard deviation = 3.6
[d]Scale mean = 19.7, standard deviation = 2.9
[e]Scale mean = 24.2, standard deviation = 6.7
[f]Scale mean = 22.2, standard deviation = 6.6
[g]Scale mean = 23.0, standard deviation = 4.1

Table 13.5g describes the *Subjective Wellbeing Index* (SWB) developed by Michalos et al. (2005), which has four items and an $\alpha = 0.87$. It is constructed by summing responses to four single-item overall life assessment statements concerning one's satisfaction with life as a whole, overall standard of living and quality of life, and one's happiness. Of the four items in the scale, satisfaction with one's overall quality of life has the highest item-total correlation, $r = 0.80$.

Table 13.6 Number of respondents and mean levels of domain and life assessment satisfaction and happiness

Satisfaction with	*N*	Mean sat.
Your house, apartment, mobile home	694	5.7
Your neighbourhood	693	5.7
Your city, town or rural area	692	5.6
Your family relations, generally	687	5.7
Your living partner	575	6.1
Your job	572	5.4
Your life as a whole	688	5.8
Your friendships	691	5.7
Your physical health	693	5.1
Your psychological health	690	5.4
Your religion or spiritual fulfillment	658	5.2
Your overall standard of living	693	5.6
Your financial security	691	5.0
Your recreation activities	692	5.1
Your level of physical activity	694	4.6
Your level of social activity	689	4.6
Air quality where you live	693	5.2
Drinking water quality where you live	689	5.5
Land pollution where you live	680	4.8
Your sense of meaning in life	690	5.5
Your self-esteem	690	5.5
Your amount of free time	686	4.9
Local primary and secondary schools	613	4.8
Your personal safety near your home	688	5.6
Federal government officials	676	3.6
Provincial government officials	677	3.6
Local government officials	670	4.0
Your overall quality of life	690	5.7
How local people treat you	692	5.7
Your access to health care	687	5.2
What you achieve in life	689	5.3
Your future security	686	5.1
Feeling part of your community	688	5.0
Your overall happiness	690	5.9

Table 13.6 lists the mean levels of domain and overall life satisfaction and happiness. Generally speaking, with the 7-point satisfaction scale and sample sizes of about 500, differences between mean scores of 0.3 or fewer percentage points are not statistically significant at the modest level of 0.05%, i.e., 19 times out of 20 one might find such differences appearing merely by chance. Of the 34 entries in the exhibit, 26 (77%) are on the positive side of the 7-point satisfaction and happiness scales. Of the 3 entries concerning satisfaction with government officials, two are

Table 13.7 Number of respondents and mean scores on respondents' lives compared to diverse standards

Your life now compared to	*N*	Mean
What you want from life	687	5.5
What others your age and sex have	692	5.1
What you deserve	684	4.6
What you need	686	4.7
What you expected it would be now	687	4.6
What you expect it to be in 5 years	688	4.8
The best in your previous experience	690	4.6

the lowest of all the scores in the table. The scores for satisfaction with federal and provincial officials are the same, 3.6, which means a little dissatisfied. Satisfaction with local government officials just reaches the scale mid-point of 4.0. The mean score for satisfaction with one's living partner (6.1) is the highest in the table and the only one in the table above 6.0. Other items with mean scores clustered at the top of the list include overall happiness (5.9) and satisfaction with life as a whole (5.8). Ignoring the scores for government officials, the cluster of items at the bottom of the list include satisfaction with one's level of social and physical activity (each 4.6), local land pollution and primary and secondary schools (each 4.8), and amount of free time (4.9). Comparing the items in Table 13.6 with their counterparts in Table 7 of Michalos and Kahlke (2008), one again finds striking similarities. In the five-communities study, 75% of 204 entries were on the positive side of the 7-point scales, with satisfaction with one's living partner again at the top (6.2), followed by overall happiness (5.9). The three government items were again at the bottom, only none reached the mid-point of the scale. Ignoring the scores for government officials, the cluster of items at the bottom of the list began again with satisfaction with one's level of social and physical activity (each 4.7), local land pollution and primary and secondary schools (each 4.8), and amount of free time and local air quality (each 4.9).

Table 13.7 lists mean scores on respondents' lives compared to seven different selfassessment standards. Mean scores reveal that respondents were on the positive side of two of the seven scales. On average, respondents scored 5.5 on the have-want scale, indicating that all things considered, their lives provided more than half of what they wanted. They also thought that their lives provided more than the lives of the average person of their sex and age in their local area (5.1). This sort of ego-centric bias has been reported by many researchers, e.g., see Michalos (1991, pp. 123–4). Regarding the other 5 standards, their scores were only in the middle range, though on the favourable side. Comparing their lives to what they expect to have in 5 years, they scored 4.8; compared to what they need, they scored 4.7. For the remaining three comparisons, they scored each the same, 4.6. Comparing the items in Table 13.7 with their counterparts in Table 8 of Michalos and Kahlke (2008), one again finds the same two clusters above and below the positive side of the scale, with the same two items at the top in the same order.

Bivariate Relationships

The main task of this section is to review 8 sets of correlational studies to discover connections among all our survey variables that seem to be interesting in themselves, suggestive of other likely relationships and potentially useful for the even more interesting multivariate investigations in the following section.

Table 13.8 lists results of correlating the average number of *hours per week* engaged in each of 22 arts-related activities *and* each activity's corresponding mean

Table 13.8 Correlations among average number of *hours per week* engaged in arts-related activities and levels of satisfaction with each activity (Act.Sat.) and seven life assessment variables: general health (GH), life satisfaction (Lsat), happiness (hap), satisfaction with overall quality of life (qolsat), satisfaction with life scale (SWLS), contentment with life assessment scale (CLAS) and subjective wellbeing (SWB)

Activity	Act. Sat.	GH	Lsat	hap	qolsat	SWLS	CLAS	SWB	$N \geq$
Age	–	ns	0.11	0.09	0.09	0.16	0.19	0.15	657
Education	–	0.22	ns	ns	ns	0.09	ns	0.09	654
House/income	–	ns	0.09	0.11	0.16	0.15	0.12	0.19	504
Body mass index	–	−0.18	ns	ns	ns	ns	ns	ns	623
Listening/music	0.09	ns	ns	ns	ns	ns	ns	ns	566
Reading novels	0.28	ns	ns	ns	ns	ns	ns	ns	390
Re/nov/sat.	1.00	0.12	0.15	0.16	0.12	ns	ns	0.15	390
Watch films dvd	ns	−0.14	ns	ns	ns	ns	ns	ns	281
Singing alone	0.25	ns	−0.12	ns	ns	ns	ns	ns	248
Singing alone sat.	1.00	ns	ns	0.21	0.13	ns	0.19	0.14	248
Read to others	0.26	ns	ns	ns	ns	ns	ns	ns	206
Read others sat.	1.00	ns	ns	0.19	ns	ns	ns	ns	206
Telling stories	0.22	ns	ns	ns	ns	−0.22	−0.18	ns	135
Tell stories sat.	1.00	ns	ns	0.21	ns	ns	ns	ns	135
Gourmet cooking	0.26	ns	ns	ns	ns	ns	ns	ns	115
Gour/cook/sat.	1.00	ns	ns	0.36	ns	ns	ns	0.19	115
Painting, drawing	0.25	ns	ns	ns	−0.19	ns	ns	ns	116
Paint/draw/sat.	1.00	0.18	ns	0.20	ns	ns	ns	ns	116
Watch TV art	ns	0.33	ns	ns	0.24	ns	ns	ns	87
Watch TV art/sat.	1.00	ns	ns	ns	ns	ns	−0.23	ns	87
Play/music/inst.	0.27	ns	ns	−0.26	ns	ns	ns	ns	66
Knit/crochet/sat.	1.00	ns	ns	ns	0.30	ns	ns	ns	56
Take/kids/arts	ns	−0.39	ns	ns	ns	ns	ns	ns	51
Take/kids/arts/sat.	1.00	ns	−0.34	ns	−0.28	ns	−0.28	−0.31	51
Arranging flowers sat.	1.00	ns	ns	0.35	0.36	0.36	0.37	0.34	44
Make clothes sat.	1.00	ns	ns	ns	0.39	ns	ns	0.41	35

$P < 0.05$

level of satisfaction (44 items total) *with* mean scores on our seven overall assessments of life, i.e., self-reported general health (GH), satisfaction with life as a whole (Lsat), happiness with life as a whole (Hap), satisfaction with the overall quality of life (qolsat), satisfaction with life as a whole index (SWLS), contentment with life assessment scale (CLAS), and subjective wellbeing (SWB). As well, the average number of *hours per week* engaged in each of the arts-related activities is correlated with each activity's corresponding mean level of satisfaction (Act.Sat. in column one of the table). We arbitrarily selected $N = 30$ as a cutoff figure and examined all zero-order linear associations (Pearson Product Moment Correlations) for activities involving that many respondents or more. The last column in the table gives the minimum sample size involved in each of the correlations for each row. The first four rows of the table give the results of correlating 4 demographic variables (age, education, household income and Body Mass Index) with the seven overall life assessments.

Our review of the results in Table 13.8 will begin with a discussion of correlations between each demographic and life assessment variable. Second, we will consider correlations between the average amount of time invested in each arts-related activity and the average amount of obtained satisfaction from that investment (results in column under Act.Sat.). Third, we will examine correlations between time invested and satisfaction obtained for each arts-related activity on the one hand with each of the seven life assessment variables on the other, taking each of the latter variables one at a time. Finally, we will give special attention to some of the variables for time invested and satisfaction obtained that had a relatively extensive impact on most of the seven life assessment variables.

Twenty-eight (4 × 7) associations between the demographic and life assessment variables were measured, and 16 (57.1%) were found to be statistically significant at the $P < 0.05$ level. (To simplify the discussion, we arbitrarily decided to use a single level of significance throughout the study.) No demographic variable was significantly correlated with every life assessment variable, although age and household income were significantly correlated with 6 of the 7. General Health scores were not correlated with age or household income, which is unusual and inconsistent with results reported in Michalos and Kahlke (2008, Table 9). On average, age was correlated with the 6 life assessment variables at $r = 0.13$, with a high of $r = 0.19$ for the Contentment with Life Assessment Scale (CLAS) and a low of $r = 0.09$ for happiness (Hap) and satisfaction with the overall quality of life (qolsat). Education and the Body Mass Index were significantly correlated with three and one of the seven life assessment variables, respectively. Generally speaking, the 4 demographic variables had weaker associations with the 7 life assessment variables in the British Columbia sample than in the five-communities sample.

Since we began with 22 arts-related activities that had at least 30 people engaged in them and each activity produced its own corresponding mean level of satisfaction, there were 22 × 2 = 44 distinct variables to correlate with 7 life assessment variables, giving a possible 308 significant correlation coefficients. Besides these 308 coefficients, there might have been 22 more indicating significant associations between each arts-related activity and its corresponding mean level of satisfaction.

The fact that there are only 22 rows of arts-related activities and/or corresponding satisfaction items in Table 13.8 shows that 22 (50.0%) of the 44 distinct variables had no significant correlations with any of the life assessment variables and/or a corresponding level of satisfaction variable. Considering only the 22 variables listed in Table 13.8, if every measurement had produced a statistically significant result then there would have been 154 (22 × 7) cells with numerical values indicating significant associations between arts-related activities and/or corresponding levels of satisfaction with each of the 7 life assessment variables plus 8 more values indicating significant associations between each activity variable and its corresponding satisfaction variable, rather than the 45 values displayed in the table. Thus, for our sample of 708 respondents, subtracting the 8 values listed in the column headed Act.Sat., there are only 37 cases out of our original possible 308 (12.0%) of the time-spent on activities variables and/or variables indicating the satisfaction obtained from those activities that had significant correlations with our 7 life assessment variables. Considering only the 22 variables listed in Table 13.8, there are 37 of 154 (24.0%) cases that had significant correlations with the 7 life assessment variables.

Since a person's engagement in arts-related activities is usually voluntary, one might expect a statistically significant positive correlation between the time spent engaged in arts-related activities and the level of satisfaction obtained from the engagement. Although there are no negative correlations in the Activity Satisfaction (Act.Sat.) column, 3 associations were not statistically significant. However, because the average number of hours per week engaged in 11 of the original 22 arts-related activities did not have statistically significant associations with any other variables, including their corresponding measures of satisfaction, these 11 are not listed in the table. There were, then, a total of 14 (63.6%) activities (3 listed in the table and 11 not listed) with statistically insignificant correlations with their corresponding mean levels of satisfaction. In all these cases, apparently the average satisfaction obtained from participation in arts-related activities cannot be the sole or even primary motivator of engagement. A similar anomaly appears in Table 13.9 regarding arts-related activities with engagement measured in number of times per year, and it was also reported in Michalos and Kahlke (2008) for the corresponding tables (Tables 13.9 and 13.10).

A casual glance at Table 13.8 suggests that there is a great variety of relationships between the average number of hours per week engaged in arts-related activities and the corresponding mean levels of satisfaction resulting from that engagement on the one hand, and the seven life assessment variables on the other. If one tried to measure the impact of arts-related activities on the perceived quality of people's lives using only one of these seven scales as one's dependent variable, one would inevitably underestimate that impact. Nine (41.0%) of the 22 arts-related activities and/or corresponding mean levels of satisfaction resulting from engagement in those activities had a significant correlation with only one life assessment variable, and five (22.7%) more had such a correlation with two life assessment variables.

Table 13.9 Correlations among average number of *times per year* engaged in arts-related activities and levels of satisfaction with each activity (Act.Sat.) and life assessment variables: general health (GH), life satisfaction (Lsat), happiness (hap), satisfaction with overall quality of life (qolsat), satisfaction with life scale (SWLS), contentment with life assessment scale (CLAS) and subjective wellbeing (SWB)

Activity	Act.Sat.	GH	Lsat	hap	qolsat	SWLS	CLAS	SWB	N ≥
Go to movies	0.22	ns	ns	ns	ns	ns	−0.12	ns	390
Go concerts	0.15	ns	ns	ns	ns	ns	ns	ns	367
Go concert sat.	1.00	ns	0.16	0.17	0.13	ns	ns	0.17	367
Go his/her site	0.15	ns	ns	ns	0.15	0.11	ns	0.14	333
Go his/her sat.	1.00	ns	ns	ns	0.14	ns	0.15	0.13	333
Go art museum	0.10	ns	ns	ns	ns	ns	ns	ns	330
Go art museum sat.	1.00	0.15	0.20	0.19	0.17	0.16	0.14	0.22	330
Go other museum sat.	1.00	0.15	0.23	0.19	0.21	0.22	0.17	0.26	284
Go public library	0.29	ns	ns	ns	ns	ns	ns	ns	283
Go public library sat.	1.00	ns	0.14	ns	ns	0.14	ns	ns	283
Go amateur theatre	0.23	0.14	ns	ns	ns	ns	ns	ns	251
Go amateur theatre sat.	1.00	0.14	0.34	0.22	0.31	0.32	0.23	0.35	251
Go prof theatre sat.	1.00	ns	0.29	0.25	0.23	0.26	0.23	0.29	243
Decorating home	0.14	ns	ns	ns	ns	ns	ns	ns	201
Decorating home sat.	1.00	ns	0.15	0.17	ns	ns	ns	ns	201
Go to school plays sat.	1.00	ns	0.22	0.23	0.17	0.22	0.18	0.24	204
Buy art work	0.14	ns	ns	ns	ns	ns	ns	ns	198
Buy art work sat.	1.00	ns	0.22	0.15	0.24	ns	0.17	0.22	198
Des. Garden sat.	1.00	ns	ns	ns	0.15	ns	0.20	ns	187
Go dancing	0.15	ns	ns	ns	ns	ns	ns	ns	173
Go dancing sat.	1.00	ns	ns	ns	0.18	ns	ns	ns	173
Wk com. Fes sat.	1.00	ns	ns	0.25	ns	ns	ns	ns	90
Give art dona sat.	1.00	ns	0.22	ns	ns	0.32	0.29	ns	84
Figure skating	0.33	ns	ns	ns	ns	ns	ns	ns	35
Figure skating sat.	1.00	ns	ns	0.39	ns	ns	ns	ns	35

$P < 0.05$

Close inspection of the seven life assessment columns in Table 13.8 reveals that the satisfaction with life index (SWLS) had the fewest number (2) of significant associations with the average number of hours per week engaged in the 22 arts-related activities and/or the corresponding mean levels of satisfaction resulting from that engagement. Two life assessment variables had 8 significant correlations with the 22 arts-related activities and/or the corresponding mean levels of satisfaction resulting from that engagement, namely, the single item measure of satisfaction with the overall quality of life (qolsat) and the single item happiness measure (Hap). On average, for the eight significant correlations with qolsat,

Table 13.10 Correlations of domain satisfaction scores with life assessment variables: general health (GH), life satisfaction (Lsat), happiness (hap), satisfaction with overall quality of life (qolsat), satisfaction with life scale (SWLS), contentment with life assessment scale (CLAS) and subjective wellbeing (SWB)

Domain sat with	GH	Lsat	hap	qolsat	SWLS	CLAS	SWB	Mean
Your house, apartment	0.11	0.43	0.38	0.44	0.39	0.38	0.51	0.38
Neighbourhood	0.12	0.36	0.34	0.41	0.37	0.32	0.47	0.34
City, town or rural area	0.11	0.34	0.28	0.38	0.33	0.30	0.40	0.31
Family relations	0.11	0.46	0.37	0.41	0.40	0.33	0.49	0.37
Living partner	0.18	0.46	0.37	0.44	0.43	0.32	0.49	0.38
Job	0.20	0.53	0.37	0.40	0.46	0.43	0.51	0.41
Friendships	0.25	0.59	0.47	0.53	0.43	0.43	0.60	0.47
Health	0.63	0.66	0.51	0.62	0.56	0.53	0.68	0.60
Religion/spirit fulfill	0.26	0.43	0.34	0.44	0.43	0.40	0.47	0.40
Financial security	0.25	0.44	0.44	0.55	0.48	0.46	0.64	0.47
Recreation activities	0.39	0.49	0.45	0.60	0.46	0.43	0.61	0.49
Environment	0.18	0.28	0.27	0.37	0.28	0.25	0.36	0.28
Sense of meaning in life	0.23	0.65	0.54	0.61	0.58	0.57	0.68	0.55
Self-esteem	0.29	0.66	0.63	0.63	0.61	0.63	0.71	0.59
Amount of free time	ns	0.35	0.32	0.40	0.32	0.33	0.39	0.35
Personal safety by home	0.19	0.41	0.35	0.50	0.38	0.31	0.50	0.38
Government officials	0.11	0.18	0.15	0.29	0.19	0.21	0.24	0.20
How locals treat you	0.25	0.56	0.44	0.63	0.50	0.48	0.64	0.50
Access to health care	0.21	0.27	0.26	0.38	0.32	0.24	0.36	0.29
Future security	0.25	0.50	0.51	0.62	0.54	0.54	0.67	0.52
Feel part of your comm.	0.19	0.54	0.49	0.58	0.54	0.51	0.63	0.50

N $\geq$ 553; $P < 0.05$

$r = 0.13$, and with Hap, $r = 0.18$. Regarding happiness, correlation coefficients ran from a positive high of $r = 0.35$ for the satisfaction obtained from arranging flowers to a negative low of $r = -0.26$ for the average number of hours per week playing music. Regarding satisfaction with the overall quality of life, correlation coefficients ran from a positive high of $r = 0.39$ for the satisfaction obtained from making clothes to a negative low of $r = -0.28$ for the satisfaction obtained from taking children to arts-related activities.

While we were prepared to find that the average amount of *time invested* in some arts-related activities was negatively associated with one or another life assessment variable (cf. Michalos and Kahlke 2008, Table 9), we were surprised to find that the average level of *satisfaction obtained* from engaging in some arts-related activities could have negative associations. Nevertheless, Table 13.8 shows that there were five such cases, involving the satisfaction obtained from watching art shows on television and taking children to arts-related activities. Remarkably, the only statistically significant associations these four arts-related satisfaction variables had with any overall life assessment variables were negative. What's more, neither of the two arts-related satisfaction variables had significant associations with the average number of hours per week invested in the corresponding arts-related activities, e.g., there was no significant correlation between the average number of hours per week spent watching art programs on television and satisfaction obtained from such activity. So, some respondents spent some time engaged in arts-related activities that generated immediate satisfaction that had no significant association with the activities themselves but was significantly and negatively related to some overall life assessment variables. How can we explain engagement in such activities and the negative impact that satisfaction from such engagement has on life assessment variables?

One might argue that one of the two arts-related activities is not a case of engaging in art at all, i.e., driving kids to some kind of artistic event or facility is not engaging in art. So, for present purposes the negative associations between satisfaction obtained from such activities and life assessment measures is irrelevant. Unfortunately, this does not address the problem that some kinds of satisfaction have a negative impact on other kinds of satisfaction. It is generally assumed, in the bottom-up explanatory model of perceived life satisfaction for example, that satisfaction from diverse sources and possibly of diverse kinds are routinely combined to produce satisfaction with life as a whole. While it is easy to understand how the time invested in driving one's kids to an art class might have a negative impact on one's life satisfaction (although we have no evidence that it did), it is far from clear why the satisfaction obtained from driving one's kids to the class should have a negative impact. Why should feeling good about driving one's kids to class have a negative impact on how one feels about one's life as a whole? Apparently the activity is some kind of a mixed blessing. One drives the kids to art class feeling pretty good about it because it makes the kids happy and is the right thing to do. Nevertheless, that pretty good feeling is not measurably significantly associated with the activity itself but has the unintended consequence of depressing one's satisfaction with the overall quality of life. The actor performs an act somewhat begrudgingly and the modest level of satisfaction obtained from it takes a heavy negative toll on the actor's overall life assessment.

There clearly are associations between time invested in activities and satisfaction obtained from the investment that were too weak to be captured by some of our measuring instruments, e.g., we have reported satisfaction obtained from arranging flowers and although it had no significant association with the time invested in the activity, it had significant correlations with several overall life assessment variables. It is theoretically possible that the reported satisfaction obtained from arranging flowers is really an effect of some kind of genetically hard-wired core affect that is somehow (wittingly or unwittingly) connected to the activity of arranging flowers. Davern et al. (2007) and Cummins et al. (2007) made an interesting case for such phenomena, although Moum (2007) and Land (2007) were not persuaded. While there must be some genetic connection to people's experiences and feelings, it is far from clear why one's genes would produce certain effects with some arts-related activities and not others. In any event, at this point we have no good genetically-based explanation for the oddities just reported.

Inspection of all the figures in the 22 rows concerning arts-related activities and corresponding levels of satisfaction reveals that there are only two cases in which as many as five significant correlations with life assessment variables appear, namely, for the satisfaction obtained from reading novels, etc. and the satisfaction obtained from arranging flowers. On average, for the five significant correlations with the satisfaction obtained from reading novels, etc., $r = 0.14$, and with the satisfaction obtained from arranging flowers, $r = 0.36$. While the flower arrangers got a much bigger average boost than the readers of novels, etc. in their life assessment scores, there may have been as few as only 44 of the former compared to as few as 390 of the latter. Regarding the satisfaction obtained from reading novels, etc., correlation coefficients ran from a high of $r = 0.16$ for happiness to a low of $r = 0.12$ for general health and satisfaction with the overall quality of life. Regarding the satisfaction obtained from arranging flowers, correlation coefficients ran from a high of $r = 0.37$ for the contentment with life assessment scale (CLAS) to a low of $r = 0.34$ for subjective wellbeing.

Considering the relative number of arts-related activities engaged in fairly frequently and/or their corresponding levels of satisfaction that were significantly correlated with Hap and/or qolsat, it seems that if one were looking for associations between such activities and/or their corresponding satisfaction *with* the perceived quality of life, one's chances for finding such associations would be maximized by using either of these two measures and minimized by using either SWLS or Lsat. Still, one's best strategy would be to use several dependent variables.

As we found in our earlier study, there was some evidence that producing art was more highly correlated with immediate satisfaction than consuming art. Of the eight variables indicating the average number of hours per week engaged in arts-related activities with significant associations, 5 referred to production (i.e., singing alone, gourmet cooking, painting and drawing, playing a musical instrument and telling stories) and 3 referred to consumption (i.e., listening to music, reading novels, etc., and reading to others). On average, the productive activities correlated at $r = 0.25$ while the consumptive activities correlated at $r = 0.21$ with the corresponding immediate satisfaction. In the most extreme case, the average number of hours per week engaged in listening to music had a correlation of $r = 0.09$ with its corresponding satisfaction, compared to the correlation of $r = 0.27$ between playing a musical instrument and its corresponding satisfaction. Of course, many more respondents could listen to music (at least 566) than produce it (possibly as few as 66).

Table 13.9 lists results of correlating the average number of *times per year* engaged in each of 19 arts-related activities and each activity's corresponding mean level of satisfaction (38 items total) *with* mean scores on our 7 overall assessments of life, and correlating the average number of times per year engaged in each of the 19 activities with each activity's corresponding mean level of satisfaction (Act. Sat.). Our cutoff figure for measuring associations was $N = 32$ simply because the activity with the next lowest number of participants had only $N = 8$. Our review of the results in this table will follow the pattern established for Table 13.8.

Beginning with 19 arts-related activities that had at least 32 respondents engaged in them and each activity's corresponding mean level of satisfaction, there were $19 \times 2 = 38$ distinct variables to correlate with 7 life assessment variables, giving a possible 266 significant correlation coefficients. Besides these 266 coefficients, there might have been 19 more indicating significant associations between each arts-related activity and its corresponding mean level of satisfaction. The fact that there are only 25 rows of arts-related activities and/or corresponding satisfaction items in Table 13.9 shows that 13 (34.2%) of the 38 distinct variables had no significant correlations with any of the life assessment variables and/or a corresponding level of satisfaction variable. Considering only the 25 variables listed in Table 13.9, if every measurement had produced a statistically significant result then there would have been 175 (25×7) cells with numerical values indicating significant associations between arts-related activities and/or corresponding levels of satisfaction with each of the 7 life assessment variables plus 10 more values indicating significant associations between each activity variable in the table and its corresponding satisfaction variable, rather than the 72 values displayed in the table. Thus, for our sample of 708 respondents, subtracting the 10 values listed in the column headed Act.Sat., there are only 62 cases out of our original possible 175 (35.4%) time-spent on activities variables and/or variables indicating the satisfaction obtained from those activities that had significant correlations with our 7 life assessment variables. Although this is not a particularly high percentage, it is larger than that concerning arts-related activities with frequency of participation counted in *hours per week*. What is perhaps even more interesting is the fact that there is only one negative correlation in Table 13.9. In our earlier study, we found that all the time spent on and the satisfaction obtained from the arts-related activities listed in the *times per year* table made a positive contribution to one or more of the overall life assessments. Here we find that only the time invested in going to movies has a negative association with one overall life assessment index, i.e., for CLAS, $r = -0.12$.

There are 10 out of a possible 19 (52.6%) statistically significant correlations in the Act.Sat. column, with an average value of $r = 0.19$, ranging from a high of $r = 0.33$ for the average number of times per year respondents engaged in figure skating (How Canadian!) to a low of $r = 0.10$ for the average number of times per year respondents went to art museums. Of course, many more people reported going to art museums (at least 330) than engaging in figure skating (perhaps as few as 35). There is again (as in Table 13.8) a great variety of relationships (i.e., heterogeneity of effects) between the average number of times per year engaged in the 19 arts-related activities and the corresponding mean levels of satisfaction resulting from that engagement on the one hand, and the 7 life assessment variables on the other.

Inspection of the 7 life assessment columns in Table 13.9 reveals that General Health (GH) had the fewest number of significant associations with the average number of times per year engaged in the 19 arts-related activities and the corresponding mean levels of satisfaction resulting from that engagement. Three of the 4 correlations with GH are with activity satisfaction variables that have significant and positive associations with *each* of the 7 life assessment variables. On average, the mean level of satisfaction obtained from visiting art museums has a correlation of $r = 0.18$ with the 7 life assessment variables, ranging from a high of $r = 0.22$ for subjective wellbeing (SWB) to a low of $r = 0.14$ for CLAS. The mean level of satisfaction obtained from visiting other museums has an average correlation of $r = 0.20$ with the 7 life assessment variables, ranging from a high of $r = 0.26$ for SWB to a low of $r = 0.15$ for GH. The mean level of satisfaction obtained from going to amateur theatre performances has an average correlation of $r = 0.27$ with the 7 life assessment variables, ranging from a high of $r = 0.35$ for SWB to a low of $r = 0.14$ for GH.

Satisfaction with the overall quality of life (qolsat) had the largest number of significant and positive associations with the average number of times per year engaged in the 19 arts-related activities and the corresponding mean levels of satisfaction resulting from that engagement. The 11 significant correlations in the qolsat column have an average of $r = 0.19$, with a high of $r = 0.31$ for the satisfaction obtained from going to amateur theatre performances to a low of $r = 0.13$ for the satisfaction obtained from going to concerts. In our earlier study, General Health had the largest number of significant and positive associations with *times per year* and corresponding satisfaction variables.

Considering the facts that the average level of satisfaction obtained from going to live amateur, professional and school theatre performances are significantly and positively correlated with 7, 6 and 6 of the life assessment variables, respectively, such theatre performances should be given special recognition. As we discovered and emphasized in our earlier study, among the 19 arts-related activities in which people participate relatively infrequently (i.e., participation is counted in times per year rather than in hours per week), live theatre is supreme in the strength of its correlation with respondents' perceived quality of life measured in diverse ways. If this is any reflection of the contribution of dramatists to the quality of human existence for over 2,500 years, they may be justifiably proud of it.

Table 13.10 lists results of correlating our 7 life assessment variables with 21 domain satisfaction variables. Three of the domain satisfaction variables are combinations of some of those listed in Table 13.6. Values for the health satisfaction variable appearing in Table 13.10 were obtained by calculating the mean of the scores on the physical and psychological health satisfaction variables. Similarly, values for the environmental satisfaction variable appearing in Table 13.10, were obtained by calculating the mean of the scores on the air, water and land quality satisfaction variables, and values for the government satisfaction variable were obtained by calculating the mean of the scores on the federal, provincial and local government officials satisfaction variables. All of the 147 correlations listed in this table are significant and positive. In the corresponding table of Michalos and Kahlke (2008, Table 11), all of the correlation coefficients are also positive and significant. Examination of the mean values of each row in the table reveals that on average for our respondents, satisfaction with one's health (mean $r = 0.60$), self-esteem (mean $r = 0.59$) and the sense of meaning in life (mean $r = 0.55$) have

Table 13.11 Correlations among seven life assessment variables: general health (GH), life satisfaction (Lsat), happiness (hap), satisfaction with overall quality of life (qolsat), satisfaction with life scale (SWLS), contentment with life assessment scale (CLAS) and subjective wellbeing (SWB)

Variable	GH	Lsat	Hap	Qolsat	SWLS	CLAS
GH	1.00					
Lsat	0.38	1.00				
Hap	0.32	0.67	1.00			
Qolsat	0.40	0.72	0.64	1.00		
SWLS	0.40	0.68	0.68	0.66	1.00	
CLAS	0.31	0.64	0.66	0.61	0.80	1.00
SWB	0.41	0.87	0.83	0.88	0.76	0.72

$N \geq 639$; $P < 0.05$

the largest correlations with the 7 life assessment variables. These were also the top three in our earlier study, with the same order and similar correlation coefficients, i.e., $r = 0.64$, $r = 0.57$ and $r = 0.54$, respectively. Smallest correlations on average were for satisfaction with government officials (mean $r = 0.20$), access to health care (mean $r = 0.29$) and the environment (mean $r = 0.28$).

Table 13.11 lists the correlations among the 7 life assessment variables, all of which are significant and positive as expected. On average and as usual, General Health (GH) has the lowest levels of association with the others, indicating that respondents recognize important differences between having good health and having a good life, generally speaking. Because happiness (Hap), satisfaction with life as a whole (Lsat) and satisfaction with the overall quality of life (qolsat) are constituents of subjective wellbeing (SWB), the former three variables have on average the highest levels of association with the latter. Considering the facts that (1) respondents recognize a difference between good health and a good life, and (2) qolsat had the greatest number of significant correlations with arts-related activities involving *infrequent* engagement and tied with Hap for having the greatest number of significant correlations with arts-related activities involving *frequent* engagement, it seems fair to say that if one were looking for associations between such activities and the perceived quality of life and if one could only have a single dependent variable, then one's chances for finding such associations would be maximized by using qolsat as that single variable.

Tables 13.12 and 13.13 display results of measuring associations among our four indexes that might provide motives for people engaging in arts-related activities, might summarize beliefs and feelings that arise as effects of experiences with arts-related activities or, as suggested earlier, most likely both. We will need longitudinal studies with panels of participants in order to properly assess these issues. Our review of these two tables will be parallel to our reviews of Tables 13.8 and 13.9, with Table 13.12 involving engagement in arts-related activities measured in *hours per week* and Table 13.13 involving engagement in arts-related activities measured in *times per year*.

Table 13.12 Correlations among average number of *hours per week* engaged in arts-related activities and levels of satisfaction with motivational indexes: index of arts as self-health enhancers (health), index of arts as self-developing activities (S-dev), index of arts as community builders (comb), index of arts as ends in themselves (ends), and demographics

Activity	Health	S-Dev	Comb	Ends	N ≥
Age	−0.08	−0.11	ns	ns	629
Education	0.16	0.09	0.15	0.13	628
Body mass index	−0.22	−0.21	−0.21	−0.14	604
Listening to music	0.10	0.13	ns	0.13	545
Listening to music satisfaction	0.28	0.24	0.17	0.22	545
Reading novels satisfaction	ns	0.12	0.15	ns	380
Singing alone satisfaction	0.32	0.33	0.15	0.16	249
Reading to others satisfaction	0.25	ns	ns	ns	206
Gourmet cooking	ns	ns	ns	−0.20	117
Gourmet cooking satisfaction	0.25	ns	ns	ns	117
Painting or drawing	ns	ns	ns	0.25	113
Painting or drawing satisfaction	0.27	0.24	ns	0.20	113
Singing in a group satisfaction	0.26	ns	ns	ns	91
Watching TV art satisfaction	0.24	ns	ns	ns	84
Playing musical instrument sat.	0.33	ns	0.31	ns	64
Arranging flowers	ns	ns	ns	0.33	43
Arranging flowers satisfaction	0.37	0.40	ns	ns	43
Writing novels etc. sat.	ns	0.48	ns	ns	30
Making clothes	ns	ns	ns	0.53	35
Teaching painting/drawing sat.	ns	ns	0.37	ns	29

$P < 0.05$

Table 13.12 lists results of correlating the average number of *hours per week* engaged in each of 22 arts-related activities *and* each activity's corresponding mean level of satisfaction (44 items total) *with* mean scores on our four motivational indexes. The fact that there are only 17 rows of arts-related activities and/or corresponding satisfaction items in Table 13.12 shows that 27 (61%) of the 44 distinct variables had no significant correlations with any of the motivational indexes. For this table, 16 associations between the 4 demographic variables and 4 motivational indexes were also measured, and 10 (62.5%) were found to be statistically significant at the $P < 0.05$ level. Household income does not appear in the table because it did not have any significant correlations with the four motivational indexes. Education and the Body Mass Index were significantly correlated with each index, positively with an average of $r = 0.13$ for the former and negatively with an average of $r = -0.20$ for the latter. Age was negatively correlated with 2 of the 4 indexes, averaging $r = -0.10$. Thus, for example, believing and/or feeling that engagement in arts-related activities make a positive contribution to one's health is significantly negatively correlated with age (r = −0.08) and Body Mass Index (r = −0.22), and positively correlated with education (r = 0.16). So, as respondents'

Table 13.13 Correlations among average number of *times per year* engaged in arts-related activities and levels of satisfaction with motivational indexes: index of arts as self-health enhancers (health), index of arts as self-developing activities (S-dev), index of arts as community builders (comb), index of arts as ends in themselves (ends)

Activity	Health	S-dev	Comb	Ends	$N \geq$
Going to movies	ns	0.14	0.13	0.12	629
Going to movies satisfaction	0.11	0.10	ns	0.16	384
Going to concerts	0.12	0.17	0.17	0.15	358
Going to concerts satisfaction	0.16	0.13	0.18	0.19	358
Attending community festivals	0.12	0.16	ns	ns	330
Attending community festivals sat.	0.16	0.19	0.20	0.12	330
Visiting historic, heritage sites	ns	0.12	ns	ns	333
Visiting historic, heritage site sat.	0.15	0.15	ns	0.13	333
Going to art museums, galleries	0.13	0.16	ns	ns	324
Go…art museums, galleries sat.	0.23	0.22	0.26	0.20	324
Go…other museums	0.15	ns	ns	ns	282
Go…other museums sat.	0.22	0.19	0.24	0.13	282
Visiting public library sat.	0.14	ns	ns	ns	280
Go…amateur live theatre	ns	0.22	0.16	ns	245
Go…amateur live theatre sat.	ns	0.13	0.26	ns	245
Go…prof. live theatre sat.	0.14	ns	ns	0.16	234
Decorating a home sat.	0.23	0.17	ns	ns	200
Volunteering in the arts sat.	ns	ns	0.46	ns	200
Go to school plays satisfaction	0.15	0.16	0.27	ns	198
Buying works of art sat.	0.17	ns	ns	0.18	200
Designing a garden sat.	0.23	ns	ns	ns	188
Making donations to arts sat.	0.22	ns	ns	ns	82

$P < 0.05$

age and BMI increased, the strength of their avowal of such beliefs and/or feelings decreased, and as their achieved level of education increased, the strength of their avowal of such beliefs and/or feelings increased, and vice versa.

Considering only the 17 non-demographic variables listed in Table 13.12, if every measurement had produced a statistically significant result then there would have been 68 (4 × 17) cells with numerical values, rather than the 30 values displayed in the table. Thus, only 44% of the time-spent on activities variables and/or variables indicating the satisfaction obtained from those activities had significant correlations with our 4 motivational indexes. (There is no comparable figure from the earlier study because the number and composition of arts-related variables and motivational indexes are different.) Inspection of the 4 motivational index columns in this table reveals that the Index of Arts as Community Builders (Comb) had the fewest number of significant associations with the average number of hours per week engaged in the 17 arts-related activities and the corresponding mean levels of satisfaction resulting from that engagement. The 5 significant correlations in the column have an average of $r = 0.23$, with a high of $r = 0.37$ for the satisfaction obtained from teaching painting or drawing to a low of $r = 0.15$ for the satisfaction obtained from reading novels, etc. and singing alone. The Index of Arts as Self-Health Enhancers (Health) had the largest number of significant associations with the average number of hours per week engaged in the 17 arts-related activities and the corresponding mean levels of satisfaction resulting from that engagement. The 10 significant correlations in the Health column have an average of $r = 0.27$, with a high of $r = 0.37$ for the satisfaction obtained from arranging flowers to a low of $r = 0.10$ for the average number of hours per week spent listening to music.

Two arts-related variables in Table 13.12 had significant and positive associations with each of the 4 motivational indexes, and 2 had significant and positive associations with 3 of the 4. Satisfaction obtained from singing alone had an average correlation of $r = 0.24$ with the 4 motivational indexes, with a high of $r = 0.33$ for S-dev and a low of $r = 0.15$ for Comb. Thus, for example, as respondents' average levels of satisfaction obtained from singing alone increased, the strength of their beliefs and/or feelings that arts-related activities contributed to their health, self-development, community building and were also enjoyed as ends in themselves increased. Satisfaction obtained from listening to music had an average correlation of $r = 0.23$ with 4 motivational indexes, with a high of $r = 0.28$ for Health and a low of $r = 0.17$ for Comb. Satisfaction obtained from painting or drawing had an average correlation of $r = 0.24$ with 3 of the 4 motivational indexes (missing Comb), with a high of $r = 0.27$ for Health and a low of $r = 0.20$ for Ends. Average number of hours per week engaged in listening to music had an average correlation of $r = 0.12$ with 3 of the 4 motivational indexes (again missing Comb), with a high of $r = 0.13$ for S-dev and Ends, and a low of $r = 0.10$ for Health.

Table 13.13 lists results of correlating the average number of *times per year* engaged in each of 19 arts-related activities and each activity's corresponding mean level of satisfaction with mean scores on our four motivational indexes (38 items total). If every measurement for Table 13.13 had produced a statistically significant result then there would have been 152 (4×38) cells with numerical values, rather than the 52 values displayed in the table. Thus, for our sample of 708 respondents, 52 of 152 (34.2%) time-spent on activities variables and/or variables indicating the satisfaction obtained from those activities had significant correlations with our four motivational indexes. One should notice first that there are no negative correlations in Table 13.13. Whether the causal arrows running from the time spent on the 19 kinds of arts-related activities and the satisfaction obtained from the engagement to beliefs and/or feelings about the arts are stronger, the same or weaker than the arrows running in the opposite direction, if there is any influence at all, it is positive.

Inspection of the four motivational index columns in Table 13.13 reveals that the Indexes of Arts as Community Builders (Comb) and as Ends in Themselves (Ends) had the fewest number of significant associations (10) with the average number of times per year engaged in the 19 arts-related activities and the corresponding mean levels of satisfaction resulting from that engagement. The Index of Arts as Self-Health Enhancers (Health) had the largest number of significant associations

Table 13.14 Correlations among motivational indexes: index of arts as self-health enhancers (health), index of arts as self-developing activities (S-dev), index of arts as community builders (comb), index of arts as ends in themselves (ends)

Index	Health	S-dev	Comb
Health	1.00		
S-dev	0.73	1.00	
Comb	0.57	0.65	1.00
Ends	0.59	0.53	0.53

$N \geq 618$; $P < 0.05$

(17) with the average number of times per year engaged in the 19 arts-related activities and the corresponding mean levels of satisfaction resulting from that engagement. The 17 significant correlations in the Health column have an average of $r = 0.17$, with a high of $r = 0.23$ for the satisfaction obtained from going to art museums, decorating a home and designing a garden to a low of $r = 0.11$ for the satisfaction obtained from going to movies.

Five arts-related time-engaged or satisfaction variables had significant correlations with all four motivational variables, and 4 more of the former had such correlations with 3 of the latter 4. First among the five, satisfaction obtained from going to art museums had an average of $r = 0.23$ for the 4 motivational indexes, with a high of $r = 0.26$ for Comb and a low of $r = 0.20$ for Ends. Satisfaction obtained from going to other kinds of museums ran second, with an average of $r = 0.20$ for the 4 motivational indexes, a high of $r = 0.24$ for Comb and a low of $r = 0.13$ for Ends. First among the 3 out of 4 group, satisfaction obtained from going to school plays had an average of $r = 0.19$ for Health, S-dev and Comb.

Table 13.14 lists the correlations among the 4 motivational indexes themselves and Table 13.15 lists the correlations among these 4 indexes and our 7 life assessment variables. The four motivational indexes in Table 13.14 are fairly strongly related, with the lowest coefficient at $r = 0.53$ between Ends, S-dev and Comb. The Index of Arts as Community Builders was modestly significantly correlated with 6 of the 7 life assessment variables at $r = 0.15$, with a high of $r = 0.24$ for General Health and a low of $r = 0.09$ for happiness (Table 13.15). General Health (GH) was the only life assessment variable significantly associated with all 4 motivational indexes.

Multivariate Relationships

Stepwise multiple regression was applied to explain the variation in scores for our 7 overall life assessment variables, and each of the next 7 Tables 13.16, 13.17, 13.18, 13.19, 13.20, 13.21 and 13.22 is laid out in the same format, with three exceptions in which one or two columns were omitted for lack of significant entries. When all columns are included, the lefthand column lists the names of the predictors. Then

Table 13.15 Correlations among motivational indexes and seven life assessment variables

Index	GH	Lsat	Hap	Qolsat	SWLS	CLAS	SWB
Health	0.21	ns	0.10	0.08	0.08	ns	ns
S-dev	0.17	ns	0.08	ns	ns	ns	ns
Comb	0.24	0.14	0.09	0.14	0.13	ns	0.13
Ends	0.17	0.09	ns	ns	ns	ns	ns

$N \geq 614$; $P < 0.05$

Table 13.16 Regressions of general health on demographics, motivation indexes, hours/times engaged and satisfaction obtained from arts-related activities and domain satisfaction

Dependent variables	Demog.	Mot. index	Hours/act. sat.	Domain sat.	All Pred
N	507	596	199	678	241
% of variance expl	8	7	4	17	20
Predictors	β	β	β	β	β
Education	0.25	*	*	*	**
Body mass index	−0.14	*	*	*	−0.13
Comm. building Ind.	*	0.19	*	*	0.14
Health enhance Ind.	*	0.10	*	*	**
Watching films dvd	*	*	−0.17	*	−0.13
Reading novels sat.	*	*	0.14	*	**
Recreat act. sat.	*	*	*	0.33	0.25
Self-esteem sat.	*	*	*	0.15	0.19

*Not in equation, **Significance level too low to enter equation

there is a column headed ‘Demog.’ containing the standardized regression coefficients (Beta values) resulting from regressing a life assessment (dependent) variable on the four demographic (explanatory, predictor or independent) variables. Standardized regression coefficients have means of zero and standard deviations of one, making comparisons of their relative influence on dependent variables easy to discern. Because standardization is sensitive to the particular variance of the variables employed in any sample, one cannot infer that relationships appearing in one sample must appear in others. The second column of figures is headed ‘Mot. Index’ and it contains the Beta values resulting from regressing the same life assessment variable on our four motivational indexes. The third column of figures is headed ‘Hrs/act.sat.’ and it contains the results of regressing the same life assessment variable on the set of hours-spent and satisfaction-obtained variables from Table 13.8 that had statistically significant correlations with that life assessment variable. The fourth column of figures is headed ‘Times/sat.’ and it contains the results of regressing the same life assessment variable on the set of times-spent and satisfaction-obtained variables from Table 13.9 that had statistically significant correlations with that life assessment variable. The fifth column of figures is headed

Table 13.17 Regressions of life satisfaction on demographics, motivation indexes, hours/times engaged and satisfaction obtained from arts-related activities and domain satisfaction

Dependent variables	Demog.	Mot. index	Hours/act. sat.	Times/sat.	Domain sat.	All pred
N	500	593	430	223	550	550
% of variance expl	1	2	3	7	66	66
Predictors	β	β	β	β	β	β
Household income	0.09	*	*	*	*	**
Comm. building Ind.	*	0.15	*	*	*	**
Reading novels sat.	*	*	0.18	*	*	**
Go other museums sat.	*	*	*	0.16	*	**
Go concert sat.	*	*	*	0.16	*	**
Future security sat.	*	*	*	*	0.10	0.10
Job sat.	*	*	*	*	0.20	0.20
Friendship sat.	*	*	*	*	0.21	0.21
Health satisfaction	*	*	*	*	0.25	0.25
Sense/mean life sat.	*	*	*	*	0.16	0.16
Self-esteem sat.	*	*	*	*	0.15	0.15

*Not in equation, **Significance level too low to enter equation

Table 13.18 Regressions of happiness on demographics, motivation indexes, hours/times engaged and satisfaction obtained from arts-related activities and domain satisfaction

Dependent variables	Demog.	Mot. index	Hours/act. sat.	Times/sat.	Domain sat.	All pred
N	505	595	235	378	669	669
% of variance expl	1	1	2	3	45	45
Predictors	β	β	β	β	β	β
Household income	0.12	*	*	*	*	**
Health enhance Ind.	*	0.11	*	*	*	**
Singing alone sat.	*	*	0.15	*	*	**
Go art museum sat.	*	*	*	0.19	*	**
Future security sat.	*	*	*	*	0.18	0.18
Recreation act. sat.	*	*	*	*	0.10	0.10
Friendships sat.	*	*	*	*	0.10	0.10
Health sat.	*	*	*	*	0.10	0.10
Self-esteem sat.	*	*	*	*	0.35	0.35

*Not in equation, **Significance level too low to enter equation

Table 13.19 Regressions of satisfaction with the overall quality of life on demographics, motivation indexes, hours/times engaged and satisfaction obtained from arts-related activities and domain satisfaction

Dependent variables	Demog.	Mot. index	Hours/act. sat.	Times/sat.	Domain sat.	All pred
N	504	596	236	361	664	664
% of variance expl	2	2	1	3	60	60
Predictors	β	β	β	β	β	β
Household income	0.16	*	*	*	*	**
Comm. building Ind.	*	0.14	*	*	*	**
Singing alone sat.	*	*	0.13	*	*	**
Go historic sites sat.	*	*	*	0.19	*	**
Local treatment sat.	*	*	*	*	0.22	0.22
Health satisfaction	*	*	*	*	0.19	0.19
Finance security sat.	*	*	*	*	0.09	0.09
Future security sat.	*	*	*	*	0.15	0.15
Sense meaning sat.	*	*	*	*	0.14	0.14
Recreation sat.	*	*	*	*	0.17	0.17
Feel part comm sat.	*	*	*	*	0.07	0.07

*Not in equation, **Significance level too low to enter equation

Table 13.20 Regressions of satisfaction with life scale (SWLS) on demographics, motivation indexes, hours/times engaged and satisfaction obtained from arts-related activities and domain satisfaction

Dependent variables	Demog.	Mot. index	Times/sat.	Domain sat.	All pred
N	487	582	308	534	534
% of variance expl	4	2	4	51	51
Predictors	β	β	β	β	β
Household income	0.12	*	*	*	**
Education	0.12	*	*	*	**
Age	0.11	*	*	*	**
Comm. building Ind.	*	0.14	*	*	**
Go other museums sat.	*	*	0.21	*	**
Sense meaning sat.	*	*	*	0.21	0.21
Job sat.	*	*	*	0.09	0.09
Health satisfaction	*	*	*	0.17	0.17
Finance security sat.	*	*	*	0.15	0.15
Feel part comm sat.	*	*	*	0.09	0.09
Self-esteem sat.	*	*	*	0.21	0.21

*Not in equation, **Significance level too low to enter equation

Table 13.21 Regressions of contentment with life assessment Scale (CLAS) on demographics, motivation indexes, hours/times engaged and satisfaction obtained from arts-related activities and domain satisfaction

Dependent variables	Demog.	Times/sat.	Domain sat.	All pred
N	493	353	538	538
% of variance expl	3	2	50	50
Predictors	β	β	β	β
Age	0.12	*	*	**
Household income	0.13	*	*	**
Singing alone sat.	*	*	*	**
Go historic site sat.	*	0.15	*	**
Job satisfaction	*	*	0.12	0.12
Health satisfaction	*	*	0.10	0.10
Self-esteem sat.	*	*	0.26	0.26
Future security sat.	*	*	0.18	0.18
Sense meaning sat.	*	*	0.16	0.16
Recreation act sat.	*	*	0.09	0.09

*Not in equation, **Significance level too low to enter equation

Table 13.22 Regressions of Subjective Wellbeing (SWB) on demographics, motivation indexes, hours/times engaged and satisfaction obtained from arts-related activities and domain satisfaction

Dependent variables	Demog.	Mot. index	Hours/act. sat.	Times/sat.	Domain sat.	All pred
N	491	583	423	374	644	644
% of variance expl	4	2	2	3	75	75
Predictors	β	β	β	β	β	β
Education	0.10	*	*	*	*	**
Household income	0.17	*	*	*	*	**
Comm. building Ind.	*	0.14	*	*	*	**
Reading novels sat.	*	*	0.15	*	*	**
Go art museum sat.	*	*	*	0.17	*	**
Local treatment sat.	*	*	*	*	0.10	0.10
Friendships sat.	*	*	*	*	0.11	0.11
Future security sat.	*	*	*	*	0.13	0.13
Health satisfaction	*	*	*	*	0.19	0.19
Finance security sat.	*	*	*	*	0.20	0.20
Sense meaning sat	*	*	*	*	0.12	0.12
Self-esteem sat.	*	*	*	*	0.14	0.14
Recreation act sat.	*	*	*	*	0.12	0.12
Feel part comm sat.	*	*	*	*	0.06	0.06

*Not in equation, **Significance level too low to enter equation

'Domain sat.' and it contains the results of regressing the same life assessment variable on the 8 variables indicating satisfaction obtained from some domain or aspect of life listed in Table 13.10 that had the largest correlation coefficients with that life assessment variable. Finally, the sixth column of figures is headed 'All Pred' and it contains the results of regressing the same life assessment variable on all of the predictors that achieved statistical significance in the previous five regressions. Because the introduction of *any* arts-related additional predictors to the set of significant domain satisfaction predictors drastically reduced the sample size (N) for the regression equation, instead of introducing these variables all together, each one was introduced separately. If it achieved statistical significance, it was maintained while the next variable was introduced and if not, it was dropped.

A quick inspection of the seven tables reveals that only two arts-related predictors achieved statistical significance in a final regression equation and only in the regression involving General Health. As well, only one demographic variable achieved statistical significance in a final equation and that was also in the regression involving General Health. This was somewhat similar to the regression results reported in Michalos and Kahlke (2008). In the latter study only the Indexes of Arts as Self-Health Enhancers and SpiritBuilding (not used in this study) achieved statistical significance in the final equation of one life assessment variable, namely, satisfaction with the overall quality of life (qolsat). In that study, on five occasions some demographic variable achieved statistical significance.

The first column of figures in Table 13.16 shows that two of our four demographic predictors remained statistically significant when pressed into service together and that collectively they explained 8.0% of the variation in self-reported General Health (GH) scores. The most influential was education, with a Beta value of $\beta = 0.25$, followed by the Body Mass Index at $\beta = -0.14$. Thus, figuratively speaking, for example, one could say that on average, for every increase of a full unit step (i.e., one standard deviation unit) of education, respondents got an increase of 25.0% of a step in self-reported General Health, with the values of all other predictors held constant. The second column of figures shows that when the four motivational indexes were used together as predictors, two remained statistically significant and they explained 7.0% of the variance in General Health scores. The Index of Arts as Community Builders (Comb) was most influential, with a Beta value of $\beta = 0.19$. The third column of figures shows that two arts-related variables from the *hours per week* set of predictors remained statistically significant and explained 4.0% of the variance in General Health scores, with the mean level of satisfaction obtained from watching dvd films having the most influence at $\beta = -0.17$. The fourth column of figures shows that two of the domain satisfaction predictors remained statistically significant and together they explained 17.0% of the variance in General Health scores. (Because the dependent variable for this table is self-reported General Health and such reports are highly correlated with satisfaction with one's own health (Michalos 2004), the latter variable was not used as a predictor of General Health.) Reported satisfaction with respondents' recreational activities was most influential, with a $\beta = 0.33$, followed by satisfaction with respondents' own self-esteem, $\beta = 0.15$. In the final column, we see that five predictors combined to explain 20.0% of the variance in General Health scores ($N = 241$), with satisfaction with respondents' recreation activity appearing most influential ($\beta = 0.25$), followed by self-esteem satisfaction ($\beta = 0.19$). Two arts-related predictors remained statistically significant in the last regression. The Index of Arts as Community Builders (Comb) had a $\beta = 0.14$ and the average number of hours per week spent watching dvd films had a $\beta = -0.13$. In Michalos and Kahlke (2008) we were able to explain 32.0% of the variance in GH scores, with satisfaction with respondents' recreational activities most influential, ($\beta = 0.28$).

The first column of figures in Table 13.17 shows that only one of our four demographic predictors remained statistically significant and it explained 1.0% of the variation in satisfaction with life as a whole (Lsat) scores. Household income had a Beta value of $\beta = 0.09$. The second column of figures shows that one of the 4 motivational indexes remained statistically significant when the 4 were used together and that by itself that one explained only 2.0% of the variance in life satisfaction scores, with the Index of Arts as Community Builders (Comb) having a Beta value of $\beta = 0.15$. The third column of figures shows that one arts-related variable from the *hours per week* set of predictors remained statistically significant and explained 3.0% of the variance in life satisfaction (Lsat) scores. Respondents' mean levels of satisfaction obtained from reading novels, etc. had a $\beta = 0.18$. The fourth column of figures shows that two arts-related variables from the *times per year* set of predictors remained statistically significant. Satisfaction obtained from going to concerts and non-art museums each had a $\beta = 0.16$, and together explained 7.0% of the variance in life satisfaction scores. The fifth column of figures shows that six of the domain satisfaction predictors remained statistically significant and together they explained 66.0% of the variance in life satisfaction scores. The most influential explanatory variable was satisfaction with one's own health ($\beta = 0.25$), followed by satisfaction with respondents' friendships ($\beta = 0.21$). The final column shows that the addition of each of the demographic and arts-related predictors (one at a time with replacement) to the six significant domain satisfaction predictors from the fifth column produced no change in our explanatory power. All the figures in columns five and six are the same, but the 5 double asterisks in the sixth column mean that in the presence of the 6 domain satisfaction predictors, no explanatory power was added by the demographic and arts-related predictors. In our earlier study, we were able to explain 71.0% of the variance in Lsat scores, with satisfaction with one's own health again most influential, ($\beta = 0.24$).

The first column of figures in Table 13.18 shows that one demographic predictor remained statistically significant and it explained 1.0% of the variation in happiness (Hap) scores. Household income had a $\beta = 0.12$. The second column of figures shows that when the four motivational indexes were used together as predictors, only one remained statistically significant and by itself explained 1.0% of the variance in happiness scores. The Index of Arts as Self-Health Enhancers had a $\beta = 0.11$. The third column of figures shows that a single arts-related variable from the *hours per week* set of predictors remained statistically significant and it explained 2.0% of the variance in happiness scores, with the mean level of satisfaction obtained from singing alone having a $\beta = 0.15$. Notice, then, that while the average number of hours per week invested in singing alone decreased respondents' satisfaction with life as a whole (Table 13.8), the mean level of satisfaction obtained from singing alone increased their happiness (Tables 13.8 and 13.18). The fourth column of figures shows that one arts-related variable from the *times per year* set of predictors remained statistically significant. The satisfaction obtained from going to art museums ($\beta = 0.19$) explained 3.0% of the variance in happiness scores. The fifth column of figures shows that 5 of the domain satisfaction variables remained statistically significant and explained 45.0% of the variance in happiness scores. The most influential explanatory variable was satisfaction with respondents' own self-esteem, $\beta = 0.35$, followed by satisfaction with their future security, $\beta = 0.18$. Again, the final column shows that the addition of each of the demographic and arts-related predictors (one at a time with replacement) to the 5 significant domain satisfaction predictors from the fifth column produced no change in our explanatory power. In our earlier study, we were able to explain 51.0% of the variance in Hap scores, with satisfaction with one's own health most influential, $\beta = 0.33$.

The first column of figures in Table 13.19 shows that one of our four demographic variables remained statistically significant and explained 2.0% of the variation in satisfaction with the overall quality of life (qolsat) scores. Household income had a $\beta = 0.16$. The second column of figures shows that one of the four motivational indexes remained statistically significant and explained 2.0% of the variance in satisfaction with the overall quality of life scores, i.e., the Index of Arts as Community Builders, $\beta = 0.14$. The third column of figures shows that a single arts-related variable from the *hours per week* set of predictors remained statistically significant, satisfaction obtained from singing alone, $\beta = 0.13$, and it explained 1.0% of the variance in satisfaction with the overall quality of life scores. The fourth column of figures shows that a single arts-related variable from the *times per year* set of predictors remained statistically significant, satisfaction obtained from going to historical sites, $\beta = 0.19$, and it explained 3.0% of the variance in satisfaction with the overall quality of life scores. The fifth column of figures shows that 7 of the domain satisfaction predictors remained statistically significant and together they explained 60.0% of the variance in satisfaction with the overall quality of life scores. The most influential explanatory variables were satisfaction with respondents' treatment by local residents, $\beta = 0.22$, followed by satisfaction with respondents' health, $\beta = 0.19$. Again, the final column shows that the addition of each of the demographic and arts-related predictors to the 7 significant domain satisfaction predictors from the fifth column produced no change in our explanatory power. In our earlier study, we were able to explain 63.0% of the variance in qolsat scores, with satisfaction with respondents' health, financial security and sense of meaning in life most influential, each $\beta = 0.16$.

The first column of figures in Table 13.20 shows that 3 of 4 demographic variables remained statistically significant and collectively explained 4.0% of the variation in scores on the 5-item Satisfaction With Life Scale (SWLS). Of the three predictors, the most influential were household income and education, each $\beta = 0.12$. The second column of figures shows that only one of the 4 motivational indexes remained statistically significant and that explained 2.0% of the variance in SWLS scores. The Index of Arts as Community Builders (Comb) had a $\beta = 0.14$. The third column of figures shows that a single arts-related variable from the *times per year* set of predictors remained statistically significant, satisfaction obtained from going to non-art museums, $\beta = 0.21$, and it explained 4.0% of the variance in SWLS scores. The fourth column of figures shows that 6 of the domain satisfaction predictors remained statistically significant and together they explained 51.0% of the variance in SWLS scores. The most influential explanatory variables were satisfaction with respondents' sense of meaning in life and self-esteem, each $\beta = 0.21$, followed by satisfaction with respondents' health, $\beta = 0.17$. Again, the final column shows that the addition of each of the demographic and arts-related predictors to the 6 significant domain satisfaction predictors from the fourth column produced no change in our explanatory power. In our earlier study, we were able to explain 48.0% of the variance in SWLS scores, with satisfaction with one's financial security most influential, $\beta = 0.22$.

The first column of figures in Table 13.21 shows that two demographic variables remained statistically significant and explained 3.0% of the variation in scores on the 5-item Contentment with Life Assessment Scale (CLAS). Of the two predictors, the most influential was household income, $\beta = 0.13$. The second column of figures shows that a single arts-related variable from the *times per year* set of predictors remained statistically significant, satisfaction obtained from visiting historic and heritage sites, $\beta = 0.15$, and explained 2.0% of the variance in CLAS scores. The third column of figures shows that 6 of the domain satisfaction variables remained statistically significant and together explained 50.0% of the variance in CLAS scores. The most influential explanatory variables were satisfaction with respondents' self-esteem, $\beta = 0.26$, followed by satisfaction with respondents' future security, $\beta = 0.18$. Again, the final column shows that the addition of each of the demographic and arts-related predictors to the 6 significant domain satisfaction predictors from the third column produced no change in our explanatory power. In our earlier study, we were able to explain 71.0% of the variance in CLAS scores, with satisfaction with respondents' financial security most influential, $\beta = 0.19$.

The first column of figures in Table 13.22 shows that two demographic variables remained statistically significant and explained 4.0% of the variation in scores on the 4-item Subjective Wellbeing Index (SWB). Of the two predictors, the most influential was household income, $\beta = 0.17$. The second column of figures shows that one of the 4 motivational indexes remained statistically significant and explained 2.0% of the variance in SWB scores. The Index of Arts as Community Builders had a $\beta = 0.14$. The third column of figures shows that a single arts-related variable from the *hours per week* set of predictors remained statistically significant, satisfaction obtained from reading novels, etc., $\beta = 0.15$, and explained 2.0% of the variance in SWB scores. The fourth column of figures shows that one arts-related variable from the *times per year* set of predictors remained statistically significant and explained 3.0% of the variance in SWB scores. Satisfaction obtained from going to art museums had a $\beta = 0.17$. The fifth column of figures shows that 9 of the domain satisfaction predictors remained statistically significant and together explained 75.0% of the variance in SWB scores. The most influential explanatory variables were satisfaction with respondents' financial security, $\beta = 0.20$, followed by satisfaction with respondents' health, b = 0.19. Again, the final column shows that the addition of each of the demographic and arts-related predictors to the 9 significant domain satisfaction predictors from the fifth column produced no change in our explanatory power. In our earlier study, we were able to explain 79.0% of the variance in SWB scores, with satisfaction with respondents' financial security most influential, $\beta = 0.25$.

Table 13.23 lists results of regressing our 7 life assessment variables on 7 mean respondent-calculated discrepancy scores. Although the predictors are drawn from multiple discrepancies theory (MDT), the whole theory is not applied here. All we have done is use the 7 basic discrepancy variables of MDT in a simple bottom-up type of linear regression of the sort applied to produce Tables 13.16, 13.17, 13.18, 13.19, 13.20, 13.21 and 13.22. On average, the 7 MDT variables explained 44.0% (vs. 48.0% in the earlier study) of the variation in life assessment scores, with a high of 59.0% for SWLS and a low of 16.0% for GH. Without GH, the average variance explained was 49.0%. The difference between the power of the MDT variables to explain General Health versus the other 6 life assessment variables (replicating results in our earlier study) suggests again that respondents recognized a difference between a healthy life and a good life, all things considered. Setting aside the GH column, in every column, the most influential variable is that indicating the

Table 13.23 Regressions of seven life assessment variables on seven mean discrepancy scores

Dependent variables	GH	Lsat	Hap	Qolsat	SWLS	CLAS	SWB
N	657	656	657	656	641	636	645
% of variance explained	16	39	43	43	59	51	58
Predictors, your life compared to	β	β	β	β	β	β	β
What you want from life	0.17	0.42	0.43	0.34	0.43	0.41	0.46
What others your age and sex have	0.18	0.12	0.08	0.21	0.15	*	0.17
What you deserve	−0.12	*	*	*	0.08	0.09	0.09
What you need	*	*	*	0.11	0.10	0.08	0.09
What you expected it to be now	*	*	0.11	*	*	0.19	0.10
What you expect it to be in 5 years	*	*	*	*	*	*	*
The best in your past experience	0.23	0.22	0.18	0.15	0.20	0.13	0.13

*Significance level too low to enter equation

perceived discrepancy between what respondents have now and what they want. On average, the Beta value for this variable is $\beta = 0.42$, with a high of $\beta = 0.46$ for SWB and a low of $\beta = 0.34$ for qolsat. The only other MDT predictor with a significant association with each of the 7 life assessment variables in the presence of all other MDT predictors is that for the gap between what respondents have now and the best they ever had in the past. On average, this predictor had a $\beta = 0.18$.

Since in every case of Tables 13.16, 13.17, 13.18, 13.19, 13.20, 13.21 and 13.22, the set of domain satisfaction predictors explained the greatest amount of variance in our life assessment variables, the column headed 'Domain sat.' in these tables is the appropriate column to compare with the results in Table 13.23 in order to assess the relative explanatory power of both sets of predictors, i.e., domain satisfaction versus discrepancy predictors. On average for the 7 life assessment variables, domain satisfaction predictors clearly explained a greater percent of the variance than discrepancy predictors, 52.0 versus 44.0% (compared to 57 and 48% in the earlier study). This is not particularly surprising or satisfying since, after all, in the former case one is using only domain satisfaction predictors to explain some sort of a more general level of satisfaction. Much more analysis will be required to make a comprehensive comparison of the relative power of MDT versus a simple domain satisfaction, bottom-up approach to explaining the variation of overall life assessment scores in the context of a plausible theory that includes arts-related variables.

Conclusion

The aims of this investigation were (1) to measure the impact of arts-related activities on the perceived quality of life of a representative sample of British Columbians aged 18 years or more in the spring of 2007, and (2) to compare the findings of this study with those of a sample of 1,027 adults drawn from 5 B.C. communities (Comox Valley, Kamloops, Nanaimo, Port Moody and Prince George) in the fall of 2006. In May and June 2007, 708 British Columbians responded to a 13-page mailed out questionnaire. The working data set was weighted by age and education to match the 2006 census statistics for the province, yielding a fairly representative sample.

Since we were aiming to get some baseline provincial figures as well as to replicate findings obtained from specifically targeted communities in different parts of the province, the best way to summarize our results is with a double column review. This is provided in Table 13.24. In broad strokes, out of 37 pairs of entries in this table, there are 10 (27.0%) in which the province-wide and five-communities results are the same. There are another 13 (35.0%) in which the results are very nearly the same. So, we have a total of 23 (62.0%) pairs with considerable similarity. While plenty of differences were identified in many of the tables in our main text, suggesting that there remains a great deal of diversity yet to be understood, the broad similarities seem to be quite remarkable.

Table 13.24 Comparisons between province-wide (2007, N = 708) and five-communities (2006, N = 1.027) results

Province-wide sample	Five-communities sample
Top 5 arts-related hours per week activities: listening to music; reading novels, short stories, plays or poetry; watching films on dvd; singing alone; reading to others	Same
Top 5 arts-related hours per week activities: average hours per week engaged = 6.9	7.0
Top 5 arts-related *hours per week* activities: average levels of satisfaction = 5.9	Same
Top 5 arts-related *times per year* activities: go to movies, concerts, community festivals, historic sites, art museums	Same
Top 5 arts-related *times per year* activities: average times per year going = 3.8	3.9
Top 5 arts-related *times per year* activities: average levels of satisfaction = 5.8	Same
First thoughts about 'arts' = painting, drawing	Same
Most important arts = music	Same
Place where first learned about arts = school	Same
Mean age when first learned = 12	12.7
Mean level of satisfaction with access to activity, information, place, access to place, price = 5.1	5.3
Mean level of satisfaction with support from city, provincial, federal government and others = 4.0	Same
Index of arts as self-health enhancers α = 0.87	0.88
Index of arts as self-developing activities α = 0.86	0.89
Index of arts as community builders α = 0.82	0.86
Index of arts as ends in themselves α = 0.71	0.77
Satisfaction with life scale (SWLS) α = 0.90	0.89
Contentment with life assessment scale (CLAS) α = 0.87	0.86
Subjective wellbeing index (SWB) α = 0.87	0.88
Average level of satisfaction on 30 domain/aspect items = 5.3	5.4
Average level of satisfaction with life as a whole, standard of living, quality of life and happiness = 5.8	Same
Top 2 discrepancy items = have/want, have/others have	Same
Demographic variable with highest average correlation with 7 life assessment variables = household income, r = 0.12	r = 0.20

(continued)

Table 13.24 (continued)

Province-wide sample	Five-communities sample
Hours per week arts-related variables with highest and second highest average correlations with 7 life assessment variables: satisfaction obtained from arranging flowers, $r = 0.25$; satisfaction obtained from taking kids to arts-related activities, $r = -0.17$	Satisfaction obtained from playing a musical instrument, $r = 0.25$; satisfaction obtained from singing in a group, $r = 0.17$
Life assessment variable with largest number of significant associations with *hours per week* arts-related variables: satisfaction with the overall quality of life tied with happiness	Satisfaction with the overall quality of life
Times per year arts-related variables with highest and second highest average correlations with 7 life assessment variables: satisfaction obtained from going to amateur theatre performances, r = 0.27; satisfaction obtained from going to professional theatre performances, r = 0.22	Satisfaction obtained from going to non-art museums, $r = 0.14$; satisfaction obtained from going to amateur theatre performances, $r = 0.13$
Life assessment variable with largest number of significant associations with *times per year* artsrelated variables: satisfaction with the overall quality of life	General health
Domain/aspect satisfaction items with highest and second highest average correlations with 7 life assessment variables: satisfaction with one's own health, $r = 0.60$; satisfaction with one's selfesteem, $r = 0.59$	Satisfaction with one's own health, $r = 0.64$; satisfaction with one's self-esteem, $r = 0.57$
Percent of variation explained in general health scores by all predictors = 20.0%, with most influential predictor = respondents' satisfaction with their recreation activities, $\beta = 0.25$	Percent of variation explained in general health scores by all predictors = 32.0%, with most influential predictor = respondents' satisfaction with their recreation activities, $\beta = 0.28$
Percent of variation explained in satisfaction with life as a whole scores (Lsat) by all predictors = 66.0%, with most influential predictor = respondents' satisfaction with their own health, $\beta = 0.25$	Percent of variation explained in satisfaction with life as a whole scores (Lsat) by all predictors = 71.0%, with most influential predictor = respondents' satisfaction with their own health, $\beta = 0.24$
Percent of variation explained in happiness scores by all predictors = 45.0%, with most influential predictor = respondents' satisfaction with their own self-esteem, $\beta = 0.35$	Percent of variation explained in happiness scores by all predictors = 51.0%, with most influential predictor = respondents' satisfaction with their own health, $\beta = 0.33$
Percent of variation explained in satisfaction with the overall quality of life scores (qolsat) by all predictors = 60.0%, with most influential predictor = respondents' satisfaction with their treatment by local residents, $\beta = 0.22$	Percent of variation explained in satisfaction with the overall quality of life scores (qolsat) by all predictors = 63.0%, with most influential predictors = respondents' satisfaction with their own health, financial security and sense of meaning in life, each $\beta = 0.19$

(continued)

Table 13.24 (continued)

Province-wide sample	Five-communities sample
Percent of variation explained in satisfaction with life scale scores (SWLS) by all predictors = 51.0%, with most influential predictor = respondents' satisfaction with their own self-esteem and sense of meaning in life, $\beta = 0.21$	Percent of variation explained in satisfaction with life scale scores (SWLS) by all predictors = 48.0%, with most influential predictor = respondents' satisfaction with their financial security, $\beta = 0.22$
Percent of variation explained in contentment with life assessment scale scores (CLAS) by all predictors = 50.0%, with most influential predictor = respondents' satisfaction with their own self-esteem, $\beta = 0.26$	Percent of variation explained in contentment with life assessment scale scores (CLAS) by all predictors = 71.0%, with most influential predictor = respondents' satisfaction with their financial security, $\beta = 0.19$
Percent of variation explained in subjective wellbeing index scores (SWB) by all predictors = 75.0%, with most influential predictor = respondents' satisfaction with their financial security, $\beta = 0.20$	Percent of variation explained in subjective wellbeing index scores (SWB) by all predictors = 79.0%, with most influential predictor = respondents' satisfaction with their financial security, $\beta = 0.25$
Average percent of variation explained in 7 life assessment variables by all domain/aspect predictors = 52.0%	Average percent of variation explained in 7 life assessment variables by all domain/aspect predictors = 57.0%
Average percent of variation explained in 7 life assessment variables by 7 MDT predictors = 44.0%	Average percent of variation explained in 7 life assessment variables by 7 MDT predictors = 48.0%

In the light of results from our two samples and in the context of all our predictors, based on the relative impact of all the arts-related activities and the satisfaction obtained from those activities on the seven overall life assessment variables, it is fair to say that such activities and their corresponding satisfaction contributed relatively little. As remarked in our earlier study, it is important to keep in mind the initial condition, "in the context of all our predictors" and the qualifier "relatively". In that context, even the usually powerful explanatory variables concerning interpersonal relations (i.e., satisfaction with one's living partner, family and friendships) had very little impact. Of the three, only satisfaction with one's friendships appeared in any final regression equation for the provincial sample and only for Lsat, Hap and SWB. This was quite different from the five-communities sample. In the latter, satisfaction with one's living partner appeared in the final equations for 6 of the 7 dependent variables (excluding General Health), satisfaction with family relations appeared in the final equations for Lsat and Hap, and satisfaction with friendships appeared in the final equations for Lsat, qolsat and SWB.

Considering domain/aspect predictors, what did most of the explanatory work for the 7 life assessment variables? Two samples with 7 final regression equations and no ties would have given us 14 possible most influential predictors. Since we had one regression with a 3-way tie for most influential predictor and one with a 2-way tie, we have 17 entries. One way to answer our question is to count the relative frequency with which various predictors occur. Using this crude measure, one finds that satisfaction with financial security had 5 firsts, followed by 4 firsts for satisfaction with respondents' own health and 3 firsts for satisfaction with respondents' own self-esteem. These predictors are understandably and often relatively heavy hitters in such exercises. Still, granting the difficulties of displacing any of the relatively heavy hitters from our final explanatory equations, it remains unclear why even arts-related activities with engagement measured in the average number of *hours per week* or *times per year* and the satisfaction obtained from such engagement were relatively weak predictors in the context of only such arts-related activities and satisfaction. Hopefully, others will be able to solve this problem in the future.

Acknowledgements We would like to express our thanks to the Social Sciences and Humanities Research Council for funding this research through the Gold Medal for Achievement in Research 2004. This project complements an earlier one also funded by the Council through its Community-University Research grants program, with Will Garrett-Petts of Thompson Rivers University Principal Investigator. We would also like to thank Joyce Henley, Office Manager of ISRE, and all the anonymous respondents who shared their time and thoughts with us to make this report possible.

Appendix: BC Arts and Quality of Life Survey, May 2007

See Table 13.25.

Table 13.25 Time spent on and levels of satisfaction with artistic activities (Total $N = 708$, unweighted data)

Particular activities	Ordered by N	Hours/week	Satisfaction
T1. Listening to music	608	13.22	6.01
T17. Reading novels, etc.	441	7.67	6.17
T37. Watching movies on video	278	4.96	5.60
T8. Singing alone	239	4.58	5.70
T21. Reading to others	195	3.27	6.03
T46. Gourmet cooking	136	4.60	6.18
T20. Telling stories	122	2.76	5.92
T5. Painting or drawing	118	5.86	5.97
T9. Singing in a group	103	2.67	6.11
T50. Watching art shows on TV	94	2.68	5.66
T2. Playing a musical instrument	85	4.91	6.05
T40. Artistic photography	66	3.11	6.34
T27. Knitting or crocheting	64	4.98	6.45
T42. Arranging flowers	57	1.37	6.38
T67. Other	50	10.00	6.65
T52. Watching concerts on TV	48	2.17	5.93

(continued)

Table 13.25 (continued)

Particular activities	Ordered by N	Hours/week	Satisfaction
T12. Taking children to arts activities	46	2.35	5.96
T19. Writing novels, etc.	45	6.18	5.89
T28. Embroidery, needlepoint	38	5.95	6.31
T16. Making quilts	32	9.75	6.29
T15. Making clothes	30	4.27	6.07
T6. Teaching painting or drawing	23	5.13	6.05
T51. Watching live theatre on TV	23	2.48	5.42
T7. Teaching singing	21	3.90	6.05
T56. Attending a class-artistic work	20	3.65	6.39
T14. Designing clothes	17	2.47	5.94
T49. Graphic designing	17	16.29	5.63
T4. Teaching—to play an instrument	15	4.27	5.20
T24. Teaching people to dance	14	2.29	5.85
T43. Creating jewelry	14	2.64	5.56
T11. Creating sculptures	13	5.38	6.30
T47. Teaching gourmet cooking	13	2.85	6.30
T53. Watching opera on TV	12	3.17	5.38
T10. Creating pottery or ceramics	11	7.00	5.78
T18. Attending a book club	11	4.45	6.00
T60. Working for pay in the arts	10	26.80	6.22
T22. Teaching creative writing	9	2.33	5.63
T3. Writing music	7	4.43	5.57
T62.Acting as an advocate for the arts	7	1.71	6.33
T58. Selling works of art	6	2.33	5.83
T25. Weaving textiles	4	13.75	6.67
T35. Non-acting work—amateur theatre	2	2.50	6.50
T26. Weaving baskets	1	4.00	7.00
T34. Acting—amateur theatre	1	6.00	–
T48. Making artistic videos or movies	1	10.00	7.00
T61. Serving as a judge for the arts	1	2.00	–
T33. Acting—professional theatre	0		
T13. Teaching sculpture	0		
Particular activities	Ordered by N	Times/year	Satisfaction
T36. Going to movies	439	5.97	5.53
T29. Going to concerts	417	3.75	6.01
T38. Going to art museums/galleries	384	3.65	5.84
T65. Visiting historic, heritage sites	367	2.97	5.93
T54. Attending community festivals	365	2.89	5.61
T39. Going to other museums	319	2.39	5.84
T66. Visiting the public library	307	9.18	5.61
T30. Going to amateur live theatre	296	2.56	5.90

(continued)

Table 13.25 (continued)

Particular activities	Ordered by N	Hours/week	Satisfaction
T31. Going to professional live theatre	293	2.80	6.14
T57. Buying works of art	224	2.33	6.12
T44. Decorating a home	220	6.08	5.75
T32. Going to school plays	211	2.13	6.00
T23. Dancing	199	5.48	5.52
T41. Designing a garden	190	4.19	6.07
T63. Making donations to the arts	111	2.62	5.79
T55. Working on community festivals	98	2.43	5.77
T59. Volunteering in the arts	53	4.94	5.94
T64. Designing, crafting furniture	49	4.16	6.02
T45. Figure skating	32	5.22	5.50
T67. Other	25	9.52	6.48
T61. Serving as a judge for the arts	8	3.00	6.14
T33. Acting—professional theatre	7	2.00	6.14
T34. Acting—amateur theatre	6	1.67	6.50
Particular activities	N	Ordered by hours/week	Satisfaction
T60. Working for pay in the arts	10	26.80	6.22
T49. Graphic designing	17	16.29	5.63
T25. Weaving textiles	4	13.75	6.67
T1. Listening to music	608	13.22	6.01
T67. Other	50	10.00	6.65
T48. Making artistic videos or movies	1	10.00	7.00
T16. Making quilts	32	9.75	6.29
T17. Reading novels, etc.	441	7.67	6.17
T10. Creating pottery or ceramics	11	7.00	5.78
T19. Writing novels, etc.	45	6.18	5.89
T34. Acting—amateur theatre	1	6.00	–
T28. Embroidery, needlepoint	38	5.95	6.31
T5. Painting or drawing	118	5.86	5.97
T11. Creating sculptures	13	5.38	6.30
T6. Teaching painting or drawing	23	5.13	6.05
T27. Knitting or crocheting	64	4.98	6.45
T37. Watching movies on video	278	4.96	5.60
T2. Playing a musical instrument	85	4.91	6.05
T46. Gourmet cooking	136	4.60	6.18
T8. Singing alone	239	4.58	5.70
T18. Attending a book club	11	4.45	6.00
T3. Writing music	7	4.43	5.57
T4. Teaching—to play an instrument	15	4.27	5.20
T15. Making clothes	30	4.27	6.07
T26. Weaving baskets	1	4.00	7.00

(continued)

Table 13.25 (continued)

Particular activities	Ordered by N	Hours/week	Satisfaction
T7. Teaching singing	21	3.90	6.05
T56. Attending a class-artistic work	20	3.65	6.39
T21. Reading to others	195	3.27	6.03
T53. Watching opera on TV	12	3.17	5.38
T40. Artistic photography	66	3.11	6.34
T47. Teaching gourmet cooking	13	2.85	6.30
T20. Telling stories	122	2.76	5.92
T50. Watching art shows on TV	94	2.68	5.66
T9. Singing in a group	103	2.67	6.11
T43. Creating jewelry	14	2.64	5.56
T35. Non-acting work—amateur theatre	2	2.50	6.50
T51. Watching live theatre on TV	23	2.48	5.42
T14. Designing clothes	17	2.47	5.94
T12. Taking children to arts activities	46	2.35	5.96
T22. Teaching creative writing	9	2.33	5.63
T58. Selling works of art	6	2.33	5.83
T24. Teaching people to dance	14	2.29	5.85
T52. Watching concerts on TV	48	2.17	5.93
T61. Serving as a judge for the arts	1	2.00	–
T62. Acting as an advocate for the arts	7	1.71	6.33
T42. Arranging flowers	57	1.37	6.38
T33. Acting—professional theatre	0		
T13. Teaching sculpture	0		
Particular activities	N	Ordered by times/year	Satisfaction
T67. Other	25	9.52	6.48
T66. Visiting the public library	307	9.18	5.61
T44. Decorating a home	220	6.08	5.75
T36. Going to movies	439	5.97	5.53
T23. Dancing	199	5.48	5.52
T45. Figure skating	32	5.22	5.50
T59. Volunteering in the arts	53	4.94	5.94
T41. Designing a garden	190	4.19	6.07
T64. Designing, crafting furniture	49	4.16	6.02
T29. Going to concerts	417	3.75	6.01
T38. Going to art museums/galleries	384	3.65	5.84
T61. Serving as a judge for the arts	8	3.00	6.14
T65. Visiting historic, heritage sites	367	2.97	5.93
T54. Attending community festivals	365	2.89	5.61
T31. Going to professional live theatre	293	2.80	6.14
T63. Making donations to the arts	111	2.62	5.79

(continued)

Table 13.25 (continued)

Particular activities	Ordered by N	Hours/week	Satisfaction
T30. Going to amateur live theatre	296	2.56	5.90
T55. Working on community festivals	98	2.43	5.77
T39. Going to other museums	319	2.39	5.84
T57. Buying works of art	224	2.33	6.12
T32. Going to school plays	211	2.13	6.00
T33. Acting—professional theatre	7	2.00	6.14
T34. Acting—amateur theatre	6	1.67	6.50

Most activities had some people indicating they spent a certain number of hours per week on it, while other people only did it a few times per year. The hours per week activities are listed first, followed by the times per year activities. The activities are listed in two orders—first from the largest number of people responding to the least and then from the largest average hours/week (or times/year) to the smallest

References

Cummins, R. A., Stokes, M. A., & Davern, M. T. (2007). Core affect and subjective wellbeing: A rebuttal to Moum and Land. *Journal of Happiness Studies, 8*(4), 457–466. doi:10.1007/s10902-007-9065-2.

Davern, M. T., Cummins, R. A., & Stokes, M. A. (2007). Subjective wellbeing as an affective-cognitive construct. *Journal of Happiness Studies, 8*(4), 429–449. doi:10.1007/s10902-007-9066-1.

Decima. (2002). *The arts in Canada: Access and availability. 2001 Research Study Final Report*, Decima Research Inc., Ottawa. Retrieved June, 2007, from http://www.pch.gc.ca/progs/arts/pubs/etude-report/arts_access.pdf.

Diener, E., Emmons, R. A., Larsen, R. J., & Griffin, S. (1985). The satisfaction with life scale. *Journal of Personality Assessment, 49*, 71–75. doi:10.1207/s15327752jpa4901_13.

DiMaggio, P., & Pettitt, B. (1999). Surveys of public attitudes toward the arts: What surveys tell us about the arts' political trials—And how they might tell us even more. *Arts Education Policy Review, 100*(4), 32–37.

Land, K. C. (2007). Comments from Kenneth C. *Land. Journal of Happiness Studies, 8*(4), 455. doi:10.1007/s10902-007-9068-z.

Lavallee, L. F., Hatch, P. M., Michalos, A. C., & McKinley, T. (2007). Development of the contentment with life assessment scale (CLAS): Using daily life experiences to verify levels of self-reported life satisfaction. *Social Indicators Research, 83*(2), 201–244. doi:10.1007/s11205-006-9054-6.

Michalos, A. C. (1985). Multiple discrepancies theory (MDT). *Social Indicators Research, 16*(4), 347–413. doi:10.1007/BF00333288.

Michalos, A. C. (1991). *Global report on student well-being, Volume 1: Life satisfaction and happiness*. New York: Springer.

Michalos, A. C. (2004). Social indicators research and health-related quality of life research. *Social Indicators Research, 65*(1), 27–72. doi:10.1023/A:1025592219390.

Michalos, A. C. (Ed.). (2005a). *Citation classics from social indicators research*. Dordrecht: Springer Publishers.

Michalos, A. C. (2005b). Arts and the quality of life. *Social Indicators Research, 71*(1–3), 11–59. doi:10.1007/s11205-004-8013-3.

Michalos, A. C., & Kahlke, P. M. (2008). Impact of arts-related activities on the perceived quality of life. *Social Indicators Research, 89*(2), 193–258. doi:10.1007/s11205-007-9236-x.

Michalos, A. C., Thommasen, H. V., Read, R., Anderson, N., & Zumbo, B. D. (2005). Determinants of health and the quality of life in the Bella Coola Valley. *Social Indicators Research, 72*(1), 1–50. doi:10.1007/s11205-004-4512-5.

Moum, T. (2007). A critique of 'Subjective wellbeing as an affective-cognitive construct. *Journal of Happiness Studies, 8*(4), 451–453. doi:10.1007/s10902-007-9067-0.

Chapter 14
What Did Stiglitz, Sen and Fitoussi Get Right and What Did They Get Wrong?

Alex C. Michalos

In the Executive Summary we are told that

> The Commission's aim has been to identify the limits of GDP as an indicator of economic performance and social progress, including the problems with its measurement; to consider what additional information might be required for the production of more relevant indicators of social progress; to assess the feasibility of alternative measurement tools, and to discuss how to present the statistical information in an appropriate way (Commission 2009, p. 7).

Along with most social indicators researchers, including many economists, I suppose the first aim was accomplished over 40 years ago at the beginning of the social indicators movement. In Michalos (1982, pp. 6–7) I gave this brief overview of the National Income and Product Accounts.

> Generally speaking, I think everyone agrees that we are much better off with than without the national accounts···In spite of all the virtues of the accounts, they are not without defects or criticism···For example, it has been objected that by concentrating on marketplace activity in which everything must have a price in order to have value, "national economic accounting has promoted a 'new Philistinism'—an approach to life based on the principle of using monetary units as the common denominator of all that is important in human life" (Gross 1966, p. 167)···It has also been objected that the accounts provide misleading measures of services (Juster 1973, p. 32), that important distinctions are disguised behind aggregated figures (Olson 1969, p. 96) and that the various indicators in the system are subject to margins of error ranging from 10 to 20% (Gross 1966, pp. 165–166). More precisely, it has even been charged that "the data errors that go into calculating the gross national product are larger than the fluctuations in GNP that most economists find significant" (*Science* 1977, p. 649). Since the reliability and validity of virtually all indicators are subject to criticism, and the fact that economists are willing to misuse indicators is clearly a fault of the former rather than the latter, I don't think these objections to national economic

Michalos, A.C.: 2011. What did Stiglitz, Sen and Fitoussi get right and what did they get wrong? Social Indicators Research, 102, pp. 117–129. © Springer Science+Business Media B.V. 2010.

A.C. Michalos (✉)
University of Northern British Columbia, Prince George, BC, Canada
e-mail: michalos@brandonu.ca

A.C. Michalos, *Development of Quality of Life Theory and Its Instruments*,
DOI 10.1007/978-3-319-51149-8_14

> accounting are devastating. They should be accepted as sound warnings and prods to increased efforts to improve our systems.

In the remaining 129 pages of that chapter, following dozens of economists, I provided detailed criticisms of all the indicators drawn from the national accounts plus many more involving diverse features of living standards, e.g., issues of equity, earnings gaps, taxes and poverty. In short, since by the 1960s practically all scholars interested in measuring economic and social progress were fully aware of the "limits of GDP", one might have thought, as I did, that assembling nearly two dozen economists to "identify" those limits was anachronistic at best. So, my first question is this. Did the Commission add any criticisms of the GDP to those that an average, non-economist social indicators researcher had heard before?

The question is admittedly a bit vague concerning the identification of the average observer and his or her knowledge, and I did not attempt to operationalize any of it or undertake a survey of the relevant researchers. All I did was study the Commission's report carefully, looking for new insights about the national accounts in general and the GDP in particular. I did not recognize any new criticisms of GDP.

It was helpful for the Commission to assign GDP figures a secondary role next to net national product (NNP), i.e., they got this right.

> ···much emphasis is usually put on GDP although net national product (which takes into account the effect of depreciation), or real household income (which focuses on the real income of households within the economy) may be more relevant. These numbers differ markedly. Then, GDP is not wrong *as such,* but wrongly used. What is needed is a better understanding of the appropriate use of each measure (Commission 2009, p. 8).

At this point in time it is too early to know if NNP will get the attention it deserves, but I hope it does.

If one tracks the progress of UN agencies crafting increasingly comprehensive systems for monitoring progress with economic, social and environmental indicators from the Paris Biosphere Conference of 1968 to the UN Conference on the Human Environment in Stockholm (1972), the UNESCO/UNEP conference in Tbilisi (1977), the Rio Declaration on Environment and Development (1992), and the UN General Assembly resolution of 2002 naming the 2005–2014 period as the UN Decade of Education for Sustainable Development, it is clear that there have been and currently are many official agencies focused on such systems. Sustainable development as the UN official documents see it is the umbrella concept to pull together the diverse activities concerning social, political, economic and environmental progress. The OECD Progress of Societies initiative should be seen against the broader background of continuous UN activities over 30 years. As well, the Stiglitz Report should be read against those activities.

Against this background, it was also helpful to read

> ···the time is ripe for our measurement system to *shift emphasis from measuring economic production to measuring people's well-being*···This means working towards the development of a statistical system that complements measures of market activity by measures centred on people's well-being and by measures of sustainability. Such a system must, of

> necessity, be plural···aggregation across dimensions···is subordinate to the establishment of a broad statistical system that captures as many of the relevant dimensions as possible. Such a system should not just measure *average* levels of well-being···but also document the diversity of peoples' experiences and the linkages across various dimensions of people's life···a good place to start is the measurement of···living standards (Commission 2009, p. 12).

This is like the position of those who developed the Human Development Index and those of us working on the Canadian Index of Wellbeing (Michalos et al. 2010). We regard the composite index as the door to the system, which is where the main work gets done with detailed linkages, possibilities for interventions, and so on.

Besides shifting the main focus from production to "income and consumption", the Commission recommended shifting the focus from per capita figures to "measures of household income and consumption" and "jointly with wealth" because

> The household perspective entails taking account of payments between sectors, such as taxes going to government, social benefits coming from government, and interest payments on household loans going to financial corporations. Properly defined, household income and consumption should also reflect in-kind services provided by government, such as subsidized health care and educational services (Commission 2009, p. 3).

Presumably this recommendation is still in the context of making the best use of the National Accounts, because it does not address the issue of the distribution or variability of income within families. To get at the latter, one would need fairly detailed household income and expenditure surveys, which have been available in many countries for many years. In spite of the importance of wealth for measuring the sustainability of wellbeing, in Canada the production and publication of wealth data has been neglected in favour of income data for most of the 40 years I have been working in social indicators research (Sharpe and Arsenault 2008; Michalos 1988). This is particularly remarkable because some Canadian researchers have devoted considerable efforts to what is called a "capital approach" to measuring sustainable development and the root notion of the approach (i.e., wealth) is financial (Smith et al. 2001). So, the Commission's emphasis on producing good measures of wealth distribution is encouraging.

While the Commission's fifth recommendation to "broaden income measures to nonmarket activities" is certainly helpful, it is unclear that its suggestion to "start with information on how people spend their time" is the right place to start. I suppose the suggestion was an endorsement of the idea of having more time-diary studies and while I am not opposed to such studies, they may not be the most cost-effective instruments for learning about non-market activities that contribute to income. Given the relative stability of time use figures (for Canada at least) and the relatively high cost of such studies, particular surveys targeted just to non-market activities that contribute to income might be a better option.

The Commission's suggestion (pp. 14–15) to use the "following key dimensions···material living standards, health, education, personal activities including work, political voice and governance, social connections and relationships, environment (present and future conditions), insecurity, of an economic as well as a physical nature" do not seem to be as comprehensive as those proposed for the Canadian Index of Wellbeing, but there is considerable overlap. My guess is that they will put arts, culture and recreation in the "activities" slot. As I have said in many other places (e.g., Michalos et al. 2010), we have considerable liberty in loading general terms with as much as we like. So we do not know exactly what will be included under the recommended general headings.

We are given an indication of some sort of commitment by the Commission to Sen's (1982, 1985, 1987) "capabilities approach" to quality of life measurement. Here are the crucial points.

> The information relevant to valuing quality of life goes beyond people's selfreports and perceptions to include measures of their "functionings" and freedoms. In effect, what really matters are the capabilities of people, that is, the extent of their opportunity set and their freedom to choose among this set, the life they value. The choice of relevant functionings and capabilities for any quality of life measure is a value judgment, rather than a technical exercise. …Measuring these features requires both objective and subjective data (Commission 2009, p. 15).

Taken together, "functionings" and "capabilities" draw Sen's approach very close to Aristotle's approach in the *Nicomachean Ethics* (1999). However, when it is said that "what really matters are the capabilities of people, that is, the extent of their opportunity set and their freedom to choose from among this set, the life they value", the distance between the approaches of Sen and Aristotle becomes sizable. As emphasized in Michalos (tbp), Aristotle

> …distinguished the "possession" or "state" of virtue from "using" or the "activity" of virtue, and insisted that the former or mere capacities for action could not be sufficient for a good or happy life. After all, he remarked, "someone may be in a state that achieves no good—if, for instance, he is asleep or inactive in some other way" (Aristotle 1999, pp. 10–11). In his view, the good life was a life of "unimpeded" action proceeding from certain appropriate states and appropriately enjoyed…All things considered, Aristotle's characterization of a good or happy life is the clearest example we have from the ancients of the view that the quality of a person's or of a community's life is a function of the actual conditions of that life and what a person or community makes of those conditions…A good or happy life…–requires internal and external gifts and good luck beyond our control, but it also requires individual and communal initiative.

This is not the place to undertake a detailed analysis of Sen and Aristotle, but a few cautionary comments may be tolerated. I suspect that Sen's view is very close to Aristotle's when he writes, for example,

> The primary feature of a person's well-being is the functioning vector that he or she achieves···Opulence does, of course, *contribute* to functioning,···Rawlsian analysis of "primary goods" has forcefully demonstrated the usefulness of that perspective compared with reliance on the mental metric of utility···A person's *capability set* can be defined as the set of functioning vectors within his or her reach. In examining the well-being aspect of a person, attention can legitimately be paid to the capability set of the person and not just to the chosen functioning vector (Sen 1985, pp. 198–201).

However, when he writes things like "I argue in favour of focusing on the capability to function, i.e., what a person can *do* or can *be,* and argue against the more standard concentration on *opulence* (as in 'real income' estimates) or on *utility* (as in traditional 'welfare economic' formulations)" (Sen 1987, p. ix), he sends a message that seems to me to be fundamentally inconsistent with his most considered, largely Aristotelian and correct view. While he emphasizes here the words "do" and "be", it is really the word "can" that is troublesome. One could hardly be said to be living a good life, all things considered (including moral goodness), if for example, one was fully free and able to pull a drowning child from the water but chose instead to continue sun bathing on the beach. Freedom to choose to live as one wants according to one's values is certainly necessary but not sufficient for a good life. One could have the resources, including freedom, to do whatever one pleases but find nothing in particular pleasing. Such a person would probably not describe himself or herself as living a good life and would not be regarded as living a good life by most people. It is indeed unfortunate that Sen's most considered and correct view is essentially mislabeled as the 'capabilities view' and often misdescribed as well as misunderstood.

The Commission's ninth recommendation strikes me as one of its most important and most likely to be ignored in the short run. It is this: "Statistical offices should provide the information needed to aggregate across quality-of-life dimensions, allowing the construction of different indexes" (p. 16). Immediately following this recommendation, they tell us that "While assessing quality-of-life requires a plurality of indicators, there are strong demands to develop a single summary measure", but they never tell us why there are, or even better, why there should be such demands. However, the reason we need appropriate aggregation functions is revealed in the Commission's relatively unclear comments on "measuring sustainability". In my view, the Commission's failure to link the requirements of an acceptable measure of wellbeing or quality of life to those of an acceptable measure of sustainability is the weakest feature of the Stiglitz report. Here are the bare essentials of the Commission's views regarding wellbeing and sustainability.

> Measuring and assessing sustainability has been a central concern of the Commission. Sustainability poses the challenge of determining if at least the current level of well-being can be maintained for future generations…The assessment of sustainability is complementary to the question of current well-being or economic performance, and must be examined separately. …confusion may arise when one tries to combine current well-being and sustainability into a single indicator. To take an analogy, when driving a car, a meter that added up in one single number the current speed of the vehicle and the remaining level of gasoline would not be any help to the driver. Both pieces of information are critical and need to be displayed in distinct, clearly visible areas of the dashboard (Commission 2009, pp. 16–17).

While it would indeed be useless to add some measure of speed to some measure of gasoline, the requirement to link an overall quality of life measure to a sustainability measure is absolutely necessary because quality of life is precisely the thing that we seek to sustain and even improve. Absent a clear vision of what it is we want to sustain, where should a sustainability analysis begin? There is no good reason to try to create every measure at the same time, but it does seem to me that there is a natural order of progression in research programs leading from a clear articulation of what it is one wants to sustain to a clear articulation of what will be required to do the job. Although one measure will not accomplish both tasks, there is a clear asymmetry of order such that the second task cannot be accomplished unless the first task is accomplished *and* directly linked to it, i.e., the possession of a good measure of the quality of life is a necessary condition for possessing a good measure of its sustainability. Given this asymmetry, it is dangerous to insist on the need to separate the two tasks unless the separation is made only in the interest of recognizing and emphasizing the order of priority.

While I do believe that some sort of aggregated measure of the most salient constituents and/or determinants of "quality-of-life dimensions" is important if one's aim is to make a comprehensive assessment of the overall quality of life, there are plenty of considerations in favour and against such measures. An extensive list may be found in Michalos et al. (2010), and more detailed reviews of alternative aggregation procedures with their respective advantages and disadvantages may be found in Nardo et al. (2005). Some readers will recall Mike Hagerty's committee in which we tried without success to get an index that all members of the International Society for Quality of Life Studies (ISQOLS) could get behind. The results of that exercise were published in Hagerty et al. (2001), and lessons learned from that exercise might have been useful for the Commission's work and others' as well.

In order to know if the current quality of life is sustainable, at a minimum one must have measures that capture the main constituents of that sort of life and their rates of change for some determinate period of time, and one must have measures of the determinants of that sort of life that includes their stock values and their rates of change for the same period. Just as one can calculate the sustainability of one's car travel by relating one's average speed to one's stock of gasoline, one could calculate the sustainability of one's quality of life by relating one's rate of usage of one's stock of determinants to the total stock available. Of course, the calculation of the sustainability of the quality of one's life is much more complicated than the calculation of the sustainability of one's car travel, but the game is the same. We have to measure what we want to sustain, what resources are required to sustain it and the rates of change of each relative to the other. In broad strokes and setting aside issues of waste absorption, our quality of life is sustainable across any period of time if the rate of use of our total stock of resources is equal to or less than the rate of resource-use required to sustain it.

According to the Commission (p. 17),

> There are two versions to the stock approach to sustainability. One version just looks at variations in each stock separately, assessing whether the stock is increasing or decreasing, with a view particularly to doing whatever is necessary to keep each above some critical threshold. The second version converts all these assets into a monetary equivalent, thereby implicitly assuming substitutability between different types of capital, so that a decrease in, say, natural capital might be offset by a sufficient increase in physical capital (appropriately weighted).

There is, in fact, at least a third approach in which one assesses the value of constituents and/or determinants of a good life by the degree to which they contribute to some sorts of mental states as reported through subjective assessments of life as a whole, e.g., life satisfaction, happiness, contentment, utility. Assuming that it is such mental states in particular that people want to sustain (a view which Aristotle, Sen and I, among others, do not share), this third approach would translate physical and other kinds of assets into a subjective wellbeing equivalent to assess benefits, costs and sustainability (Diener et al. 2009). While the Commission does accept the necessity of adopting "a pragmatic approach that combines a monetary indicator···and a set of physical indicators devoted to environmental issues" (p. 62), it never includes subjective assessments in the mix of sustainability measures. The closest it comes to including subjective assessments in the mix is in comments like the following.

> In order to measure sustainability, what we need are indicators that tell us the sign of the change [positive or negative] in the quantities of the different factors that matter for future well-being. Putting the sustainability issue in these terms compels recognition that sustainability requires the simultaneous preservation or increase in several 'stocks': quantities and qualities not only of natural resources but also of human, social and physical capital. Any approach that focuses on only a part of these items does not offer a comprehensive view of sustainability (pp. 77–78).

As we will see below, the Commission does not seem to fully appreciate the range of issues involved in human and social capital, nor the necessity of statistical offices investigating the full range of issues.

Given the current status of what we know about what matters most to most people in most countries and what we know about how to measure those things, one can only agree with the Commission when it is asserted that

> ···the commission regards its report as opening a discussion rather than closing it···a global debate around the issues and recommendations raised in this report provides an important venue for a discussion of···what we···care about··· At the national level, round-tables should be established···to identify and prioritise those indicators···the commission hopes that this report will provide the impetus not only for this broader discussion, but for on-going research into the development of better metrics··· (p. 18).

In its discussion of problems concerning the "measurement of government-provided services", the Commission makes a quite general point that is applicable also to goods and worth emphasizing and endorsing here, namely,

> Improving the volume measures of outputs does not dispense with the need to improve – and publish – the volume measures of inputs. Only if both the outputs and inputs of service production are well captured will it be possible to estimate productivity change and undertake productivity comparisons across countries (p. 28).

These remarks merit attention because some scholars have suggested that comprehensive reports of what matters to people should focus only on output or outcome measures. Setting aside the fact that what one regards as an input or an output indicator is largely determined by one's measurement purposes, one cannot begin to assess the sustainability of what matters most unless one has both kinds of measures.

All members of the team working on the Canadian Index of Wellbeing will be pleased to read that "…of course, widening the scope of asset and production measures brings with it more imputations" (p. 29). We found that as we moved from the domain of living standards with its relatively vast store of measures and data to the domains of health, community vitality, democratic engagement, leisure and culture, we were faced with increasingly great gaps in data availability that required considerable boldness in making more and more imputations in order to construct time series trends over several years (Michalos et al. 2010).

Regarding the "key dimensions" listed above (i.e., material living standards, health, education, etc.), the Commission addresses "cross-cutting issues" such as the importance of measuring "*inequalities* in individual conditions in the various dimensions of life", assessing the "*relationship* between the various dimensions of quality of life" and the need to "*aggregate* the rich array of measures in a parsimonious way" (pp. 54–56). With respect to the problem of aggregation, the Commission issues a profound challenge to official statistical agencies.

> The search for a scalar measure of quality of life is often perceived as the single most important challenge faced by quality-of-life research. While this emphasis is partly misplaced-the informational content of any aggregate index will always reflect the quality of the measures used in its construction—the demands in this field are strong, and statistical offices should play a role in answering them (p. 56).

My impression, based on anecdotes and informal discussions among quality-of-life researchers in many countries rather than on careful research, is that there are relatively few statistical offices with much enthusiasm for taking on all the problems of constructing aggregate quality-of-life indexes. In fact, on the page following the apparent challenge just quoted, the Commission tells us that "…rather than focusing on constructing a single summary measure of quality of life, statistical systems should provide the data required for computing various aggregate measures according to the philosophic perspective of each user" (p. 57).

This suggestion is misguided for two reasons. First, it is counter-productive to recommend that research priority should be given to individual indicators that might find their way into an aggregated composite because in all statistical offices priority is already given to such indicators. It is precisely this bias for producing individual indicators within relatively discrete silos containing apparently closely related statistical time series that has made it so difficult for people working in statistical offices to even imagine composite measures linking the information in diverse silos. Second, the absence of adequately resourced specific programs of development of composite indexes prevents researchers from raising important questions concerning, for example, the completeness or incompleteness of current stocks of statistical time series, links in the form of causal interactions or mere correlations among the indicators housed in different silos, the collection of redundant indicators needlessly absorbing scarce resources and the failure to collect important data whose availability might reveal serious limitations and/or distortions of our understanding of the quality of our lives.

Later in the report, the Commission begins to articulate some of what was just written in the previous paragraph, but it is immediately followed by a note of caution.

> …the challenge of providing a more parsimonious description of QoL than the one provided by scores of non-monetary indicators is real…the most likely consequences of producing only sub-domain indicators could well be that GDP will remain the dominant indicator, and that statistics produced with no concern for a synthesis will fail to supply appropriate data. On the other hand, the search for a synthetic indicator risks embroiling statistical institutions in political debates that put their neutrality at risk (p. 207).

Apart from the two good reasons to avoid any suggestion of prioritizing research programs in statistical offices, there is, nevertheless, a very good reason to devote adequate resources to developing reliable and valid individual indicators within their traditional silos and to developing aggregate/composite indexes of such indicators simultaneously. The fact is that we need both kinds of statistical instruments to address the full array of issues that arise when one takes seriously such questions as 'What matters most to most people?', 'How can we measure what matters most?' and 'How can we measure the sustainability of what matters most?'.

At the end of Chap. 2, on "Conceptual approaches to measuring quality of life", the Commission tells us that "Measures of subjective well-being provide key information about people's quality of life." and it recommends (among other things) that "Statistical offices should incorporate questions to capture people's life evaluations, hedonic experiences and priorities in their own surveys" (p. 58). This is ok as far as it goes, but it does not go far enough. Statistical offices must be as aggressive in exploring the full range of subjective determinants and constituents of wellbeing as they are in exploring the full range of objective determinants and constituents. Thus, the following sorts of things should be on their research agenda: generic feelings of positive or negative affect; specific feelings of fear, joy and contentment; attitudes of racism, sexism, classism and homophobia; beliefs in progress and democratic process; knowledge of natural sciences, arts and current events; personal standards for evaluation like equity, justice, moral virtue and beauty; motives like vengeance or the pursuit of wealth; needs for love, friendship, social and self esteem; wants for luxury items, leisure activities or just free time; personal assessments of one's own happiness, satisfaction with life as a whole or domains/aspects of life (job, marriage, housing), satisfaction with the overall quality of one's life or one's overall wellbeing. Researchers do not have direct, sensible access to other people's felt affect, attitudes, beliefs, knowledge, motives, values, evaluation standards, needs, wants and personal assessments of happiness, etc., although it is precisely such attributes that supremely characterize our species and human agency in particular.

If we are going after comprehensive assessments of human wellbeing, we must obtain much more information than can be reasonably categorized under the three headings of "people's life evaluations, hedonic experiences and priorities". My impression is that relatively few people in national statistical offices around the world are remotely interested in undertaking research addressing the issues listed in the previous paragraph, preferring instead to leave such things to academics. The main problems with this status quo approach to subjective indicators are that (1) academics do not have access to the same level of resources that statistical offices have (so academics' sample sizes, frequency of surveys, levels of analyses, for example, are in relatively shorter supply), (2) public officials pay more attention to analyses coming from their statistical offices than from academics, (3) many academics prefer to use data collected by statistical offices rather than collect their own, and therefore (4), relatively deep, theory-driven survey research leading to greater understanding of people's assessments of the quality of life will continue to be overwhelmed by relatively shallow, atheoretical research (depending on one's definition of 'theory' (Michalos 2006)) and, what is worse, (5) public policy will continue to be made on relatively half-baked research (i.e., research purporting to explain important aspects of our lives on the basis of incorrectly specified equations lacking crucial explanatory variables) and (6) people will continue to suffer the consequences.

Given the rough state but considerable promise of ecological footprint analyses, I would encourage the many advocates of that approach to continue their research. However, I agree with the Commission's remark that "···much of the information that it conveys about national contributions to non-sustainability is imbedded in a simpler indicator, the carbon footprint, which is therefore one good candidate for monitoring humanity's pressure on the climate,···" (p. 79). (An excellent critique of ecological footprint analyses may be found in Crummey and Victor 2008.)

Regarding what the Commission calls "environmental sustainability", which seems to be some sort of mixture of environmental aspects of economic sustainability, we are told that "···at this stage of the debate, economists do not have any particular qualification for suggesting what the right choices are. This is why we will not propose any closed list of these indicators here" (p. 79). We are not told why those who formed the Commission could not come up with a short list of environmental/ecological experts to serve on it. One would have thought that at this point in time the necessity of considering the natural environment in any reasonable assessment of the sustainability of human wellbeing, quality of life or progress would have been obvious. Unfortunately, it does not appear to have been obvious to those who formed the Commission. So, the best the group could do was to offer some suggestions to put some appropriate material on a dashboard sometime.

The under-representation of environmental/ecological experts on the Commission is matched by the under-representation of non-economist social scientists, and the limited results are revealed in Chap. 2 on "Quality of life". To begin with, we are told that

> The Commission's goal in this area has not been to reach a shared understanding of what 'quality of life' means but, rather, to identify areas where credible measures, based on clear conventions and definitions, could be established. As a result, this report does not aim to be comprehensive: attention is limited to areas where members of the Commission had specific competencies and where available indicators allow drawing a more comprehensive assessment of QoL (p. 143).

In a footnote we are told that "The term 'quality of life' is used in this chapter to refer to those aspects of life that shape human well-being beyond the command of economic resources" (p. 143).

In a footnote on p. 208 we find the remark that "the social indicator movement was particularly active in the 1960s and 1970s. Key contributions from this research are gathered in the journal, *Social Indicators Research,* founded in 1974, which publishes research dealing with measurement of the quality of life". As you can imagine, the Editor and Founder of that journal, which since its first issue in 1974 has carried the subtitle "An International and Interdisciplinary Journal for Quality-of-Life Measurement", would naturally want to have a look at the references for Chap. 2. Of the 161 references listed, there was one to *Social Indicators Research,* i.e., one useful paper in a series containing at the time of the Commission's work about 90 volumes, with about 30 articles per volume or roughly 2700 articles covering 35 years of research! One might have expected something useful could be found in *Citation Classics from Social Indicators Research* (Michalos 2005), the collection of papers reviewing the first 30 years of the journal's publication. As well, the overview of the past, present and future of "the quality-of-life movement" by Sirgy et al. (2006) might have been useful, or the later global surveys in the collection by MØller et al. (2008). Health-related quality of life research reported in *Quality of Life Research* over the past 18 years was entirely neglected. Taken together, all these omissions are enough to make an interested reader suspicious of the criteria of selection of issues to be discussed and places to look for useful information concerning those issues.

In its critique of the method of "aggregating averages across domains" to obtain a single value for a composite index, the Commission mentions 4 limitations: (1) such values "cannot track the accumulation of disadvantages by certain groups", (2) "the choice of weights for various domains" remains unclear and/or arbitrary, (3) "the interpretation of *changes* in these aggregate indicators" remains unexplained, and (4) "the approach does not allow for a diversity of viewpoints about the relative importance of various dimensions of QoL" (pp. 208–209). Interested readers may find 18 additional relatively familiar alleged disadvantages plus a dozen advantages of composite indexes in Michalos et al. (2010). Regarding the 4 limitations mentioned above, while the Commission's discussion would lead one to believe that they are peculiar to multidimensional indexes, each of these applies to the unidimensional GDP values as well. We have already noticed the Commission's insistence on taking account of inequalities and/or inequities in the distribution of GDP, i.e., issue (1), and treating money spent or made on preventing or redressing evils as having or producing the same value as money spent or made on obtaining goods (issue 2).

Issue (3) is essentially a variant of (2) insofar as one cannot fully comprehend what a particular numerical change means without examining the causes for the changes, e.g., a nice upward spike in GDP per capita that is caused by selling one's last supply of drinking water would be a sign of disaster rather than progress. Similarly, the history of the development of the composition of GDP right up to the debates going on today about "greening" it are just examples of issue (4). (Incidentally, given the number of times in the Commission's report that the problem of assigning weights to indicators is mentioned, some references to the early work of Andrews and Withey (1976) showing the relative unimportance of "importance weights" to judgments of perceived quality of life and to the more recent work of Hagerty and Land (2007) showing that agreements and disagreements about weights assigned to objective indicators will be largely overwhelmed by the correlations among indicators and "much rarer than expected" except in some relatively extraordinary circumstances.)

It would be foolish to under-emphasize or fail to address the technical, political and any other kinds of problems presented in the development of composite indexes representing multidimensional phenomena, but it is a demonstrable mistake to suppose that many if not most of the problems with such indexes are unique to them. It is also a mistake to suppose that a small set of diverse dimensions with their individual values conveniently displayed in a dashboard-like figure can solve the fundamental problem that a composite is supposed to solve, namely, the reduction of a multi-dimensional to a uni-dimensional space. The most one can hope for from a dashboard of indicators with no aggregation mechanism is some kind of a cost-benefit dominance of values, i.e., one counts the number of indicator values showing positive movement compared to the number showing negative movement, assumes movements of the same size in the right or wrong direction are equally important, and creates policies and programs to address the apparent state of affairs (Michalos 1970, 1978, 1980a, b, 1981a, b, 1982, 1997). As the list of publications will show, I have used and defended such decision-making rules largely on pragmatic grounds for many years. The main point I want to make here is that one should not make a virtue out of pragmatic necessity. A dashboard model with an aggregation mechanism has been developed by Jochen Jesinghaus and his colleagues at the Joint Research Centre in Italy, but this model was not discussed in the Commission's report. (See the Millennium Development Goals Indicators Dashboard at http://esl.jrc.it/dc/mdg_unsd for more on this option.)

If at the end of many work days of many people over many years the best we can get is cost-benefit dominance or near-dominance decision making, then so be it. We will have to live with it. However, at this point in time, I would prefer to accept the wisdom of one of my favourite philosophers and former manager of the New York Yankees, Yoggi Berra, when he said, "It ain't over till it's over." If we invest enough resources, maybe we can come close to a workable composite index representing the multidimensional space of a sustainable good quality of life. The Commission on the Measurement of Economic Performance and Social Progress had an opportunity to take us a few steps closer to that goal, but for one reason or another failed. According to Gertner (2010, p. MM60),

> "Joe has a little bit of the pragmatism that pushed Mahbub," [ul Haq, creator of the Human Development Index] Sen said, referring to Stiglitz, who was the driving force behind the commission's work. "You can see when push comes to shove, he'd say, 'For God's sake, let's do something that changes the world.'"

I hoped they would, and I still hope that others might yet do it. Roughly adding up the score considering what the Commission got right and wrong, I counted 10 right and 11 wrong. In baseball, that would give it a batting average of 10/21 = 0.476, which in baseball would be excellent. Unfortunately for the

Commission, I doubt that it is reasonable to assess their success by the standards of baseball players. Considering the opportunity and resources given to the Commission, a success rate of slightly less than chance is hardly a triumph. If anyone in the future is offered the same opportunity and resources, which I suppose is unlikely in the near future, I hope they will remember and keep reminding each other that human beings are complex organisms living in very complex social, political, economic and environmental conditions, and that a plausible measure of progress will almost certainly have to be very complex. So it will take time and other resources, and most of all, patience to develop. We should expect progress to be slow, but help to keep it moving.

References

Andrews, F. M., & Withey, S. B. (1976). *Social indicators of well-being*. New York: Plenum Press.

Aristotle. (1999). *Nicomachean ethics* (2nd ed., T. Irwin, Trans.). Indianapolis: Hackett Publishing Company.

Commission. (2009). In J. E. Stiglitz, A. Sen, & J.-P. Fitoussi (Eds.), *Report by the commission on the measurement of economic performance and social progress*. Paris: Commission.

Crummey, E., & Victor, P. (2008). *Statistics Canada's ecological footprint workshop: Final report,* March 1 (Draft obtained from P. Victor, Professor of Environmental Studies, York University).

Diener, E., Lucas, R. E., Schimmack, U., & Helliwell, J. F. (2009). *Well-being for public policy*. Oxford: Oxford University Press.

Gertner, J. (2010). The rise and fall of the G.D.P. *New York Times, Sunday Magazine,* May 16, p. MM60.

Gross, B. M. (1966). The state of the nation: Social systems accounting. In R. A. Bauer (Ed.), *Social indicators*. Cambridge: The M.I.T. Press.

Hagerty, M. R., Cummins, R. A., Ferriss, A. L., Land, K. C., Michalos, A. C., Peterson, M., et al. (2001). Quality of life indexes for national policy: Review and agenda for research. *Social Indicators Research, 55*(1), 1–96.

Hagerty, M. R., & Land, K. C. (2007). Constructing summary indices of quality of life: A model for the effect of heterogeneous importance weights. *Sociological Methods and Research, 35,* 455–496.

Juster, F. T. (1973). A framework for the measurement of economic and social performance. In M. Moss (Ed.), *The measurement of economic and social performance*. New York: National Bureau of Economic Research.

Michalos, A. C. (1970). Cost-benefit versus expected utility acceptance rules. *Theory and Decision, 1,* 61–88.

Michalos, A. C. (1978). *Foundations of decision making*. Ottawa: Canadian Library of Philosophy.

Michalos, A. C. (1980a). *North American social report: A comparative study of the quality of life in Canada and the USA from 1964 to 1974, volume one foundations, population and health.* Dordrecht: D. Reidel.

Michalos, A. C. (1980b). *North American social report: A comparative study of the quality of life in Canada and the USA from 1964 to 1974, volume two, crime, justice and politics.* Dordrecht: D. Reidel.

Michalos, A. C. (1981a). *North American social report: A comparative study of the quality of life in Canada and the USA from 1964 to 1974, volume three, science, education and recreation*. Dordrecht: D. Reidel.

Michalos, A. C. (1981b). *North American social report: A comparative study of the quality of life in Canada and the USA from 1964 to 1974, volume four, environment, transportation and housing*. Dordrecht: D. Reidel.

Michalos, A. C. (1982). *North American social report: A comparative study of the quality of life in Canada and the USA from 1964 to 1974, volume five, economics, religion and morality*. Dordrecht: D. Reidel.

Michalos, A. C. (1988). A case for a progressive annual net wealth tax. *Public Affairs Quarterly, 2*, 105–140.

Michalos, A. C. (1997). Combining social economic and environmental indicators to measure sustainable human well-being. *Social Indicators Research, 40*, 221–258.

Michalos, A. C. (Ed.). (2005). *Citation classics from social indicators research: The most cited articles edited and introduced by Alex C. Michalos*. Dordrecht: Springer.

Michalos, A. C. (2006). Logic, philosophy of science and the quality of life. In *The encyclopedia of life support systems* (UNESCO, online encyclopedia).

Michalos, A. C., et al. (2010). *An approach to the canadian index of wellbeing*. Toronto: Atkinson Charitable Foundation.

Michalos, A. C. (tbp). The good life: Eighth century to fourth century BCE. In K. Land (Ed.), *Handbook of social indicators and quality of life research*. Dordrecht: Springer.

MØller, V., Huschka, D., & Michalos, A. C. (Eds.). (2008). *Barometers of quality of life around the globe: How are we doing?*. Dordrecht: Springer Science and Business Media B.V.

Nardo, M., Saisana, M., Saltelli, A., & Tarantola, S. (2005). *Tools for composite indicators building*. Ispra, Italy: Joint Research Centre European Commission.

Olson, M. (1969). Community values, social measurement and transportation policy. In Highway Research Board (Ed.), *Transportation and community values*. Washington: National Academy of Science-National Academy of Engineering.

Science. (1977). *Game theorist Morgenstern Dies* (p. 649).

Sen, A. (1982). *Choice welfare and measurement*. Oxford: Blackwell.

Sen, A. (1985). Well-being, agency and freedom: The Dewey lectures 1984. *Journal of Philosophy, 82*(4), 169–221.

Sen, A. (1987). *Commodities and capabilities*. Oxford: Oxford University Press.

Sharpe, A., & Arsenault, J.-F. (2008). *Living standards domain of the Canadian index of wellbeing*. Toronto: Atkinson Charitable Foundation.

Sirgy, M. J., Michalos, A. C., Ferriss, A. L., Easterlin, R. A., Patrick, D., & Pavot, W. (2006). The quality-of-life (QOL) research movement: Past, present and future. *Social Indicators Research, 76*(3), 343–466.

Smith, R. C., Simard, C., & Sharpe, A. (2001). *A proposed approach to environment and sustainable development indicators based on capital. Memorandum prepared for the national round table on the environment and the economy's environment and sustainable development indicators initiative*. Ottawa: NRTEE.

Chapter 15
Progress in Measuring Knowledge, Attitudes and Behaviours Concerning Sustainable Development Among Tenth Grade Students in Manitoba

Alex C. Michalos, P. Maurine Kahlke, Karen Rempel, Anu Lounatvuori, Anne MacDiarmid, Heather Creech and Carolee Buckler

Introduction

The aim of this paper is to present additional progress since Michalos et al. (2011, 2012), on the development of standardized measures of tenth grade students' knowledge, attitudes and behaviours concerning sustainable development as those

---

Michalos, A.C., Kahlke, P.M., Rempel, K., Lounatvuori, A., MacDiarmid, A., Creech, H., & Buckler, C.: 2015. Progress in measuring knowledge, attitudes and behaviours concerning sustainable development among tenth grade students in Manitoba. Social Indicators Research, 123, pp. 303–336. © Springer Science+Business Media B.V. 2014.

A.C. Michalos (✉)
University of Northern British Columbia, Prince George, BC, Canada
e-mail: michalos@brandonu.ca

P. Maurine Kahlke
9005 College Drive, Coldstream, BC V1B 2P7, Canada
e-mail: pmhatch@shaw.ca

K. Rempel · A. Lounatvuori
Faculty of Education, Centre for Aboriginal and Rural Education Studies, Brandon University, Brandon, MB R7A 6A9, Canada
e-mail: Rempelk@brandonu.ca

A. Lounatvuori
e-mail: lounatvuoria@brandonu.ca

A. MacDiarmid
Manitoba Education and Advanced Learning, 1567 Dublin Ave., Winnipeg, MB R3E 3J5, Canada
e-mail: Anne.MacDiarmid@gov.mb.ca

A.C. Michalos, *Development of Quality of Life Theory and Its Instruments*,
DOI 10.1007/978-3-319-51149-8_15

concepts are understood by United Nations Educational, Scientific and Cultural Organization (UNESCO), the lead agency for the UN Decade for Education for Sustainable Development 2005–2014 (DESD).

One of the challenges that has been identified during the DESD is that of monitoring and evaluation, and in particular assessing whether efforts invested in education for sustainable development (ESD) can lead to positive learning outcomes in students. There has been limited evidence to date that ESD can influence knowledge, attitudes and behaviours that will contribute to sustainable development (Michalos et al. 2012). A rare example is the 2008–2009 International Civics and Citizenship Study (ICCS) across 38 countries, in which researchers found a positive correlation between teaching about citizenship and the subsequent participation of students in active citizenship (joining student organizations, volunteering in the community, and so forth) (Schulz et al. 2010). However, the ICCS does not explore outcomes across all the dimensions of sustainability—social, economic, and environmental—nor has there yet been an attempt at developing any standardized measures for assessment of the outcomes of ESD. Other examples of such explorations are difficult to find in the research literature.

The Grade 10 research was therefore structured with two objectives in mind:

1. To increase the precision of standardized measures of the knowledge, attitudes and behaviours of Manitoban tenth grade students towards sustainable development.
2. To obtain evidence of changes in knowledge, attitudes and behaviours among students that might be correlated to current investments in education for sustainable development (ESD).

Definition of Education for Sustainable Development (ESD)

The UN DESD has led to the exploration and implementation of new forms of teaching and learning that will support the evolution of more sustainable societies (UNESCO 2012). At its heart, ESD is about what and how people learn in order to live more responsibly and respectfully on the planet (CMEC 2014). Among the many definitions of ESD, UNESCO considers that ESD is learning that "empowers everyone to make informed decisions for environmental integrity, economic

H. Creech
International Institute for Sustainable Development, 161 Portage Ave. E., 6th Floor, Winnipeg, MB R3B 0Y4, Canada
e-mail: hecreech@gmail.com

C. Buckler
Manitoba Education, 1567 Dublin Avenue, Winnipeg, MB R3E 3J5, Canada
e-mail: Carolee.Buckler@gov.mb.ca

viability and a just society for present and future generations, while respecting cultural diversity" (UNESCO 2013).

ESD is considered by many to be an umbrella framework that connects a number of UN initiatives and types of education including, for example, the Dakar commitments in 2000 to Education for All (EFA), the Millennium Development Goal (MDG) for universal primary education, the UN Literacy Decade 2003–2012, The UN Secretary General's Global Education First Initiative (GEFI), the Tbilisi +35 Intergovernmental conference on environmental education (2012), and the inclusion of ESD in the outcomes of the 2012 UN Conference on Sustainable Development (Rio+20) (Wals 2009, pp. 8–10, 25–30; GEFI nd; Tbilisi +35 2012; UN 2012). Articles 8 and 9 of the Bonn Declaration, which was accepted by the delegates at the UNESCO World Conference on Education for Sustainable Development in Bonn, Germany (31 March–2 April, 2009) emphasize the richness of ESD.

> 8. ESD is based on values of justice, equity, tolerance, sufficiency and responsibility. It promotes gender equality, social cohesion and poverty reduction and emphasizes care, integrity and honesty, as articulated in the Earth Charter. ESD is underpinned by principles that support sustainable living, democracy and human well-being. Environmental protection and restoration, natural resource conservation and sustainable use, addressing unsustainable production and consumption patterns, and the creation of just and peaceful societies are also important principles underpinning ESD.
>
> 9. ESD emphasizes creative and critical approaches, long term thinking, innovation and empowerment for dealing with uncertainty, and for solving complex problems. ESD highlights the interdependence of environment, economy, society, and cultural diversity from local to global levels, and takes account of past, present and future (UNESCO 2009).

As the commitment periods for EFA, the MDGs, and other initiatives come to an end in 2015, global consultations on a post 2015 development agenda and the setting of new sustainable development goals (SDGs) are underway. Most encouraging is the consideration of ESD in the post 2015 thematic consultation on education (UNICEF, UNESCO 2013) and in the outcome document of the UN Open Working Group on sustainable development goals (UN 2010, Goal 4). These new discussions represent a significant reinforcement of views that education is essential to the building of more sustainable societies. As countries continue efforts initiated during the DESD to equip their citizens with the knowledge, perspectives and skills needed for today and into the future, it will be important to provide them with measurement and assessment tools so that they may learn whether and how their efforts are making a difference.

Education for Sustainable Development in Manitoba

In 2004, the provincial Ministry of Education declared ESD to be one of the Ministry's top priorities and developed a provincial ESD Action Plan (2004–2008) that directed the first steps in fostering teaching and learning for sustainability in elementary and secondary classrooms; with follow-up actions in subsequent years designed to maintain momentum on reorienting the provincial education system towards sustainability.

The action plan was designed to support educators in their efforts to teach about and for sustainability. The action plan committed the Ministry to a suite of actions including:

- Benchmarking of sustainability outcomes in the curriculum;
- Integrating sustainable development concepts into new curricula;
- Holding in-service teacher training workshops and other projects to enhance teaching and learning for sustainability;
- Providing information, best practices, and learning resources on ESD.

Since 2004, Manitoba has taken an integrated approach to the implementation of sustainable development across the curriculum rather than developing a standalone course. In 2008, correlation charts were prepared that aligned ESD and ESD learning outcomes across the existing curriculum; professional development workshops were then conducted in the following years to help teachers understand sustainability, ESD, and how to use the correlation charts in their teaching practice. ESD is now embedded in the K-12 curriculum with specific outcomes benchmarked in science, social studies, health and physical education as well as Technical Vocational education. Curriculum revision occurs on an as-needed basis when research or pedagogy provide new understandings in a subject area. When curriculum is revised the ESD learning outcomes are embedded and are benchmarked and posted for educators when finalized.

However, the province considers that several other factors have influenced change in the education system, in addition to the benchmarking of learning outcomes and changes in curricula.

- An ESD website was established in 2008 as a hub for resources and information for educators.
- Two grants have been consistently provided over the years by the Ministry to support engagement by the schools and School Divisions, the ESD categorical Grant provided to School Divisions in the fall of each year and the ESD Action Project grant which provides 20 grants annually for up to $2,000. These grants support all aspects of sustainability implementation such as covering teacher release time, professional development, educational resources, and supporting older schools to green their facilities, through reducing water use, minimizing waste, the greening of school-grounds and sustainable transportation.
- The Eco-Globe Schools recognition program was established in 2008 to profile and acknowledge individual school commitment and innovation for sustainability.
- From 2007 to 2010 Manitoba Education offered the Sustainability and Education Academy (SEdA) to provide learning opportunities for senior level officials of schools and school divisions on how to integrate sustainable development into all aspects of the K-12 education system (e.g. governance,

facilities and operations, curriculum, teaching and learning, capacity building and partnerships). In partnership with SEdA, Manitoba Education and Advanced Learning released the Whole System Domain Framework to School Divisions in 2012 to track progress.
- The province has encouraged schools to put in place Sustainable Development action plans to reinforce sustainability as a "whole school" approach, one that extends beyond the curriculum and addresses the entire planning and management of the school facility. The Guide for Sustainable Schools in Manitoba supports schools in this process and to develop annual ESD school plans.

The turning point in ESD adoption is considered to be 2010, after the final SEdA, when demand for ESD professional development increased significantly, school divisions began to promote ESD as a priority, pedagogy was shifting, and schools began to look to the early adopters for ideas and guidance on ESD implementation (MacDiarmid 2014).

In order to determine if these ESD efforts were making a difference in Manitoba, in 2009 Manitoba Education partnered with the International Institute for Sustainable Development on a study to acquire a measure of students' understanding, attitudes and behaviours favourable to sustainable development. This led to the first survey of Grade 10 students (Michalos et al. 2011): the cohort completed the survey instrument in 2010, at a time when they would have benefitted from only a year or two of exposure to the province's correlation exercises, curriculum revisions and capacity building for ESD across school divisions, and without the full emphasis on whole school sustainability action plans.

The following paper presents the results of the 2014 survey of a second cohort: This group of Grade 10 students has now had an exposure to ESD throughout most of their years of formal education. Comparisons made later in this paper to the results from the first cohort will contribute to understanding whether ESD is making a difference in the education system of Manitoba.

Structure of the Paper

The structure of the paper is as follows. In the next section "Questionnaire, Methods and Sample Statistics" we briefly describe the questionnaire, sampling methods and sample demographic statistics. Section "Descriptive Statistics" provides descriptive statistics for the three sets of sentences concerning knowledge, attitudes and behaviours, including rank orderings of the sentences in each set according to their numbers of valid responses, percentages of respondents giving responses that are favourable for sustainable development, mean scores, percentages of 'don't know' and 'don't understand' responses, and simple missing values. In section "Section A: Knowledge" we describe the three indexes, namely, the *Index of Knowledge of SD, Index of Favourable Attitudes Toward SD* and *Index of Favourable Behaviours Toward SD.* Section "Indexes of Knowledge, Attitudes and

Behaviours" reviews correlations among the indexes and results of regressing the Behaviours Index on the other two. The paper ends with a brief summary in section "Bi-variate and Multi-variate Relations".

Questionnaire, Methods and Sample Statistics

Survey Instrument

A three-page questionnaire was developed that contained three sets of sentences which might describe respondents' knowledge, attitudes and behaviours concerning SD. The complete questionnaire with on-scale means, numbers and percentages of responses is reproduced in "Appendix 1". "Appendix 2" contains on- and off-scale numbers and percentages including those for 'don't know', 'don't understand' and simply missing values for sentences in Sections A–C identified only by the sentence numbers.

Standardized measures of respondents' knowledge, attitudes and behaviours were crafted for each attribute, with 20 items in Section A, 15 in Section B and 16 in Section C, respectively. In each Section, respondents were asked to indicate their level of agreement or disagreement with each sentence on a Likert-type scale running from 'strongly agree' (=1), through 'neutral' (=3) to 'strongly disagree' (=5). For the sentences in Section A, 'strongly agree' and 'agree' responses indicate that the respondent's knowledge is consistent with themes regarded as necessary and/or favourable for sustainable development. For most of the sentences in Sections B and C, 'strongly agree' and 'agree' responses indicate that the respondent's attitudes and behaviours, respectively, are supportive and/or favourable for sustainable development. A few sentences were worded negatively as a hedge against erroneous responses, e.g., always checking the same response category resulting from fatigue, boredom, lack of understanding or somewhat playful malice (Sudman and Bradburn 1983). Such sentences are clearly identified for analytic purposes and where necessary, responses are reverse-coded so that percentages indicating views favourable to sustainable development are used correctly.

While on-scale responses give us information about students' levels of agreement, disagreement or neutrality regarding sentences in each section, off-scale responses are equally important because they indicate that students did not know how to respond or did not understand the sentence. For any given on-scale response, it is possible that students were not entirely sure how to respond and/or did not fully understand the sentence being considered, but we have no way of measuring levels of such response nuances. However, as we will show shortly, off-scale responses provide useful guides to diverse difficulties with some sentences.

Following these three sections, there was a set of demographic questions concerning gender, age, cultural/ethnic background, school name and school division.

Survey Process

The questionnaire and appropriate letters of permission received approval from the Brandon University Research Ethics Committee in November 2013. In June and September 2013 an email letter was sent from the Sustainable Development Coordinator of the Manitoba Ministry for Education to the Superintendents of all 36 School Divisions in the province. The letter briefly reviewed the history and purposes of our earlier surveys and the new survey, and requested cooperation to ensure successful completion of the initiative. Superintendents who agreed to participate received a formal consent letter from Brandon University research team. The consent letter confirmed the School Division's participation, asked the superintendents to identify the participating schools as well as the permission to contact the principals of these schools. When the principals were contacted they were also asked to provide their consent to identify and contact teachers. Teachers were asked to provide their consent to participate by distributing consent forms to parents and students. With the consent of principals, teachers, parents and students, a representative from our research team contacted schools and teachers, and arranged to have students complete our questionnaire online using a password protected Survey Monkey or a paper version. Data collection took place from December 2013 to May 2014. Teachers were given the option to distribute the survey instrument through an electronic link or using a paper copy. Completed paper copies were returned to the Centre for Aboriginal and Rural Education Studies. Graduate students entered the survey data from the paper copies on to the Survey Monkey site. When all of the data were entered into Survey Monkey, the data were exported SPSS for final cleaning and analysis.

In sum, from the 36 School Divisions, 22 superintendents gave permission to conduct the survey, 60 principals (of 99 contacted) agreed and 57 schools participated. Permissions were required from parents of students completing the questionnaire and an opt-in procedure was used. Students took home a form requesting permission and returned it before being allowed to complete the questionnaire.

After removing cases corrupted in one way or another, there were 1,108 cases in the working dataset, or <1% of the roughly 16,000 students enrolled in Grade 10 in the 2013–2014 school year.

Demographic Characteristics of the Survey Group

Of the 1,057 students who identified their gender, 48.4% were female and 51.6% male (see "Appendix 1"). The mean age was 15.7 years, and ranging from 13 to

22 years. Grade 10 students in Manitoba, according to the Department of Education, are usually between 15 and 16 years of age. Of the 1,061 students who identified their "cultural, ethnic or national background", 53.8% simply wrote 'Canadian', 15.4% 'First Nations', 8.7% 'Asian', 6.3% Metis and 5.5% 'European', and. Of the 22 participating School Divisions, only 23.4% of respondents came from Winnipeg, 56.0% from rural and 20.6% from northern and remote areas. This sample should not be regarded as representative of tenth graders in School Divisions across the whole province. Although it would be possible to add weights to responses to obtain sample sizes more representative of the Manitoba tenth grade school population, we have not adopted that strategy because completion of the questionnaire was entirely voluntary and we suspect that the students who took the time to complete our questionnaire are probably not like those who did not bother with regard to issues surrounding sustainable development. Apart from this suspicion, we know that we did not have participation from all school districts or all schools in some districts. So, many students did not have the opportunity to opt in or out.

Descriptive Statistics

In this section we provide two sets of observations: the first on the responses themselves and what they might tell us about the levels of student knowledge, attitudes and behaviours and the second on what the responses mean for the construction of the standardized measures. There is much more information in the tables than we could conveniently summarize in our overview. As different people reflect on the results reported here, we hope that they will find ways to improve our understanding of the strengths and limitations of the specific sentences used in each section. With more work we should be able to improve our understanding of what sentences best describe the knowledge, attitudes and behaviours concerning SD that we hope to nourish in our students today and adult citizens tomorrow.

Because rank order scores are ordinal numbers, strictly speaking the mathematical functions of addition and so on are not applicable. So one might prefer to rank order the support indicated for each sentence by the percentage of respondents strongly agreeing (or disagreeing for negatively worded sentences) or perhaps the total percentage of favourable responses (i.e., percent strongly agreeing plus percent agreeing, or disagreeing for negatively worded sentences). However, because quite a bit of information is lost by neglecting the responses that are unfavourable or neutral, one might prefer to treat the rank order numbers as if they were cardinal. This has the particular advantage of allowing one to use mean or average scores as summary measures of favourable or unfavourable responses. Given these options, for each sentence, we have provided both percentages of respondents strongly agreeing (or disagreeing in cases of reverse-coding) and mean scores of all responses. Mean scores have been calculated as the average of all the on-scale scores divided by the number of respondents responding on scale, with 1 being highest and 5 being lowest on the scale. Our own preference is for mean scores.

To simplify our discussion, hereafter expressions like 'Section A Sentence #5' will be abbreviated to 'A.S5'.

Section A: Knowledge

Table 15.1 presents a summary of the on-scale responses (the Likert scale of 1–5 from strongly agree to strongly disagree) to the first section of the survey instrument that presented 20 sentences describing aspects of sustainability that one might expect a Grade 10 student to know, plus one sentence saying "I have taken a course in which sustainable development was discussed". According to the new learning outcomes developed by the Department of Education for Kindergarten through to Grade 12 students, by Grade 10, students should have received instruction in the basic social, environmental and economic dimensions of sustainability in their social studies, geography, technical vocational and science classes. And yet, of the 902 respondents for this item, only 50.3% agreed or strongly agreed that they had taken a course in which "sustainable development" was discussed. In section "Bi-variate and Multi-variate Relations" below we will explore what might lie behind this data point; and we will investigate the differences in responses for those who agreed or strongly agreed versus those who disagreed or strongly disagreed.

Reading across the first row, one finds that the overall average score of 1.66 (out of 5) for A.S12 (Conservation of fresh water is necessary for SD) gives it a first place rank among mean scores. Eighty-six percent of respondents agreed or strongly agreed with A.S12, which ranks it first place in terms of these two categories indicating favourable responses for sustainable development. "Appendix 2" shows that 49.5% strongly agreed.

The sentences were crafted to reflect a range of themes on the environmental, social and economic dimensions of sustainability. Three of the first five ranked responses were on statements explicitly concerned with environmental issues, namely, A.S12, A.S2 on protecting the environment and A.S5 on atmosphere and climate change. Two of the top five were on social issues, A.S15 on human rights and A.S10 on good quality education for all. Two of the five bottom ranked responses were on statements explicitly concerned with social issues (A.S4 on a culture of peace and A.S19 on the quality of life) and two were on economic issues (A.S on economic development and A.S20 on how the economy works). The last ranked item was A.S17 on the United Nations' Millennium Development Goals. It is noteworthy that for every statement in the table, more than 50% of students gave a response that was favourable for knowledge of sustainable development.

Table 15.2 reveals key issues with several sentences when the off-scale responses (don't know, don't understand or didn't answer) are also considered. Examining the table, we find that the sentence ranked first on both measures of

Table 15.1 Summary, Section A: Ranking with valid entries (on scale responses of 1–5), ordered by mean score on knowledge sentences

Sentence	Mean	% strongly agree or agree	% strongly disagree or disagree	*N* valid entries
12. Conservation of fresh water is necessary for SD	1.66	86.0	4.3	1,019
15. SD requires respect for human rights	1.73	84.9	4.5	1,021
2. Protecting the environment is necessary for SD	1.74	83.4	2.7	1,038
5. Human actions are contributing to changes in our atmosphere and climate systems	1.85	77.8	6.0	1,012
10. SD requires access to good quality education for everyone	1.91	79.3	5.9	1,015
14. Respect for cultural diversity (variety of cultures) is necessary for SD	1.92	78.4	5.7	999
1. Improving people's opportunities for long and healthy lives contributes to SD	1.98	77.1	2.9	950
11. SD requires businesses to behave responsibly to their employees, customers and suppliers	2.01	75.0	5.6	997
8. Gender equality is important to SD	2.03	72.1	10.5	1,000
16. SD requires shifting to the use of renewable resources as much as possible	2.03	71.3	5.3	948
13. 'Maintaining biodiversity' means maintaining the number and variety of living organisms. This is necessary for SD	2.07	68.5	6.3	934
7. Good citizenship is necessary for SD	2.10	70.4	6.9	1,005
9. The elimination of poverty is necessary for SD	2.10	70.4	7.8	975
18. SD requires people to learn new things throughout their lives	2.10	70.4	5.9	1,009
6. SD requires individuals to reduce all kinds of waste	2.11	69.0	7.3	984
4. A culture of peace where people settle conflicts by discussion is necessary for SD	2.12	68.4	8.2	991
19. SD requires people to reflect on what it means to improve the quality of life	2.12	69.6	6.5	998
3. Economic development is necessary for SD	2.20	67.2	6.3	990
20. SD requires that people understand how the economy works	2.28	62.7	9.0	988
17. SD requires achieving the United Nations' Millennium Development Goals	2.38	55.0	8.2	737
21. I have taken a course in which sustainable development was discussed	2.72	50.3	30.0	902

Table 15.2 Section A: Rankings including off scale responses

Rank	Sentence no.	% don't know	Sentence no.	% don't underst.	Sentence no.	% missing N = 1,108	Sentence no.	N all entries
1	17	14.9	17	18.0	21	0.7	1	1,108
2	21	10.6	13	9.3	10	0.6	2	1,108
3	6	6.6	1	8.6	17	0.6	3	1,108
4	9	6.3	16	8.3	6	0.5	4	1,108
5	20	6.3	21	7.2	7	0.5	5	1,108
6	11	6.0	4	5.5	8	0.5	6	1,108
7	13	6.0	9	5.2	9	0.5	7	1,108
8	16	5.7	3	5.1	11	0.5	8	1,108
9	19	5.6	8	4.6	12	0.5	9	1,108
10	1	5.4	14	4.6	14	0.5	10	1,108
11	3	5.3	5	4.4	15	0.5	11	1,108
12	7	5.3	6	4.2	16	0.5	12	1,108
13	18	5.3	20	4.1	20	0.5	13	1,108
14	4	4.7	19	4.0	4	0.4	14	1,108
15	8	4.7	7	3.5	13	0.4	15	1,108
16	14	4.7	12	3.5	18	0.4	16	1,108
17	10	4.6	11	3.4	19	0.4	17	1,108
18	5	4.1	10	3.2	1	0.3	18	1,108
19	15	4.1	15	3.2	2	0.3	19	1,108
20	12	4.0	18	3.2	3	0.3	20	1,108
21	2	3.2	2	2.8	5	0.2	21	1,108

confusion about the sentence meaning was A.S17 (SD requires achieving the United Nations' Millennium Development Goals.), with 14.9% 'don't know' and 18.0% 'don't understand' responses, respectively. The millennium development goals (MDGs) have been a central international building block for global sustainability, and figured prominently in the long term planning of UN agencies (including UNESCO) as well as other multilateral and bilateral development assistance agencies. Granting that the MDGs will not be achieved by the end of the Decade of ESD (2015), their achievement nevertheless has been an important theme of ESD and SD. The sentence ranked second on the 'don't know' response and fifth on the 'don't understand' response was A.S21 (I have taken a course in which SD was discussed), with 10.6% 'don't know' and 7.2% 'don't understand' responses, respectively. There were no other sentences that ranked in the top five items on both measures of confusion.

Section B: Attitudes

Table 15.3 presents a summary of the responses to the second section of the survey instrument, that presented 15 statements describing attitudes towards sustainability that one might expect a Grade 10 student to hold. The table lists the on-scale responses (the Likert scale of 1–5 from strongly agree to strongly disagree) with reverse coding for negative statements.

The first row of Table 15.3 tells us that B.S13 (Males and females should have equal access to all kinds of education and employment.) had the lowest (i.e., most favourable) mean score, the third highest percentage of students agreeing or strongly agreeing (85.9%), and the third largest number of valid responses (1,013). Statement B.S1 (Every person should receive education that teaches the knowledge, values and skills necessary for sustainable living in a community.) had the second lowest mean score (1.65), the highest percentage of students agreeing or strongly agreeing (88.2%) and the largest number of valid responses (1,029). Statement B.S2 (The present generation should make sure that the next generation can live in communities that are at least as healthy as those that exist today.) had the third lowest mean score (1.68), the second highest percentage of students agreeing or strongly agreeing (86.1%) and the second largest number of valid responses (1,020).

At the bottom of the rank order, we find the four sentences for which disagreeing or strongly disagreeing would represent favourable attitudes toward sustainable development. For such items, we reverse-coded responses so that they would be consistent with our regular-coded items, i.e., so that larger percentages would indicate more favourable responses. At the very bottom we see that B.S5 (We don't need stricter laws and regulations to protect the environment.) had the highest mean score (2.81), indicating that it was the statement that had on average the least support. This was followed by B.S.14 (It is alright to use as much water as we want, as long as it is available.) at 2.77, then B.S4 (As long as resources are available, using more than we need now doesn't threaten the health and welfare of future generations.) at 2.56 and B.S8 (Understanding and addressing the problems of climate change is not important.) at 2.49. For this table, 13 of 15 (86.6%) of statements had more than 50% of responses indicating favourable attitudes toward sustainable development.

Table 15.4 reveals key issues with several sentences when the off-scale responses (don't know, don't understand or didn't answer) are also considered. The first row shows that B. S7 (SD will not be possible until wealthier nations stop exploiting workers in poorer nations.) had the largest percentages of students responding 'don't know' (9.7%) or 'don't understand' (8.1%). There is only one other case in which the same statement had the same rank order number. B.S.11 (Citizens should be well-informed and actively participate in democratic processes like voting.) ranked fifth for 'don't know' (7.1%) and 'don't understand (4.1%). One would have thought that the four statements requiring reverse coding

Table 15.3 Summary, Section B: Ranking with valid entries (on scale responses of 1–5), ordered by mean score on attitudes sentences

Sentence	Mean	% strongly agree or agree	% strongly disagree or disagree	*N* valid entries
13. Males and females should have equal access to all kinds of education and employment	1.56	85.9	4.0	1,013
1. Every person should receive education that teaches the knowledge, values and skills necessary for sustainable living in a community	1.65	88.2	2.8	1,029
2. The present generation should make sure that the next generation can live in communities that are at least as healthy as those that exist today	1.68	86.1	3.6	1,020
6. It is important to find ways to reduce poverty	1.83	82.3	4.4	1,008
15. Household tasks should be equally shared among members of the household regardless of gender	1.99	73.1	7.8	963
11. Citizens should be well-informed and actively participate in democratic processes like voting	2.09	69.4	6.8	959
3. Manufacturers should discourage the use of disposables	2.23	63.0	10.4	919
9. Use of fuel-efficient vehicles should be encouraged by governments	2.25	65.8	13.9	975
7. SD will not be possible until wealthier nations stop exploiting workers in poorer nations	2.26	61.8	10.2	886
12. People who pollute our land, air or water should pay for damage done to communities and the environment	2.28	62.3	14.1	988
10. Governments should adopt SD as a national priority	2.34	58.3	10.7	933
8. Understanding and addressing the problems of climate change is not important[a]	2.49	56.0	23.3	984
4. As long as resources are available, using more than we need now doesn't threaten the health and welfare of future generations[a]	2.56	53.4	27.6	967
14. It is alright to use as much water as we want, as long as it is available[a]	2.77	47.3	30.6	983
5. We don't need stricter laws and regulations to protect the environment[a]	2.81	46.1	33.3	988

[a]Reverse scored

Table 15.4 Section B: Rankings including off scale responses

Rank	Sentence no.	% don't know	Sentence no.	% don't underst.	Sentence no.	% missing N = 1,108	Sentence no.	N all entries
1	7	9.7	7	8.1	10	2.7	1	1,108
2	10	8.4	3	7.5	9	2.3	2	1,108
3	15	7.8	4	4.7	11	2.3	3	1,108
4	3	7.6	10	4.7	12	2.3	4	1,108
5	11	7.1	11	4.1	15	2.3	5	1,108
6	9	6.6	6	3.3	7	2.2	6	1,108
7	12	6.4	8	3.2	8	2.1	7	1,108
8	4	6.3	9	3.2	13	2.1	8	1,108
9	5	6.3	14	3.2	14	2.1	9	1,108
10	8	6.0	15	3.0	3	2.0	10	1,108
11	14	6.0	5	2.9	4	1.7	11	1,108
12	6	4.1	13	2.9	5	1.6	12	1,108
13	2	4.0	1	2.7	6	1.6	13	1,108
14	13	3.6	2	2.4	1	1.5	14	1,108
15	1	2.9	12	2.2	2	1.5	15	1,108

(B.S4, 5, 8 and 14) would have been near the top of the rank orders for 'don't know' and 'don't understand', but only B.S4 was in the top five with 4.7% responding 'don't understand'.

Section C: Behaviours

Table 15.5 presents a summary of the responses to the third section of the survey instrument that presented 16 statements describing behaviours supportive of sustainability that one might expect a Grade 10 student to demonstrate. The table lists the on-scale responses (the Likert scale of 1–5 from strongly agree to strongly disagree) with reverse coding for negative statements.

C. S16 (I give men and women, boys and girls the same level of respect.) had the lowest mean score (1.83) and the highest percentage of responses agreeing or strongly agreeing with it (78.4%). It was followed by C.S4 (When I use the computer or phone for social networking or gaming I always treat everyone as respectfully as I would in person.) with a mean of 2.26 and 65.6% agreeing or strongly agreeing with it. In third place was C.S14 (I usually examine problems from many points of view.) with a mean of 2.36 and 58.6% agreeing or strongly agreeing with it. At the bottom end of the rank order, C.S9 (Even when I have the option, I do not always compost.) had the highest mean score (3.28), followed by

Table 15.5 Summary, Section C: Ranking with valid entries (on scale responses of 1–5), ordered by mean score on behaviour sentences

Sentence	Mean	% strongly agree or agree	% strongly disagree or disagree	*N* valid entries
16. I give men and women, boys and girls the same level of respect	1.83	78.4	7.3	1,019
4. When I use the computer or phone for social networking or gaming I always treat everyone as respectfully as I would in person	2.26	65.6	14.4	1,010
14. I usually examine problems from many points of view	2.36	58.6	12.4	994
3. At home I recycle as much as I can	2.45	57.8	20.5	1,021
15. I have thought quite a bit about how to live sustainably	2.60	46.9	18.5	966
6. I try to do things that will help people living in poverty	2.64	45.1	17.8	972
5. I always make lifestyle choices that are good for my health	2.65	46.2	21.8	1,015
1. I choose to walk or bike to places instead of using a motor vehicle	2.67	45.9	24.2	1,008
8. I do not think about how I might be damaging the natural environment[a]	2.84	41.3	30.4	1,014
7. I pick up litter when I see it in a park or a natural area	2.91	36.8	30.6	1,011
12. I participate in democratic activities related to student life at my school	2.91	39.0	33.0	927
11. I have changed my personal lifestyle to reduce waste	2.96	32.8	31.8	981
10. I try to avoid buying goods from companies with poor track records on caring for their workers or the environment	2.98	32.1	32.2	868
13. I volunteer to work with local charities or environmental groups	2.98	35.3	36.5	971
2. I never waste water	3.05	31.2	38.7	1,027
9. Even when I have the option, I do not always compost[a]	3.28	24.4	46.5	933

[a]Reverse scored

C.S2 (I never waste water.) at 3.05 and C.S13 (I volunteer to work with local charities or environmental groups.) at 2.98.

There were only four statements of the 16 with more than 50% agreeing or strongly agreeing with it, namely, C.S16, C.S4, and C.S14 as we just saw and C.S3 (At home I recycle as much as I can.), with a mean of 2.45 and 57.8% agreeing or strongly agreeing with it. While it is encouraging to find that most students know about and have attitudes favourable toward sustainable development, we had hoped

Table 15.6 Section C: Rankings including off scale responses

Rank	Sentence no.	% don't know	Sentence no.	% don't underst.	Sentence no.	% missing N = 1,108	Sentence no.	N all entries
1	10	13.3	9	6.4	10	3.2	1	1,108
2	12	7.8	12	5.6	3	3.1	2	1,108
3	15	7.3	10	5.2	4	3.1	3	1,108
4	13	7.2	6	2.6	14	3.1	4	1,108
5	6	6.9	15	2.6	1	3.0	5	1,108
6	9	6.5	14	2.5	12	3.0	6	1,108
7	11	6.5	13	2.3	2	2.9	7	1,108
8	1	4.8	11	2.1	5	2.9	8	1,108
9	14	4.7	4	1.9	8	2.9	9	1,108
10	7	4.2	7	1.8	9	2.9	10	1,108
11	8	4.0	16	1.7	11	2.9	11	1,108
12	4	3.9	5	1.6	13	2.9	12	1,108
13	5	3.9	8	1.6	15	2.9	13	1,108
14	16	3.4	3	1.4	16	2.9	14	1,108
15	3	3.3	1	1.3	6	2.8	15	1,108
16	2	3.2	2	1.2	7	2.7	16	1,108

to find more evidence of changes in behaviours as well: the world will not change unless people's behaviour is consistent with what they know and how they feel.

Table 15.6 presents the off-scale responses (don't know, don't understand or didn't answer) for the behaviours section. Of all 16 statements in the table, statement C.S10 (I try to avoid buying goods from companies with poor track records on caring for their workers or the environment.) had the most 'don't know' responses (13.3%). Adding the 5.2% of 'don't understand' responses for this statement, it is clear that students had more trouble with this statement than any of the others. It is unclear why. Statement C.S12 (I participate in democratic activities related to student life at my school.) ranked second for both 'don't know' and 'don't understand' responses, at 7.8 and 5.6%, respectively. Again, we do not know what was particularly confusing about this statement.

Indexes of Knowledge, Attitudes and Behaviours

Table 15.7 lists Indexes of Knowledge of, and Favourable Attitudes and Behaviours Toward Sustainable Development, with numbers of respondent cases used in the calculations, Cronbach alpha reliability coefficients, scale means and item-total correlations. Each of the indexes was built on the sentences in Sections A–C. It should be noted that as a result of missing values for one reason or another

Table 15.7 Indexes of Knowledge of, Favourable Attitudes and Behaviours Toward Sustainable Development, with numbers of respondents, Cronbach alphas, scale means and item-total correlations

Knowledge Index		Favourable Attitudes Index		Favourable Behaviours Index	
N	492	*N*	598	*N*	622
Alpha	0.91	Alpha	0.81	Alpha	0.81
Scale mean	1.96	Scale mean	2.16	Scale mean	2.68
SD	0.17	SD	0.40	SD	0.38
Item no.	Item-total. cor.	Item no.	Item-total cor.	Item no.	Item-total cor.
A1	0.532	B1	0.474	C1	0.444
A2	0.558	B2	0.491	C2	0.526
A3	0.525	B3	0.408	C3	0.405
A4	0.538	B4 rev.	0.378	C4	0.419
A5	0.500	B5 rev.	0.348	C5	0.487
A6	0.544	B6	0.483	C6	0.591
A7	0.512	B7	0.355	C7	0.572
A8	0.462	B8 rev.	0.404	C8 rev.	−0.017
A9	0.569	B9	0.402	C9 rev.	−0.117
A10	0.639	B10	0.441	C10	0.419
A11	0.551	B11	0.379	C11	0.612
A12	0.526	B12	0.323	C12	0.507
A13	0.552	B13	0.529	C13	0.499
A14	0.599	B14 rev.	0.410	C14	0.443
A15	0.601	B15	0.409	C15	0.536
A16	0.545			C16	0.390
A17	0.490				
A18	0.512				
A19	0.609				
A20	0.461				

(as indicated in "Appendix 2"), our sample sizes for results reported in Tables 15.7, 15.8 and 15.9 are smaller than those in Tables 15.1, 15.2, 15.3, 15.4, 15.5 and 15.6.

The first two columns of Table 15.7 tell us that for the 20-item *Index of Knowledge of SD,* there were 492 valid cases used in the calculation that produced a Cronbach reliability coefficient of $\alpha = 0.91$. Generally speaking, alpha coefficients above 0.70 are regarded as acceptable and those above 0.80 as relatively high. Alpha coefficients measure the intercorrelations among the sentence items in a set

Table 15.8 Correlations *(N)* among Indexes for Knowledge of, Favourable Attitudes, and Behaviours Toward Sustainable Sevelopment, $p < 0.0001$

Index	Knowledge	Attitudes
Attitudes	0.66 (371)	
Behaviours	0.46 (367)	0.35 (456)

Table 15.9 Regressions of Favourable Behaviours Index on Knowledge and Favourable Attitudes Indexes

N	302
Of variance explained	25
Predictors ↓	Betas ↓
Knowledge	0.36
Attitudes	0.19

based on pairwise correlations, and more precisely they measure "the proportion of variance attributable to common sources" (Viswanathan 2005, p. 27).

This 20-item index had a scale mean of 1.96 (out of 5) and a SD of 0.17. Its average item-total correlation was $r = 0.54$, with a range from $r = -0.461$ to $r = 0.639$. Comparing results here with those of the 20-item Knowledge Index in Michalos et al. (2012), one finds some improvement. The Knowledge Index in the earlier study had an $\alpha = 0.89$ and an average item-total correlation of $r = 0.51$. The fact that our average item-total correlation was also higher in this study than in the pilot shows that we have managed to reduce the random error in our index scores.

The second two columns of Table 15.7 tell us that for the 15-item *Index of Attitudes Favourable Toward SD,* there were 598 valid cases used in the calculation that produced a Cronbach reliability coefficient of $\alpha = 0.81$. This 15-item index had a scale mean of 2.16 and a standard deviation of 0.40. Its average item-total correlation was $r = 0.42$, with a range from $r = 0.323$ to $r = 0.529$. Comparing these results with those of the 15-item attitude index in Michalos et al. (2012), one finds that the earlier study had better results. The attitude index in that study had an $\alpha = 0.84$ and an average item-total correlation of $r = 0.46$.

Finally, the last two columns of Table 15.7 tell us that for the 16-item *Index of Behaviours Favourable Toward SD*, there were 622 valid cases used in the calculation that produced a Cronbach reliability coefficient of $\alpha = 0.81$. This index had a scale mean of 2.68 and a SD of 0.38. Its average item-total correlation was $r = 0.42$. Comparing these results with those of the 14-item behaviours index in Michalos et al. (2012), one finds a mixed result. The attitude index in the earlier study had a scale mean of 2.83, and $\alpha = 0.83$ and an average item-total correlation of $r = 0.46$.

Because the mean scores on the three indexes represent the best summary of the overall performance of our tenth grade respondents, it is fair to say that on average the 2014 respondents performed better than the 2010 respondents insofar as the

2014 group had scores indicating more knowledge of, and more favourable attitudes and behaviours toward sustainable development. Granting that the two samples are not representative of total population of tenth grade students in Manitoba, that they are not well-matched samples and that there still seems to be problems with sentences requiring reverse coding, it does appear that some progress has been made from the earlier to the later study. With a bit more fine-tuning of the attitude and behaviour indexes and increased involvement from school divisions, schools, teachers, students and parents in completing questionnaires, we will be able to produce a reliable and valid baseline measure of the success of efforts to teach what students ought to learn about sustainable development.

Bi-variate and Multi-variate Relations

Table 15.8 lists the Pearson Product-Moment Correlations among our three indexes. The Knowledge and Attitudes Indexes have a relatively high association ($r = 0.66$) compared to the associations between the Knowledge and Behaviours Indexes ($r = 0.46$) and Attitudes and Behaviours Indexes ($r = 0.35$). These correlations are all highly significant at $p < 0.0001$.

Table 15.9 summarizes the results of regressing the Behaviour Index on the other two Indexes, mindful of our need to make individual "sustainable behaviours become daily habits" and our assumption that knowledge and favourable attitudes should be our main instruments of transformation. If knowledge and favourable attitudes were sufficient to explain respondents' behaviours, then the second column and row entry of Table 15.9 would have 100% instead of the 25% found there. Based on a sample of 302 respondents, our assumption leaves about 75% of the variation in Behavioural Index scores unexplained. The Beta (β) values are standardized regression coefficients, with means of zero and SDs of one. Figuratively speaking, they may be interpreted as percentages of a full step, i.e., when the values of all but one predictor in an equation are held constant and the value of the unbound predictor moves one full step, the value of the dependent variable will move a certain percentage of a step. Thus, the last row of the table tells us that if the Knowledge Index score increased by one full step (one standard deviation unit), then the Favourable Behaviours Index score would increase by 36% of a step. Comparing the Beta value entries in the last and second last rows, we see that knowledge is more influential than attitudes. The regression analysis has the benefit of revealing the relative influence of each predictor in the presence of the other. In Michalos et al. (2012) the Knowledge and Favourable Attitudes Indexes could only explain 21% of Favourable Behaviours scores, with attitudes more influential than knowledge.

Differences Between Groups Based on Recognition of the Term "Sustainable Development"

In section "Descriptive Statistics" we noted our surprise at finding that, although all tenth grade students were supposed to have had some instruction in issues of sustainable development, only 50.3% of our respondents agreed or strongly agreed that they had "taken a course in which sustainable development was discussed". Thirty percent disagreed or strongly disagreed that they had taken such a course.

In discussions with the Ministry of Education, it became clear that while these students have had instruction in the themes and issues of sustainable development, the term "sustainable development" itself is rarely used. It appears only in the grade 8 and 10 Physical Education/Health Education learning outcomes. In the social studies curriculum, the term does not appear at all (although terms such as environmental stewardship, sustainability, citizenship, and social justice are used). This suggests that while students may have attained knowledge of the many dimensions of sustainable development, they may not, in many cases, have recognized their learning as being explicitly about "sustainable development". As we will see below, however, the recognition factor may be correlated to stronger performance on knowledge, attitudes and behaviours.

Tables 15.10, 15.11 and 15.12 show results of measuring differences in performance between the two groups.

Table 15.10 shows that for the Knowledge Index there were statistically significant differences between the mean scores of the two groups for 9 of the 20 statements (45%) and in each case the group of students who agreed or strongly agreed that they had taken a course in which sustainable development had a superior mean score.

Table 15.11 shows that for the Attitudes Index there were statistically significant differences between the mean scores of the two groups for 5 of the 15 statements (33.3%) and in three cases the group of students who agreed or strongly agreed that they had taken a course in which sustainable development was discussed had a superior mean score. The other two cases involved statements requiring reverse coding and we suspect that this feature of the statements created some confusion. As well, we suspect there may have been more respondents in the group of students who agreed or strongly agreed that they had taken a course in which SD was discussed who had an acquiescence bias, which is a tendency to agree with a statement independent of its content. Of the 45 regularly coded items of the three indexes in all but one case (B.S13) the group of students who agreed or strongly agreed that they had taken a course in which SD was discussed had a superior mean score; whereas in all cases of the six reverse-coded items this group had an inferior mean score. This could happen if more respondents in this group had an acquiescence bias, because by usually agreeing with the statement they would be answering in a less favourable way toward sustainable development for the reverse-coded items.

Table 15.10 Section A: Mean differences between groups claiming to have had or not to have had a course including discussions of sustainable development

Sentence	Mean diff.	Mean (*N*) of sentence for A21 grouping		Statistically significant difference
		Have not had course	Have had course	
1. Improving people's opportunities for long and healthy lives contributes to SD	0.07	1.99 (236)	1.92 (414)	*ns*
2. Protecting the environment is necessary for SD	0.20	1.81 (259)	1.61 (443)	$^{**}p < 0.01$
3. Economic development is necessary for SD	0.22	2.27 (248)	2.05 (429)	$^{**}p < 0.01$
4. A culture of peace where people settle conflicts by discussion is necessary for SD	0.07	2.12 (257)	2.05 (429)	*ns*
5. Human actions are contributing to changes in our atmosphere and climate systems	0.14	1.88 (258)	1.74 (433)	*ns*
6. SD requires individuals to reduce all kinds of waste	0.18	2.18 (251)	2.00 (426)	$^{*}p < 0.05$
7. Good citizenship is necessary for SD	0.08	2.11 (253)	2.03 (435)	*ns*
8. Gender equality is important to SD	0.02	2.02 (252)	2.00 (434)	*ns*
9. The elimination of poverty is necessary for SD	0.20	2.21 (248)	2.01 (430)	$^{*}p < 0.05$
10. SD requires access to good quality education for everyone	0.07	1.93 (251)	1.86 (438)	*ns*
11. SD requires businesses to behave responsibly to their employees, customers and suppliers	0.16	2.08 (250)	1.92 (431)	$^{*}p < 0.05$
12. Conservation of fresh water is necessary for SD	0.10	1.70 (256)	1.60 (439)	*ns*
13. 'Maintaining biodiversity' means maintaining the number and variety of living organisms. This is necessary for SD	0.10	2.06 (236)	1.96 (410)	*ns*
14. Respect for cultural diversity (variety of cultures) is necessary for SD	0.10	1.96 (251)	1.86 (433)	*ns*
15. SD requires respect for human rights	0.07	1.76 (257)	1.69 (437)	*ns*
16. SD requires shifting to the use of renewable resources as much as possible	0.13	2.03 (235)	1.90 (418)	*ns*
17. SD requires achieving the United Nations' Millennium Development Goals	0.40	2.62 (156)	2.22 (347)	$^{***}p < 0.001$
18. SD requires people to learn new things throughout their lives	0.24	2.20 (253)	1.96 (438)	$^{**}p < 0.01$
19. SD requires people to reflect on what it means to improve the quality of life	0.28	2.26 (253)	1.98 (432)	$^{***}p < 0.001$
20. SD requires that people understand how the economy works	0.44	2.53 (256)	2.09 (439)	$^{***}p < 0.001$

Table 15.11 Section B: Mean differences between groups claiming to have had or not to have had a course including discussions of sustainable development

Sentence	Mean diff.	Mean (*N*) of sentence for A21 grouping		Statistically significant difference
		Have not had course	Have had course	
1. Every person should receive education that teaches the knowledge, values and skills necessary for sustainable living in a community	0.04	1.64 (257)	1.60 (436)	*ns*
2. The present generation should make sure that the next generation can live in communities that are at least as healthy as those that exist today	0.08	1.67 (258)	1.59 (433)	*ns*
3. Manufacturers should discourage the use of disposables	0.23	2.30 (233)	2.07 (403)	$*p < 0.05$
4. As long as resources are available, using more than we need now doesn't threaten the health and welfare of future generations[a]	−0.25	2.36 (247)	2.61 (418)	$*p < 0.05$
5. We don't need stricter laws and regulations to protect the environment[a]	−0.12	2.71 (251)	2.83 (422)	*ns*
6. It is important to find ways to reduce poverty	0.07	1.82 (256)	1.75 (433)	*ns*
7. SD will not be possible until wealthier nations stop exploiting workers in poorer nations	0.12	2.30 (225)	2.18 (395)	*ns*
8. Understanding and addressing the problems of climate change is not important[a]	−0.29	2.26 (252)	2.55 (421)	$**p < 0.01$
9. Use of fuel-efficient vehicles should be encouraged by governments	0.04	2.25 (244)	2.21 (420)	*ns*
10. Governments should adopt SD as a national priority	0.15	2.39 (233)	2.24 (411)	*ns*
11. Citizens should be well-informed and actively participate in democratic processes like voting	0.14	2.11 (247)	1.97 (415)	ns
12. People who pollute our land, air or water should pay for damage done to communities and the environment	0.19	2.36 (253)	2.17 (419)	*p < 0.05
13. Males and females should have equal access to all kinds of education and employment	−0.04	1.50 (257)	1.54 (426)	*ns*
14. It is alright to use as much water as we want, as long as it is available[a]	0.12	2.66 (249)	2.78 (418)	*ns*
15. Household tasks should be equally shared among members of the household regardless of gender	0.21	2.06 (246)	1.85 (411)	$*p < 0.05$

[a]Reverse scored

Table 15.12 shows that for the Behaviours Index there were statistically significant differences between the mean scores of the two groups for 10 of the 16 statements (62.5%) and, as we found with the Knowledge Index, in each case the

Table 15.12 Section C: Mean differences between groups claiming to have had or not to have had a course including discussions of sustainable development

Sentence	Mean diff.	Mean (*N*) of sentence for A21 grouping		Statistically significant difference
		Have not had course	Have had course	
1. I choose to walk or bike to places instead of using a motor vehicle	0.15	2.79 (250)	2.64 (431)	*ns*
2. I never waste water	0.26	3.24 (259)	2.98 (432)	$^{**}p < 0.01$
3. At home I recycle as much as I can	0.27	2.61 (256)	2.34 (434)	$^{**}p < 0.01$
4. When I use the computer or phone for social networking or gaming I always treat everyone as respectfully as I would in person	0.10	2.29 (249)	2.19 (428)	*ns*
5. I always make lifestyle choices that are good for my health	0.37	2.90 (255)	2.53 (432)	$^{***}p < 0.001$
6. I try to do things that will help people living in poverty	0.41	2.88 (251)	2.47 (417)	$^{***}p < 0.001$
7. I pick up litter when I see it in a park or a natural area	0.48	3.23 (257)	2.75 (425)	$^{***}p < 0.001$
8. I do not think about how I might be damaging the natural environment[a]	−0.15	2.70 (254)	2.85 (431)	*ns*
9. Even when I have the option, I do not always compost[a]	−0.01	3.30 (237)	3.31 (404)	*ns*
10.1 try to avoid buying goods from companies with poor track records on caring for their workers or the environment	0.44	3.25 (233)	2.81 (370)	$^{***}p < .001$
11. I have changed my personal lifestyle to reduce waste	0.47	3.26 (257)	2.79 (424)	$^{***}p < 0.001$
12. I participate in democratic activities related to student life at my school	0.63	3.29 (231)	2.66 (404)	$^{***}p < 0.001$
13. I volunteer to work with local charities or environmental groups	0.51	3.31 (250)	2.80 (415)	$^{***}p < 0.001$
14. I usually examine problems from many points of view	0.16	2.45 (252)	2.29 (428)	*ns*
15. I have thought quite a bit about how to live sustainably	0.27	2.76 (248)	2.49 (418)	$^{**}p < 0.01$
16. I give men and women, boys and girls the same level of respect	0.04	1.78 (254)	1.74 (427)	*ns*

[a]Reverse scored

group of students who agreed or strongly agreed that they had taken such a course had a superior mean score. Taken together, these results send mixed signals. It is not the case that everyone who recognizes that they have had a relevant course in which sustainable development was discussed performs better than everyone who lacks such recognition. Still, most of those who recognize they have had a relevant course in which sustainable development was discussed do tend to perform better.

Observations on the Survey Findings

The results for the 2014 cohort, with their longer, sustained exposure to ESD, have improved over the 2010 group of students across all measures of knowledge, attitudes and choices. This suggests that the province's investment in ESD is leading to the desired results in a significant percentage of Manitoban students. Furthermore, it suggests that the sustained exposure throughout many years and levels of schooling leads to stronger results, compared to a limited exposure over only 1 or 2 years.

A correlation is beginning to be seen between sustainability-related levels of knowledge and choices favourable to sustainability: in at least 25% of the response group, knowledge is fairly clearly linked to positive choices, moreso perhaps than attitudes. Our findings should provide some encouragement to Manitoba's Ministry of Education and others working in formal, K-12 education: while the shaping of attitudes and values is challenging and may lie beyond the scope of formal education, it is clearly within the mandate of ministries of education to strengthen the knowledge base, and our research is beginning to suggest that strengthening the knowledge base itself contributes to the adoption of more sustainable choices and actions. Nevertheless, the fact that only 25% of the variation in our Favourable Behaviours Index scores could be accounted for by our Knowledge Index and Favourable Attitudes Index indicates that we are still far from having a complete explanation of why some students behave in ways that are favourable to sustainable development and others do not.

Students who recognized that they had heard the term "sustainable development" demonstrated a stronger knowledge of sustainable development, more supportive attitudes and appeared to be more likely to adopt sustainability-related behaviours. This opens up an interesting line of discussion about whether one needs to "call a spade a spade", and use the term "sustainable development" in classrooms, beyond mainstreaming various dimensions throughout the curriculum.

The researchers were intrigued that the top two behaviours in the survey are connected to an understanding of "respect" ("I give men and women, boys and girls the same level of respect"; "When I use the computer or phone for social networking or gaming I always treat everyone as respectfully as I would in person"). It may be worth exploring whether teaching about the environmental dimensions of sustainable development should be couched in the concepts and language of "respect", as it may resonate with students and connect with other behaviours aligned with the social dimensions of sustainability. Such an approach would be consistent with the way that many practitioners and policy makers are now talking about ESD in the context of building responsible and respectful societies (UNESCO 2012).

Knowledge of the social and environmental dimensions of sustainability appears to be stronger than that of the economic dimensions, with the economic statements "Economic development is necessary for SD" and "SD requires that people understand how the economy works" scoring among the bottom four of the 21 knowledge statements. This may suggest a gap in how the economic dimension of sustainable development has been benchmarked in the learning outcomes or covered in the curriculum.

Finally, the researchers were concerned about the high level of off-scale responses (don't know/don't understand) to the question on democratic activities ("Citizens should be well-informed and actively participate in democratic processes like voting"). There may well be a weakness in how the statement was phrased; perhaps an emphasis on democratic processes closer to the daily lives of students, such as student councils in schools might improve the level of understanding of the question. But the number of off-scale responses also opens questions about whether there may be a growing "democratic deficit" among students—that participation in democracy is something that students simply don't understand or aren't aware of. Given the importance of access to information and democratic processes to sustainable development (whether at the local level, nationally or among nations at the international level), these may be areas for attention in learning outcomes and curriculum.

Conclusion

The aim of this paper was to develop standardized measures of tenth grade students' knowledge, attitudes and behaviours concerning sustainable development as those concepts are understood in the United Nations Educational, Scientific and Cultural Organization (UNESCO Education Sector 2006) and to test the hypothesis that knowledge and favourable attitudes toward SD would lead to favourable behaviours. The survey questionnaire used in this study was a refined version of the student questionnaire used Michalos et al. (2011). While further work on the questionnaires and indexes is still necessary, some clear and important progress was made over our earlier study. Questions and opportunities for further research lie in several directions: undertaking a survey of a third cohort of Grade 10 students in 2–3 years time, using a refined survey instrument to see whether performance continues to improve; deploying the survey in other jurisdictions to compare and provide further validation of the approach; and finally, to resurvey those who participated in the 2010 and 2014 surveys to see whether they are retaining and strengthening their knowledge, attitudes and behaviours supportive of sustainable development.

Acknowledgements This Project was supported by the Government of Manitoba and the Centre for Aboriginal and Rural Education Studies, Faculty of Education, Brandon University. We are grateful for the support and collaboration with Manitoba Education and Advanced Learning, and would like to thank all the teachers and administrators who helped us undertake this survey and especially all the students who took the time to complete our questionnaire. As well, in our data collection, we benefited from help of our students Jessica Murray and Erin Paupanekis.

Appendix 1

Summary for Student Sustainable Development Survey, 2014: Valid Answers (1–5) in %'s.

Information

In the 1987 United Nations report on Environment and Development, *sustainable development* (SD) was described as "development that meets the needs of the present without compromising the ability of future generations to meet their own needs". We are interested in your understanding of the meaning of sustainable development, from what you have learned at school and from all other sources.

Instructions

Section A: For each sentence below in the space provided, please indicate with an appropriate number whether you strongly agree (1), agree (2), are neutral (3), disagree (4) or strongly disagree (5) with it. If you do not have an opinion, write (6) or do not understand the question, write (7).

Sentence	1–7
1. Improving people's opportunities for long and healthy lives contributes to SD	
2. Protecting the environment is necessary for SD	
3. Economic development is necessary for SD	
4. A culture of peace where people settle conflicts by discussion is necessary for SD	
5. Human actions are contributing to changes in our atmosphere and climate systems	
6. SD requires individuals to reduce all kinds of waste	
7. Good citizenship is necessary for SD	
8. Gender equality is important to SD	
9. The elimination of poverty is necessary for SD	
10. SD requires access to good quality education for everyone	

(continued)

(continued)

Sentence	1–7
11. SD requires businesses to behave responsibly to their employees, customers and suppliers	
12. Conservation of fresh water is necessary for SD	
13. 'Maintaining biodiversity' means maintaining the number and variety of living organisms. This is necessary for SD	
14. Respect for cultural diversity (variety of cultures) is necessary for SD	
15. SD requires respect for human rights	
16. SD requires shifting to the use of renewable resources as much as possible	
17. SD requires achieving the United Nations' Millennium Development Goals	
18. SD requires people to learn new things throughout their lives	
19. SD requires people to reflect on what it means to improve the quality of life	
20. SD requires that people understand how the economy works	
21. I have taken a course in which sustainable development was discussed	

Section A: Summary

Sentence	N	M	1 strongly agree (%)	2 agree (%)	3 neutral (%)	4 disagree (%)	5 strongly disagree (%)	6 don't know	7 don't underst. + missing
1	950	1.98	28.6	48.5	19.9	2.0	0.9	60	95 + 3
2	1,038	1.74	46.9	36.5	13.9	1.5	1.2	36	31 + 3
3	990	2.20	21.5	45.7	26.5	4.1	2.2	59	56 + 3
4	991	2.12	29.7	38.7	23.4	5.9	2.3	52	61 + 4
5	1,012	1.85	45.5	32.3	16.3	3.3	2.7	45	49 + 2
6	984	2.11	29.1	39.9	23.7	5.2	2.1	73	46 + 5
7	1,005	2.10	28.9	41.5	22.8	4.6	2.3	59	39 + 5
8	1,000	2.03	39.1	33.0	17.4	6.8	3.7	52	51 + 5
9	975	2.10	29.6	40.8	21.7	5.6	2.2	70	58 + 5
10	1,015	1.91	36.7	42.6	14.8	4.4	1.5	51	35 + 7
11	997	2.01	31.6	43.4	19.4	4.0	1.6	67	38 + 6
12	1,019	1.66	53.8	32.2	9.8	2.5	1.8	44	39 + 6
13	934	2.07	32.1	36.4	25.2	4.6	1.7	67	103 + 4
14	999	1.92	37.7	40.7	15.8	3.2	2.5	52	51 + 6
15	1,021	1.73	48.7	36.2	10.6	2.6	1.9	45	36 + 6
16	948	2.03	33.4	37.9	23.4	3.2	2.1	63	92 + 5
17	737	2.38	17.0	38.0	36.8	6.2	2.0	165	199 + 7
18	1,009	2.10	27.4	43.0	23.8	4.0	1.9	59	36 + 4
19	998	2.12	27.3	42.3	23.9	4.6	1.9	62	44 + 4
20	988	2.28	21.6	41.1	28.3	6.3	2.7	70	45 + 5
21	902	2.72	18.8	31.5	19.6	19.4	10.6	118	80 + 8

Mean calculations are not reverse calculated here

Section B: Again, for each sentence below in the space provided, please indicate with an appropriate number whether you strongly agree (1), agree (2), are neutral (3), disagree (4) or strongly disagree (5) with it. If you do not have an opinion, write (6) or do not understand the question, write (7).

Sentence	1–7
1. Every person should receive education that teaches the knowledge, values and skills necessary for sustainable living in a community	
2. The present generation should make sure that the next generation can live in communities that are at least as healthy as those that exist today	
3. Manufacturers should discourage the use of disposables	
4. As long as resources are available, using more than we need now does not threaten the health and welfare of future generations	
5. We don't need stricter laws and regulations to protect the environment	
6. It is important to find ways to reduce poverty	
7. SD will not be possible until wealthier nations stop exploiting workers in poorer nations	
8. Understanding and addressing the problems of climate change is not important	
9. Use of fuel-efficient vehicles should be encouraged by governments	
10. Governments should adopt SD as a national priority	
11. Citizens should be well-informed and actively participate in democratic processes like voting	
12. People who pollute our land, air or water should pay for damage done to communities and the environment	
13. Males and females should have equal access to all kinds of education and employment	
14. It is alright to use as much water as we want, as long as it is available	
15. Household tasks should be equally shared among members of the household regardless of gender	

Section B: Summary

Sentence	N	M	1 strongly agree (%)	2 agree (%)	3 neutral (%)	4 disagree (%)	5 strongly disagree (%)	6 don't know	7 don't underst. + missing
1	1,029	1.65	51.1	37.1	9.0	1.5	1.3	32	30 + 17
2	1,020	1.68	51.0	35.1	10.4	1.6	2.0	44	27 + 17
3	919	2.23	27.2	35.8	26.6	7.4	3.0	84	83 + 22
4	967	3.44	10.3	17.3	18.9	25.1	28.3	70	52 + 19
5	988	3.19	14.1	19.2	20.5	25.6	20.5	70	32 + 18
6	1,008	1.83	40.6	41.7	13.4	2.7	1.7	45	37 + 18
7	886	2.26	25.3	36.5	28.1	7.0	3.2	108	90 + 24
8	984	3.51	7.9	15.4	20.6	29.5	26.5	66	35 + 23
9	975	2.25	28.7	37.1	20.3	7.7	6.2	73	35 + 25
10	933	2.34	22.1	36.2	31.1	6.9	3.8	93	52 + 30

(continued)

(continued)

Sentence	N	M	1 strongly agree (%)	2 agree (%)	3 neutral (%)	4 disagree (%)	5 strongly disagree (%)	6 don't know	7 don't underst. + missing
11	959	2.09	30.7	38.7	23.9	4.8	2.0	79	45 + 25
12	988	2.28	30.1	32.2	23.7	8.1	6.0	71	24 + 25
13	1,013	1.56	63.6	22.3	10.2	2.4	1.6	40	32 + 23
14	983	3.23	13.8	16.8	22.1	26.9	20.4	67	35 + 23
15	963	1.99	38.9	34.2	19.1	4.8	3.0	86	33 + 26

Mean calculations are not reverse calculated here

Section C: Using the same 5-point (plus 2) scale from Sections A and B, what is your level of agreement with the following possible descriptions of your own behaviour?

Sentence	1–7
1. I choose to walk or bike to places instead of using a motor vehicle	
2. I never waste water	
3. At home I recycle as much as I can	
4. When I use the computer or phone for social networking or gaming I always treat everyone as respectfully as I would in person	
5. I always make lifestyle choices that are good for my health	
6. I try to do things that will help people living in poverty	
7. I pick up litter when I see it in a park or a natural area	
8. I do not think about how I might be damaging the natural environment	
9. Even when I have the option, I do not always compost	
10. I try to avoid buying goods from companies with poor track records on caring for their workers or the environment	
11. I have changed my personal lifestyle to reduce waste	
12. I participate in democratic activities related to student life at my school	
13. I volunteer to work with local charities or environmental groups	
14. I usually examine problems from many points of view	
15. I have thought quite a bit about how to live sustainably	
16. I give men and women, boys and girls the same level of respect	

Section C: Summary

Sentence	N	M	1 strongly agree (%)	2 agree (%)	3 neutral (%)	4 disagree (%)	5 strongly disagree (%)	6 don't know	7 don't underst. + missing
1	1,008	2.67	19.4	26.5	29.9	16.5	7.7	53	14 + 33
2	1,027	3.05	10.6	20.6	30.1	30.6	8.1	36	13 + 32
3	1,021	2.45	23.8	34.0	21.7	14.3	6.2	37	16 + 34
4	1,010	2.26	29.8	35.8	19.9	7.7	6.7	43	21 + 34
5	1,015	2.65	15.9	30.3	31.9	16.9	4.9	43	18 + 32
6	972	2.64	13.0	32.1	37.1	13.7	4.1	76	29 + 31
7	1,011	2.91	9.9	26.9	32.5	23.1	7.5	47	20 + 30
8	1,014	3.16	6.9	23.5	28.3	29.5	11.8	44	18 + 32
9	933	2.72	12.5	34.0	29.0	17.8	6.6	72	71 + 32
10	868	2.98	12.1	20.0	35.6	22.2	10.0	147	58 + 35
11	981	2.96	9.7	23.1	35.4	24.7	7.1	72	23 + 32
12	927	2.91	11.9	27.1	28.0	24.2	8.8	86	62 + 33
13	971	2.98	12.0	23.3	28.2	27.7	8.8	80	25 + 32
14	994	2.36	21.4	37.2	29.0	8.7	3.7	52	28 + 34
15	966	2.60	14.8	32.1	34.6	14.9	3.6	81	29 + 32
16	1,019	1.83	48.5	29.9	14.3	5.0	2.3	38	19 + 32

Mean calculations are not reverse calculated here

Description of Sample

The following questions are used to describe the sample of students who have taken part in this survey and for statistical purposes.

D1. Are you: 48.4% Female 51.6% Male $N = 1{,}057$.

D2. Your present age: ———— years $N = 1{,}045$, $M = 15.7$. *Age ranged from 13 to 22 years.*

D3. How would you name your cultural, ethnic or national background? (e.g., Chinese, Cree, Métis, English Canadian, Greek, etc.) $N = 1{,}061$.

Ethnicity	Percentage (%)	Frequency
African	2.5	27
American	0.8	9
Asian	8.7	92
Australia/Oceania	0.1	1
Canadian	53.8	571
Caribbean	0.1	1
Central American/Mexico	1.0	11
European	5.5	58

(continued)

(continued)

Ethnicity	Percentage (%)	Frequency
First Nations	15.4	163
French Canadian	0.7	7
Metis	6.3	67
Middle Eastern	1.0	11
South American	0.8	8
Other	3.3	35

D4. What is the name of your School Division? $N = 1{,}069$.

School division	Percentage (%)
Beautiful Plains	5.5
Brandon	14.1
Evergreen	0.9
Flin Flon	1.6
Frontier	17.5
Hanover	0.7
Kelsey	2.1
Lakeshore	2.0
Lord Selkirk	6.3
Mountain View	3.9
Mystery Lake	3.6
Park West	2.2
Pine Creek	0.9
Prairie Spirit	2.2
Rolling River	4.5
Southwest Horizon	4.2
Turtle Mountain	0.8
Turtle River	3.4
Winnipeg	23.5

D5. What is the name of your School? $N = 1{,}063$ (Table includes School Groupings).

School name	% of tot.	School group	Of group	Group of total data
Alonsa School	1.0	Rural	1.8	
Arborg Collegiate	0.1	Rural	0.2	
Ashern Central School	1.0	Rural	1.8	
Birtle Collegiate	2.0	Rural	3.5	
Boissevain School	0.8	Rural	1.5	

(continued)

(continued)

School name	% of tot.	School group	Of group	Group of total data
Carberry Collegiate	2.0	Rural	3.5	
Cartwright School	1.3	Rural	2.4	
Crocus Plains High School	3.7	Rural	6.6	
Deloraine School	1.4	Rural	2.5	
Elton Collegiate	0.1	Rural	0.2	
Ethelbert School	0.7	Rural	1.2	
Falcon Beach School	0.3	Rural	0.5	
Gilbert Plains Collegiate	1.7	Rural	3.0	
Glenboro School	0.9	Rural	1.7	
Glenella School	0.4	Rural	0.7	
Goose Lake High School	1.6	Rural	2.9	
Hamiota Collegiate	0.1	Rural	0.2	
Hartney School	0.5	Rural	0.08	
Landmark Collegiate	0.8	Rural	1.3	
Little Black River School	0.8	Rural	1.3	
Lord Selkirk Regional Comprehensive School	6.3	Rural	11.3	
Lundar School	0.9	Rural	1.7	
Melita School	0.9	Rural	1.7	
Minegoziibe Anishinabe School	1.0	Rural	1.8	
Minnedosa Collegiate	2.5	Rural	4.5	
Neepawa Area Collegiate	3.6	Rural	6.4	
Pierson School	0.6	Rural	1.0	
Rivers Collegiate	1.8	Rural	3.2	
Riverton Collegiate	0.8	Rural	1.5	
Rorketon School	1.1	Rural	2.0	
Shoal Lake School	0.3	Rural	0.5	
Ste. Rose School	2.0	Rural	3.5	
Vincent Massey Collegiate	10.1	Rural	18.0	
Wanipigow School	1.4	Rural	2.5	
Waskada School	0.8	Rural	1.3	
William Morton Collegiate Institute	0.8	Rural	1.3	
School group rural				56.0, $N = 595$
Children of the Earth High School	1.2	Winnipeg	5.2	
Churchill High	4.7	Winnipeg	20.1	
Ecole Churchill	0.7	Winnipeg	2.8	
Kelvin High School	13.5	Winnipeg	57.4	
R.B. Russell Vocational	1.4	Winnipeg	6.0	
St. John's High School	2.0	Winnipeg	8.4	

(continued)

(continued)

School name	% of tot.	School group	Of group	Group of total data
School group Winnipeg				23.4, *N* = 249
Cormorant Lake School	0.8	Northern/remote	3.7	
Frontier Collegiate Institute	9.9	Northern/remote	47.9	
Gillam School	0.8	Northern/remote	3.7	
Grand Rapids School	0.1	Northern/remote	0.5	
Hapnot Collegiate Institute	1.5	Northern/remote	7.3	
Helen Betty Osborne Ininiw Education Resource Centre	0.6	Northern/remote	2.7	
Joseph H. Kerr School	0.5	Northern/remote	2.3	
Leaf Rapids Education Centre	0.4	Northern/remote	1.8	
Margaret Barbour Collegiate Institute	1.7	Northern/remote	8.2	
Mary Duncan School	0.4	Northern/remote	1.8	
Mel Johnson School	0.1	Northern/remote	0.5	
Oscar Blackburn School	0.4	Northern/remote	1.8	
R.D. Parker Collegiate	3.7	Northern/remote	17.8	
School group northern/remote				20.6, *N* = 219

Appendix 2

Summary for Student Sustainable Development Survey, 2014: Valid AND Don't Know and Don't Understand Answers in %'s

Section A: Summary

Sentence	N	1 strongly agree (%)	2 agree (%)	3 neutral (%)	4 disagree (%)	5 strongly disagree (%)	6 don't know (%)	7 don't underst. (%)	Missing (%)
1	1,108	24.5	41.6	17.1	1.7	0.8	5.4	8.6	0.3
2	1,108	44.0	34.2	13.0	1.4	1.1	3.2	2.8	0.3
3	1,108	19.2	40.8	23.6	3.7	2.0	5.3	5.1	0.3
4	1,108	26.5	34.7	20.9	5.2	2.1	4.7	5.5	0.4
5	1,108	41.5	29.5	14.9	3.0	2.4	4.1	4.4	0.2
6	1,108	25.8	35.5	21.0	4.6	1.9	6.6	4.2	0.5
7	1,108	26.2	37.6	20.7	4.2	2.1	5.3	3.5	0.5
8	1,108	35.3	29.8	15.7	6.1	3.3	4.7	4.6	0.5
9	1,108	26.1	35.9	19.1	5.0	1.9	6.3	5.2	0.5
10	1,108	33.7	39.0	13.5	4.1	1.4	4.6	3.2	0.6

(continued)

(continued)

Sentence	N	1 strongly agree (%)	2 agree (%)	3 neutral (%)	4 disagree (%)	5 strongly disagree (%)	6 don't know (%)	7 don't underst. (%)	Missing (%)
11	1,108	28.4	39.1	17.4	3.6	1.4	6.0	3.4	0.5
12	1,108	49.5	29.6	9.0	2.3	1.6	4.0	3.5	0.5
13	1,108	27.1	30.7	21.2	3.9	1.4	6.0	9.3	0.4
14	1,108	34.0	36.7	14.3	2.9	2.3	4.7	4.6	0.5
15	1,108	44.9	33.4	9.7	2.4	1.7	4.1	3.2	0.5
16	1,108	28.6	32.4	20.0	2.7	1.8	5.7	8.3	0.5
17	1,108	11.3	25.3	24.5	4.2	1.4	14.9	18.0	0.6
18	1,108	24.9	39.2	21.7	3.6	1.7	5.3	3.2	0.4
19	1,108	24.5	38.1	21.6	4.2	1.7	5.6	4.0	0.4
20	1,108	19.2	36.6	25.3	5.6	2.4	6.3	4.1	0.5
21	1,108	15.3	25.6	16.0	15.8	8.7	10.6	7.2	0.7

Section B: Summary

Sentence	N	1 strongly agree (%)	2 agree (%)	3 neutral (%)	4 disagree (%)	5 strongly disagree (%)	6 don't know (%)	7 don't underst. (%)	Missing (%)
1	1,108	47.5	34.5	8.4	1.4	1.2	2.9	2.7	1.5
2	1,108	46.9	32.2	9.6	1.4	1.8	4.0	2.4	1.5
3	1,108	22.6	29.7	22.0	6.1	2.5	7.6	7.5	2.0
4	1,108	9.0	15.1	16.5	21.9	24.7	6.3	4.7	1.7
5	1,108	12.5	17.1	18.3	22.8	18.3	6.3	2.9	1.6
6	1,108	36.9	37.9	12.2	2.4	1.5	4.1	3.3	1.6
7	1,108	20.2	29.2	22.5	5.6	2.5	9.7	8.1	2.2
8	1,108	7.0	13.7	18.3	26.2	23.6	6.0	3.2	2.1
9	1,108	25.3	32.7	17.9	6.8	5.4	6.6	3.2	2.3
10	1,108	18.6	30.5	26.2	5.8	3.2	8.4	4.7	2.7
11	1,108	26.5	33.5	20.7	4.2	1.7	7.1	4.1	2.3
12	1,108	26.8	28.7	21.1	7.2	5.3	6.4	2.2	2.3
13	1,108	58.1	20.4	9.3	2.2	1.4	3.6	2.9	2.1
14	1,108	12.3	14.9	19.6	23.8	18.1	6.0	3.2	2.1
15	1,108	33.8	29.7	16.6	4.2	2.6	7.8	3.0	2.3

Section C: Summary

Sentence	N	1 strongly agree (%)	2 agree (%)	3 neutral (%)	4 disagree (%)	5 strongly disagree (%)	6 don't know (%)	7 don't underst. (%)	Missing (%)
1	1,108	17.7	24.1	27.2	15.0	7.0	4.8	1.3	3.0
2	1,108	9.8	19.1	27.9	28.3	7.5	3.2	1.2	2.9
3	1,108	21.9	31.3	20.0	13.2	5.7	3.3	1.4	3.1
4	1,108	27.2	32.7	18.1	7.0	6.1	3.9	1.9	3.1
5	1,108	14.5	27.8	29.2	15.5	4.5	3.9	1.6	2.9
6	1,108	11.4	28.2	32.6	12.0	3.6	6.9	2.6	2.8
7	1,108	9.0	24.5	29.7	21.1	6.9	4.2	1.8	2.7
8	1,108	6.3	21.5	25.9	27.0	10.8	4.0	1.6	2.9

(continued)

(continued)

Sentence	N	1 strongly agree (%)	2 agree (%)	3 neutral (%)	4 disagree (%)	5 strongly disagree (%)	6 don't know (%)	7 don't underst. (%)	Missing (%)
9	1,108	10.6	28.6	24.5	15.0	5.6	6.5	6.4	2.9
10	1,108	9.5	15.7	27.9	17.4	7.9	13.3	5.2	3.2
11	1,108	8.6	20.5	31.3	21.8	6.3	6.5	2.1	2.9
12	1,108	9.9	22.7	23.5	20.2	7.4	7.8	5.6	3.0
13	1,108	10.6	20.4	24.7	24.3	7.7	7.2	2.3	2.9
14	1,108	19.2	33.4	26.0	7.8	3.3	4.7	2.5	3.1
15	1,108	12.9	28.0	30.1	13.0	3.2	7.3	2.6	2.9
16	1,108	44.6	27.5	13.2	4.6	2.1	3.4	1.7	2.9

References

CMEC. (2014). UN decade of education for sustainable development. Canada's submission to the UN's DESD final report. 2014, Council of Ministers of Education, Canada (not yet published).

Global Education First Initiative (GEFI). Retrieved August 13, 2014, from http://www.globaleducationfirst.org.

MacDiarmid, A. (2014). Personal correspondence, 7 Aug 2014.

Michalos, A. C., Creech, H., McDonald, C., & Hatch Kahlke, P. M. (2011). Measuring knowledge, attitudes and behaviours concerning education for sustainable development: Two exploratory studies. *Social Indicators Research, 100*(3), 391–413.

Michalos, A. C., Creech, H., Swayze, N., Kahlke, P. M., Buckler, C., & Rempel, K. (2012). Measuring knowledge, attitudes and behaviours concerning sustainable development among tenth grade students in Manitoba. *Social Indicators Research, 106*(2), 213–238.

Schulz, W., Ainley, J., Fraillon, J., Kerr, D., & Losito, B. (2010). *ICCS 2009 International Report: Civic knowledge, attitudes, and engagement among lower-secondary school students in 38 countries*. Amsterdam: International Association for the Evaluation of Educational Achievement.

Sudman, S., & Bradburn, N. M. (1983). *Asking questions: A practical guide to questionnaire design*. San Francisco: Jossey-Bass.

Tbilisi +35. (2012). Intergovernmental conference on environmental education and sustainable development. Tbilisi Communique: Educate today for a sustainable future. Retrieved August 13, 2014, from https://cmsdata.iucn.org/downloads/tbilisi_story_komunike_small.pdf.

UNESCO. (2009). *Bonn seclaration. UNESCO world conference on education for sustainable development, Bonn, Germany*. Retrieved August 5, 2014, from http://www.esd-world-conference-2009.org/fileadmin/download/ESD2009_BonnDeclaration080409.pdf.

UNESCO. (2012). *Shaping the education of tomorrow: 2012 full length report on the UN decade of education for sustainable development*. Paris: UNESCO.

UNESCO. (2013). Education for sustainable development (ESD): A sound investment to accelerate African development. Retrieved August 5, 2014, from https://en.unesco.org/events/education-sustainable-development-esd-sound-investment-accelerate-african-development.

UNESCO Education Sector. (2006). *Framework for the UNDESD International Implementation Scheme*. Paris: UNESCO.

UNICEF, UNESCO. (2013). Making education a priority in the post—2015 development agenda: Report of the global thematic consultation on education in the post-2015 development agenda. Retrieved August 13, 2014, from http://www.unicef.org/education/files/Making_Education_a_Priority_in_the_Post-2015_Development_Agenda.pdf.

United Nations. (2012). Conference on Sustainable Development. The future we want: outcome document. Retrieved August 13, 2014, from http://sustainabledevelopment.un.org/futurewewant.html.

United Nations. (2014). Open Working Group on Sustainable Development Goals. Outcome document. Retrieved August 13, 2014, from http://sustainabledevelopment.un.org/focussdgs.html.

Viswanathan, M. (2005). *Measurement error and research design*. Thousand Oaks: Sage.

Wals, A. (2009). *Review of contexts and structures for education for sustainable development 2009*. Paris: UNESCO.

Chapter 16
Social Indicators Research: The Little Red Hen 40 Years Later

Alex C. Michalos

In August 1978 at the 9th World Congress of Sociology in Uppsala, Sweden, I presented a paper explaining the birth of this journal in 1973 and its early development. That paper was published in Michalos (2005). Among other things, it began with the comment "As I remember it, there's a children's story about a Little Red Hen who repeatedly tried to get others to help with the chores and repeatedly found herself saying 'Very well, I'll do it myself.' That's about how I began SIR".

Since a detailed development story is told in that essay and that book has a robust discussion and republication of the most frequently cited articles in the first 30 years of the journal's life, there is no need to repeat that material here. In this short essay I only want to usher the Little Red Hen out gracefully, express some thanks to others and wish the new Editor the very best of luck.

When I thought about what I should say here, it occurred to me to have a look at Volume One, Number One of the journal to see how I introduced it. To my surprise, I found that I did not write an introduction. That reminded me of a remark I heard on the radio when I was a graduate student in Chicago driving home from my night job in the accounting department of St. Joseph's Hospital. The preacher of an evangelical church said "My daughter is always asking me about rehearsing, but I told her I don't need no rehearsing. Like the angels of the Lord, I just come out singing."

I had a second surprise when I read the material on the back cover of the journal describing what we now call its aim and scope. Much of it, as you will see, I might have written today.

> *Social Indicators Research* is a quarterly journal intended to serve as a 'central clearing house' for research dealing with descriptive, evaluative and prescriptive problems related to

---

Michalos, A.C.: 2013. Social Indicators Research: The Little Red Hen Forty Years later. Social Indicators Research, 115, pp. 1–4. © Springer Science+Business Media B.V. 2014.

A.C. Michalos (✉)
University of Northern British Columbia, Prince George, BC, Canada
e-mail: michalos@brandonu.ca

A.C. Michalos, *Development of Quality of Life Theory and Its Instruments*,
DOI 10.1007/978-3-319-51149-8_16

> the measurement of the quality of life. Since the United Nations took an active interest in the 1950s in measuring 'levels of living', there has been an increasing amount of research in this field. These days, the field of investigation that the United Nations designated by 'levels of living' is more likely to be called the area of social indicators, social reporting, social systems accounting, social bookkeeping or quality-of-life measurement. It is this multi-named and enormously complex area, or more precisely, *set* of areas to which this journal is devoted.
>
> The quality of one's life is affected by the conditions in which one lives as well as by the activities one engages in and the motives and attitudes that one has toward all of these. The conditions in which one lives are, broadly speaking, physical or psychosocial. The study of the contribution of physical conditions to the quality of human existence takes us into the areas of human (physical) health, population, shelter, transportation and natural environmental quality. The study of the contribution of psycho-social conditions to the quality of human existence takes us into the areas of social customs and morality, mental health, law enforcement, politics, education, religion, the media and arts, science and technology, economics, poverty and welfare. Furthermore, we must be concerned with the interaction of these conditions and human action, motives and attitudes at work, at play and for ordinary nurture or maintenance.

What began as a quarterly journal with 4 issues per year became in 2004 a journal publishing 5 volumes per year with 3 issues per volume. As I write this essay, we have completed not 40 volumes as originally envisioned but 114 volumes and will complete volume 119 by the end of 2014. While there are other journals whose scope overlaps that of SIR, none of them matches our level of production. It is fair to say that SIR is not only the first journal devoted to research on the quality of life but also the most distinguished journal in its field.

The first Editorial Board had 39 members from 19 countries. None of those 39 members is on the current board, which has 68 members from 21 countries.

Roughly 24 years after we launched SIR, I initiated the *Social Indicators Research Book Series,* a direct descendent of the journal. I have always regretted the fact that the idea for the series came to me so many years later than the journal. We might have contributed much more if we had started earlier. As I write this, there are 52 volumes in this series.

Sixteen years after launching this series, we launched the *Quality of Life in Asia Book Series,* which currently has three volumes. This time the "we" applies to myself as Editor in Chief and two co-editors, Daniel T.L. Shek and Doh Chull Shin.

As early as 2003 I began having discussions with representatives of Kluwer Academic Publishers to create an encyclopedia of quality of life research that would provide a comprehensive summary of work in the field over the past 50 years and suggest directions for research over the next 10 years or so. In January 2014, Springer will publish my 12 volume *Encyclopedia of Quality of Life and Well-Being Research* which is the culmination of those discussions.

The basic working assumption for all my journals (seven founded or co-founded) and other editorial projects came to me from a professor when I was a graduate student at the University of Chicago. I don't remember his name, but what he said was that editors should "try to help people get into the conversation". Of course, we have to keep one eye on keeping up our quality standards, but our job as he and I see it is to help bring authors up to those standards so they can have their voices heard and their ideas fairly assessed. That is, the job is not basically that of a gatekeeper but of a helpmate or, to use Socrates's word, a midwife. In this respect, editing a scholarly journal or any other kind of scholarly work is very much like teaching. While I am just completing my 40th year of editing this journal, I completed 40 years of university teaching in 2001.

Reflecting on all the excellent scholarly work published in the journal and its direct descendents, I think it is fair to say that the Little Red Hen has had a high level of reproductive success. Nathan Keyfitz, an old friend, fine demographer and sometime Board Member of SIR, wrote that the model of the corpus of science as a building with individual scholars contributing blocks of one sort or another should be replaced by a biological model. From this point of view, he wrote,

> What is old dies and is biodegraded and so provides the raw material for new life. If nothing ever died the natural world would have long ago filled up and evolution would have come to a stop. Knowledge can evolve because with a short delay after one reaches the peak of his or her productivity, each year sees some forgetting, some shrinkage in the references of one's work. The Index of Citations shows in its year to year changes the phenomena of birth and death as they apply to books and articles, and hence to the scholar who wrote them…The teachers' good work is incorporated in the work of others, so losing its identity, just as in biology each creature loses its identity as it is biodegraded into the stuff out of which other creatures grow. Nothing is lost but the atoms are reshuffled, the ideas reassembled, sooner or later without any reference to their original inventor. In short, sooner or later any contribution one of us may make, whether as a teacher or innovative scholar, dies as such and, though biodegraded, is combined with other materials to make the anonymous base from which new knowledge springs.Among living creatures one generation creates the next, and then the created replace their creators; among us one generation teaches the next, and then the taught supplant their teachers (Keyfitz 2003, pp. 130–131).

Usually when I tell Nathan's story, I remark that we all suppose that the work of some of our colleagues is closer to fertilizer than they imagine, but we need not dwell on this. Like so many other ideas he had, I think Nathan had the right idea about scholarly work and the scholarly communities to which we all belong.

Finally, then, I would like to thank many people who have contributed to the success of SIR and its descendents. It is of course impossible to remember and mention everyone by name. Regardless of my omissions, the paragraphs that follow provide evidence that this Little Red Hen was never as alone as I thought.

All of my Board Members, past and present, and many unrecognized peer reviewers have been essential to our work. Ken Land has been on the Board since 1979, has never turned down a manuscript to review and has always provided thoughtful and helpful comments even on papers that appeared very farfetched. If I gave a medal for extraordinary service, he would certainly get it. When I was working on my *Citation Classics* volume, I noticed that Land's help received a footnote acknowledgement in four of the top ten most frequently published articles.

We would have had no product at all unless hundreds of authors over the years had submitted their manuscripts to us, had them published and cited by other authors. So they deserve our thanks.

The journal was initiated by D. Reidel of Dordrecht, was taken over by Kluwer Academic Publishing and finally by Springer. As one would expect, then, many different people in these organizations had a hand in producing it. I think the production manager with the longest connection to the journal is Jos Walbeek. For 23 years, Jos has been like a steady, reliable lighthouse shining over and guiding all our work through sometimes rough seas. People submit manuscripts in all kinds of shapes and diverse, frequently changing technology has been applied to turning them into standard-looking scholarly publications. So it is vitally important for editors to have production managers who are extremely patient and efficient. I have been lucky to have Jos.

Astrid Huizer, Myriam Poort, Esther Otten, Miranda Dijksman and Radha Shankar also have had an immediate impact on the work of the journal. They are listed here by the order of the length of time I worked with them, beginning with Astrid 18 years ago. Their help has been generously given and essential to our success.

I am delighted to have my friend Filomena Maggino take over the editorship. Her expertise, patience, attention to details, entrepreneurial skills and deep interest in quality of life research will certainly contribute to the journal's continued reproductive success. I wish her and all those responsible for the production of *Social Indicators Research* in the future the very best of luck.

References

Keyfitz, N. (2003). Nathan Keyfitz on Mr. Somerville and others. In A. C. Michalos (Ed.), *The best teacher I ever had* (pp. 126–130). London: Althouse Press.

Michalos, A. C. (Ed.). (2005). *Citation classics from social indicators research*. Dordrecht: Springer.

Chapter 17
Michalos-Zumbo Well-Being Index

Bruno D. Zumbo and Alex C. Michalos

Synonyms

Measure of subjective well-being; Well-being, Michalos-Zumbo Index

Definition

The direct monitoring of key ► attitudes, expectations, ► feelings, aspirations, and ► values in a population is necessary for an understanding of ► social change and the ► quality of life. A direct monitoring of this sort can be achieved in social surveys using the Michalos-Zumbo Well-being Index (Michalos and Zumbo 1999, 2000). Zumbo and Michalos (2008) present a detailed statistical framework and results for the first psychometric study of the Index, a summary of which is provided herein—the Michalos-Zumbo Index was called the Subjective Well-being Index in an earlier publication.

Zumbo, B.D., & Michalos, A.C.: 2014. Michalos-Zumbo Well-Being Index. In A.C. Michalos (Ed.) Encyclopedia of Quality of Life and Well-Being Research (pp. 4032–4036). © Springer Science+Business Media B.V. 2014.

B.D. Zumbo
Department of ECPS & Department of Statistics, Institute of Applied Mathematics, University of British Columbia, Vancouver, BC, Canada

A.C. Michalos (✉)
University of Northern British Columbia, Prince George, BC, Canada
e-mail: michalos@brandonu.ca

A.C. Michalos, *Development of Quality of Life Theory and Its Instruments*,
DOI 10.1007/978-3-319-51149-8_17

Description

The Michalos-Zumbo Well-being Index (also called the MZWI) was developed for the purposes of tracking the perceived quality of life and studying its correlates and determinants with such life domains as health status, satisfaction with family, and job. The Index consists of four statements, each on a 7-point rating scale (see Fig. 17.1). The first three statements ask respondents to rate their level of satisfaction based on their overall standard of living, whole lives, and overall quality of life, in which '1' indicates respondents are very dissatisfied and '7' indicates respondents are very satisfied. The last statement asks respondents to rate their overall level of happiness, in which '1' indicates respondents are very unhappy and '7' indicates respondents are 'very happy'. These responses are then combined into a simple ► composite index (the sum of questions 1–4) ranging from 4 to 28, in which a high score on the index reflects a greater self-perceived well-being.

Descriptive well-being categories for the Michalos-Zumbo Index total score were derived by dividing respondents' total score into the top and bottom 10th percentiles, as well as the middle 50% of the distribution of sample of survey respondents (Zumbo and Michalos 2008). These categories correspond, somewhat,

Please indicate how satisfied you are with each of the following aspects of your life. If the item does not apply to you, just skip over it. Indicate whether you are (1) very dissatisfied, (2) somewhat dissatisfied, (3) a little dissatisfied, (4) about evenly balanced, (5) a little satisfied, (6) somewhat satisfied, (7) very satisfied with each of the following:

How satisfied are you with

(circle your response)

	Very Dissat.			Even Balance			Very Satis.
1. Your overall standard of living	1	2	3	4	5	6	7
2. Your life as a whole	1	2	3	4	5	6	7
3. Your overall quality of life	1	2	3	4	5	6	7

4. Considering your life as a whole, would you describe it as (1) very unhappy, (2) somewhat unhappy, (3) a little unhappy, (4) an even mix of happiness and unhappiness, (5) a little happy, (6) somewhat happy, or (7) very happy?

Very Unhappy			Even Balance			Very Happy
1	2	3	4	5	6	7

Fig. 17.1 Michalos-Zumbo well-being index

with the item anchors: (a) 4–15 Very dissatisfied with one's life, (b) 16–19 Somewhat dissatisfied, (c) 20–24 Middling, (d) 25–26 Somewhat satisfied, and (e) 27–28 Very satisfied with one's life.

Psychometric Characteristics

As described by Zumbo and Michalos (2008), the psychometric properties were investigated for a sample of 388 community-dwelling adults living in the city of Prince George, British Columbia, of which 160 identified as female (mean age 43 years, SD = 13.34, with a range of 18–79 years), 223 identified as male (mean age of 48 years, SD = 12.30, with a range from 19 to 85 years), and five did not identify as either male or female. In terms of the education level, the sample of respondents was slightly more educated compared to the 2001 Statistics Canada census data of Prince George. A cross-tabulation of gender with education level revealed nearly twice as many males than females had completed a diploma or certificate, whereas nearly twice as many females than males had completed some university courses. The average household income was $69,880 CND (females $63,891 and males $73,973).

The dimensionality of the Index items was investigated in two steps. Step 1: given that the item responses were on a rating scale, a ► principal component analysis of the polychoric correlation matrix was computed using PRELIS 2.30 (Jöreskog and Sörbom 2002) to establish a pointer to a reasonable number of ► latent variables (factors) that are represented in the item response data. The results pointed to one salient factor with the first principal component accounting for 76.5% of the generalized multivariate variance. Step 2: Given the results of Step 1, a one factor model was fit using PRELIS, with MINRES estimation, and the loadings on this first factor were all above 0.73, indicating that the index is strongly unidimensional. In addition, the resulting residual correlation matrix showed small residual values (relative to the original polychoric correlations) suggesting that the data fit a one-factor model. Ordinal coefficient alpha was 0.897. This can be interpreted that at least 89.7% of the observed variation is attributable to individual differences among survey respondents on the latent variable, the variable being measured—i.e., the total score on the scale. Given that coefficient alpha is a marginal reliability estimate; akin to an average over the continuum of the index, nonparametric ► item response theory was used to compute the conditional reliability function.

Figure 17.2 depicts the conditional reliability plot for the Michalos-Zumbo Index. One can see in Fig. 17.2 that the scale reliability varies from approximately 0.70–0.92, and that the index, therefore, measures less precisely for respondents who report being very dissatisfied to somewhat dissatisfied with their life and performs best at the high end of the total score continuum. Please note that there are few individuals who scored 28 on the scale; so the curve at that end of the continuum should not be considered accurate.

Fig. 17.2 Conditional reliability plot of the Michalos-Zumbo well-being index

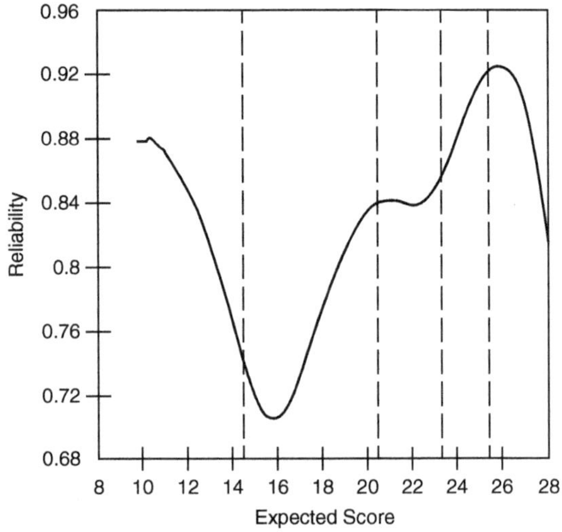

Gender differences were investigated using multi-group exploratory factor anlaysis. The Index was found to be essentially unidimensional with all loadings greater than 0.70 for both male and female respondents. The factor congruence coefficient was 0.997 indicating that the factors are similar for males and females. The one minor difference that was apparent is that item #3, the quality of life item, loaded less for females (males = 0.92, females = 0.79 factor loadings). This suggests that there is either more ► measurement error in this item for female respondents or that some specific factor is being tapped for female respondents that is not being tapped for male respondents. A well-known statistical limitation of ► factor analysis is that one cannot ascertain which reason it is from the modeling itself. Differential item functioning analysis using nonparametric item response theory was used to confirm the gender differences suggested in the multi-group exploratory factor analysis. The results indicate that the items performed the same for males and females calling into question the specific factor explanation.

We report ► concurrent validity evidence by investigating the relationship between the Michalos-Zumbo Well-being Index and a widely used measure of subjective well-being, Diener's ► Satisfaction with Life Scale, (SWLS; Diener et al. 1985). Diener's SWLS scale is a five-item self-report scale designed to measure global cognitive judgments of one's life. The SWLS items are, like the Index, on a 7-point response scale. We therefore estimated the correlation between our Index and the SWLS using latent variable structural equation modeling based on the joint polychoric correlation matrix of the items from both scales. The resultant correlation between the latent variables is 0.873. Although the correlation between Diener's measure and our Index is substantial, it also indicates that approximately 24% of the variation in our Index is distinct from Deiner's scale. Thus, this lends support to the unique contribution of our Index to the literature.

Table 17.1 Correlation of the Michalos-Zumbo index and satisfaction with various life domains

Variable	Correlation with the Michalos-Zumbo index
Satisfaction with	
Your financial security	0.827
Your self-esteem	0.824
Your living partner	0.709
Your health	0.686
Your job	0.663
Your recreation activities	0.662
Your friendships	0.625
Your religion or spiritual fulfilment	0.529
Your family relations, generally	0.462
Your personal safety	0.379

Assessing the assumption that measures like SWLS and MZWI are sensitive to changes in the circumstances of one's life measured by selfperceptions of change, Michalos and Kahlke (2010b) conducted a longitudinal panel study of 462 adult residents of British Columbia covering 3 points in time in 2005, 2006 and 2007. Among other things, it was found that measuring year-by-year changes in respondents' life circumstances by reports of their own perception, SWLS and MZWI scores were consistent with perceived changes 92% and 74% of the time, respectively.

To demonstrate the use of our Index to investigate correlates and determinants with such life domains we turned to the correlation of our Index with the reported satisfaction with various life domains. As traditionally done in the research literature the satisfaction with the various life domains is reported on a single question using a 7-point satisfaction response scale thus, as described by Zumbo and Michalos (2008) a newly developed correlation coefficient was necessitated to quantify the relationship between the latent variable represented by our Index and the ordinal item response for the life domain. Table 17.1 lists the correlations of the Michalos-Zumbo Index and the satisfaction with ten commonly studied life domains. The domains are listed in decreasing magnitude of the correlations. All the correlations are statistically significant. The largest correlations are with satisfaction with financial security, and with the respondents own satisfaction with their selfesteem. The smallest correlations (although they are still statistically significant) are with satisfaction with personal safety and satisfaction with family relations.

Using an array of domain satisfaction predictors including those in Table 17.1 above and a representative sample of 1,027 adult British Columbians taken in the spring of 2007, Michalos and Kahlke (2010a) found that 51% of the variance in SWLS scores could be explained and that the two most influential predictors were satisfaction with respondents' own self-esteem and satisfaction with their sense of meaning in life, each with a $\beta = 0.21$. Seventy-five percent of the variance in MZWI scores could be explained and the most influential predictor was satisfaction with respondents' financial security ($\beta = 0.20$). Generally speaking, compared to SWLS, MZWI had statistically significant associations with more arts-related activities than SWLS scores.

Cross-References

- Good Health Versus a Good Life
- Measurement Methods
- Subjective Well-Being (SWB).

References

Diener, E., Emmons, R. A., Larsen, R. J., & Griffin, S. (1985). The satisfaction with life scale. *Journal of Personality Assessment, 49,* 71–75.

Jöreskog, K. G., & Sörbom, D. (2002). *LISREL (Version 8.53) [Computer software].* Chicago: Scientific Software International.

Michalos, A. C., & Kahlke, P. M. (2010a). Arts and the perceived quality of life in British Columbia. *Social Indicators Research, 96,* 1–39.

Michalos, A. C., & Kahlke, P. M. (2010b). Stability and sensitivity in perceived quality of life measures: Some panel results. *Social Indicators Research, 98,* 403–434.

Michalos, A. C., & Zumbo, B. D. (1999). Public services and the quality of life. *Social Indicators Research, 48,* 125–156.

Michalos, A. C., & Zumbo, B. D. (2000). Criminal victimization and the quality of life. *Social Indicators Research, 50,* 245–295.

Zumbo, B. D., & Michalos, A. C. (2008). Advances in psychometric methods for measuring the subjective aspects of well-being. In *Proceedings of the 44th Conference of the Societá Italiana di Statistica (SIS; Statistical Society of Italy),* Cosenza, Italy.

Appendix

History in Photographs

See Figs. A.1, A.2, A.3, A.4, A.5, A.6, A.7, A.8, A.9, A.10 and A.11.

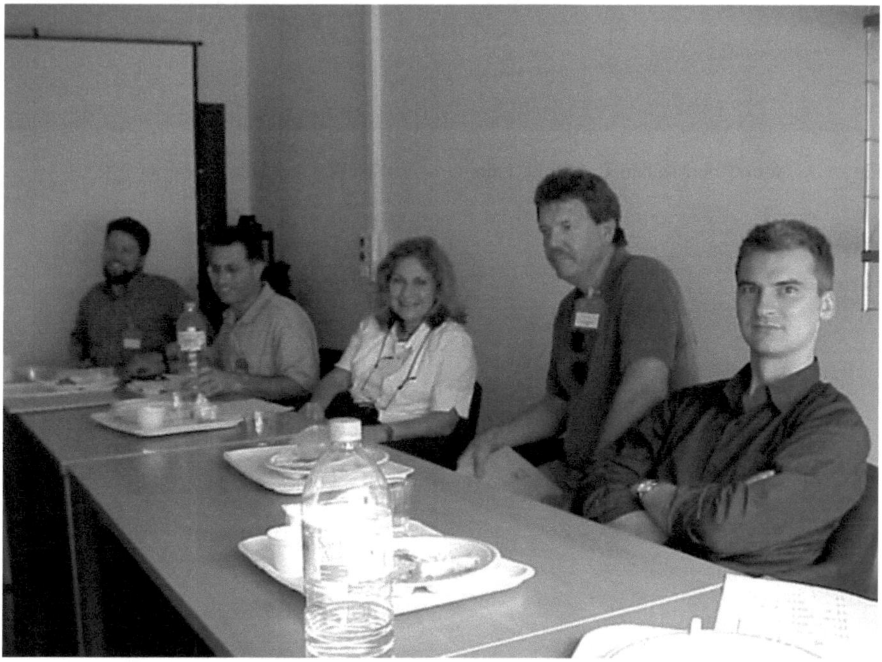

Fig. A.1 Members of ISQOLS meeting at Girona, Spain in 2000. From *right* Andrew Clark, Don Rahtz, Elaine Sherman, M. Joseph Sirgy and Aaron Ahuvia

A.C. Michalos, *Development of Quality of Life Theory and Its Instruments*,
DOI 10.1007/978-3-319-51149-8

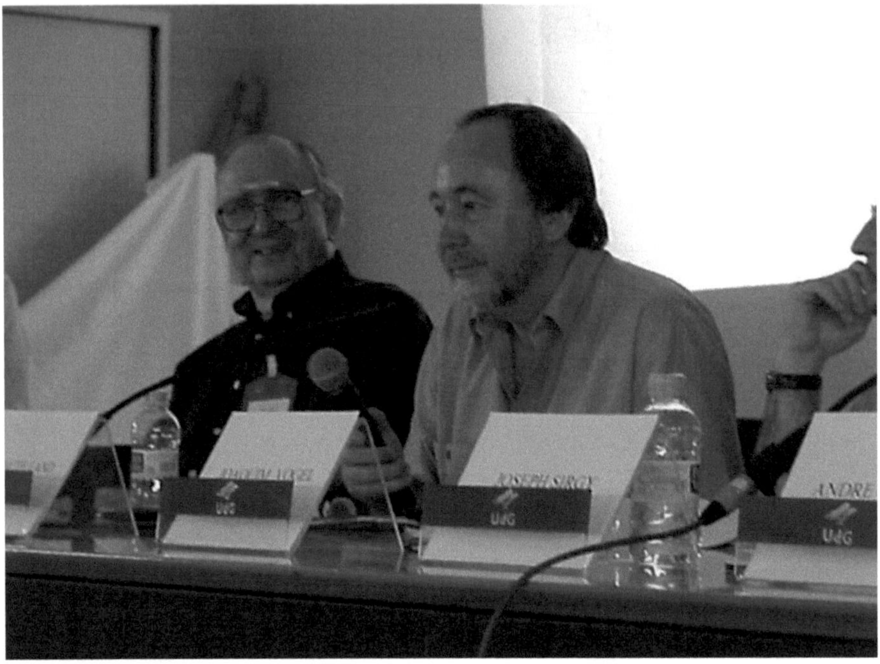

Fig. A.2 Abbott Ferriss and Robert A. Cummins at ISQOLS meeting in Girona 2000

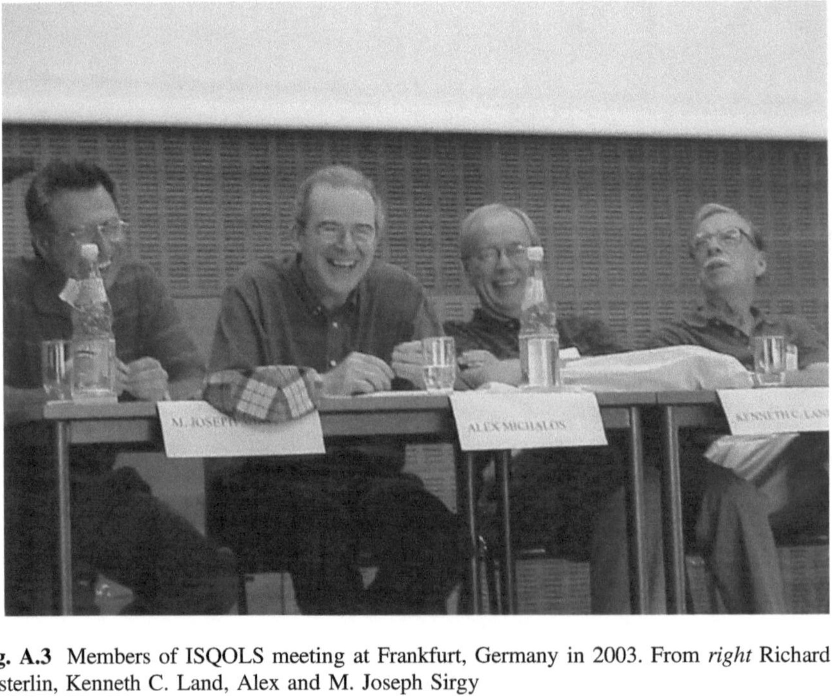

Fig. A.3 Members of ISQOLS meeting at Frankfurt, Germany in 2003. From *right* Richard A. Easterlin, Kenneth C. Land, Alex and M. Joseph Sirgy

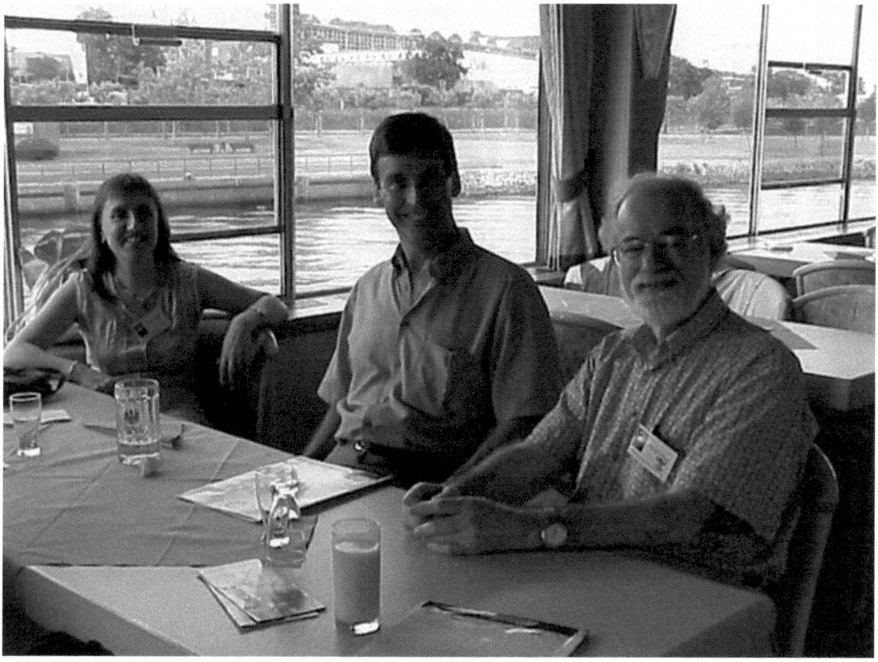

Fig. A.4 Graciela Tonon, Ferran Casas and Richard J. Estes at ISQOLS meeting in Frankfurt 2003

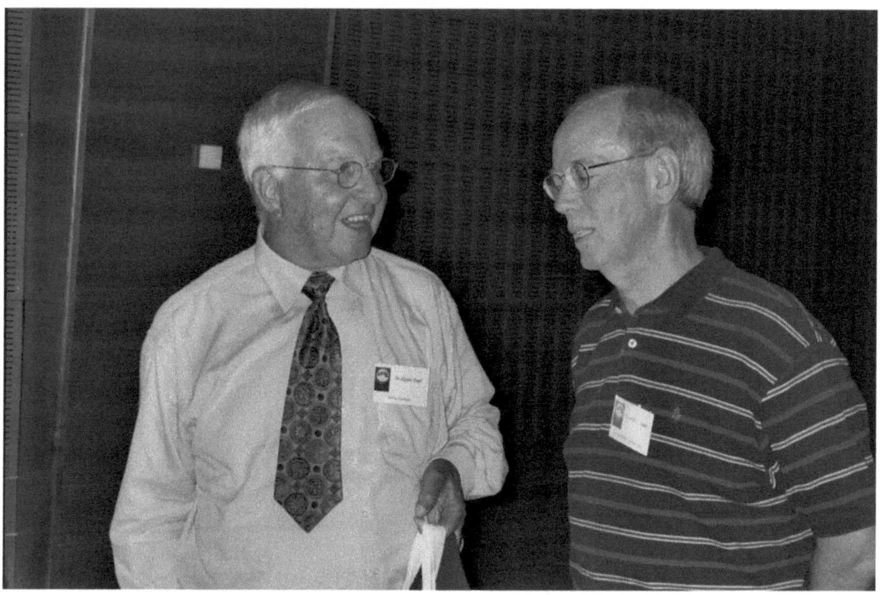

Fig. A.5 Wolfgang Zapf and Kenneth C. Land at ISQOLS meeting in Frankfurt 2003

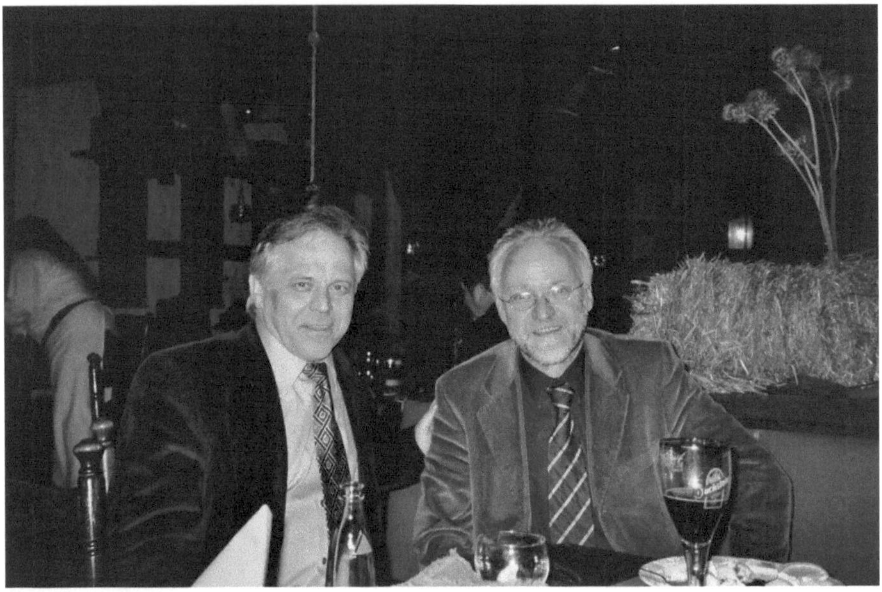

Fig. A.6 Wolfgang Glatzer and Ruut Veenhoven at ISQOLS meeting in Frankfurt 2003

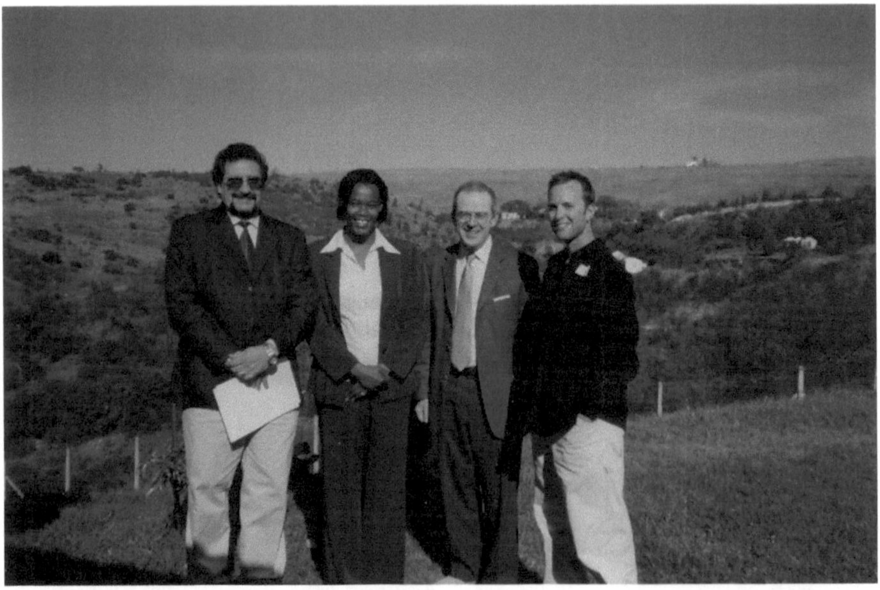

Fig. A.7 Attie Coetser, Stella Kwizera, Alex and unknown at South Africa Roving Conference on Quality of Life Measurement at Rhodes University campus in Grahamstown, South Africa in 2004

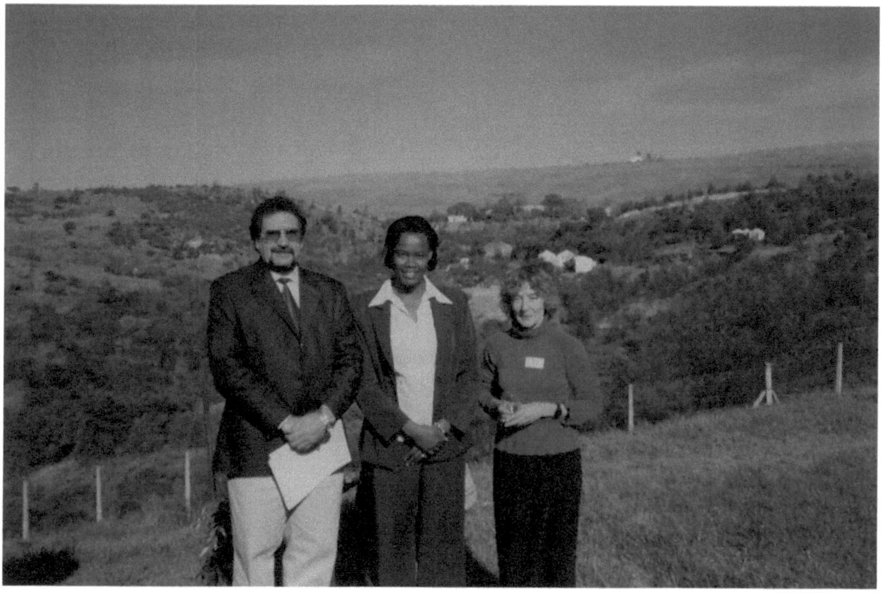

Fig. A.8 Attie Coetser, Stella Kwizera and Valerie Moller at the Roving Conference

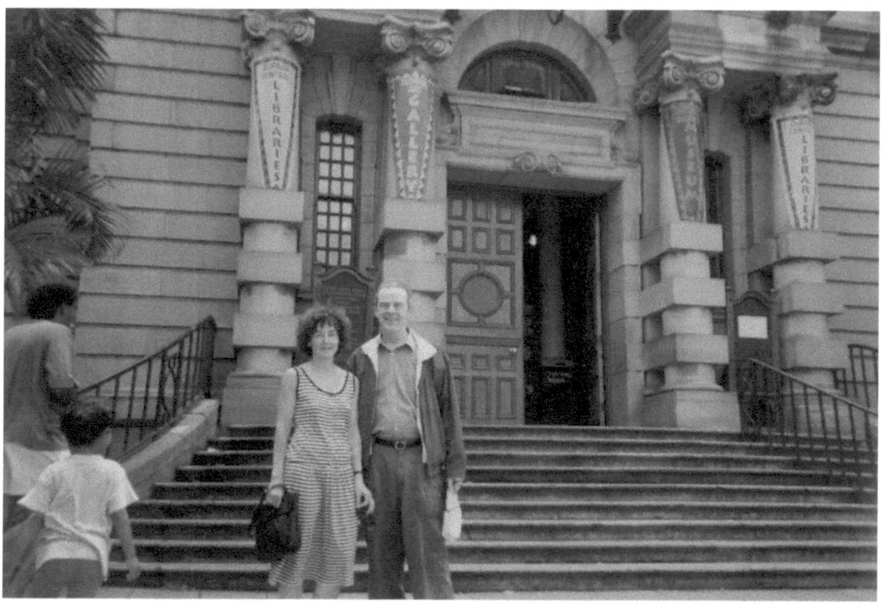

Fig. A.9 Valerie Moller and Alex at Rhodes University for Roving Conference in 2004

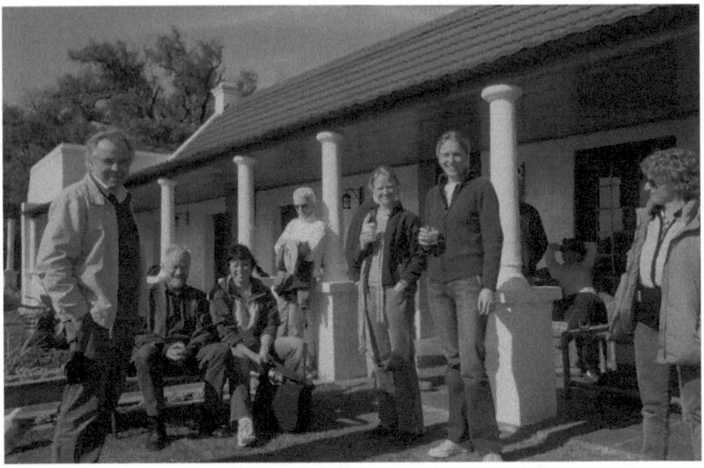

Fig. A.10 Participants in ISQOLS meeting at Grahamstown, South Africa in 2006. From *left* Wolfgang Glatzer, Ruut Veenhoven, Esther Otten, unknown, Peggy Schyns, Welmoed Spahr and Filomena Maggino

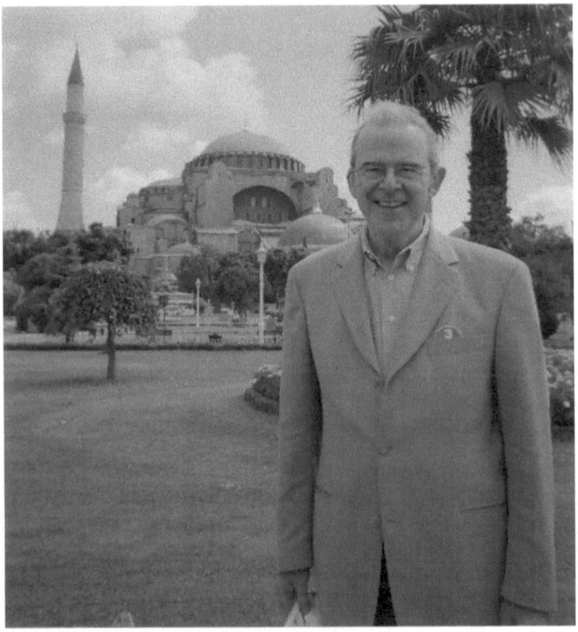

Fig. A.11 Alex at OECD Conference on Measuring and Fostering the Progress of Societies in Istanbul, Turkey in 2007, cite of the Istanbul Declaration

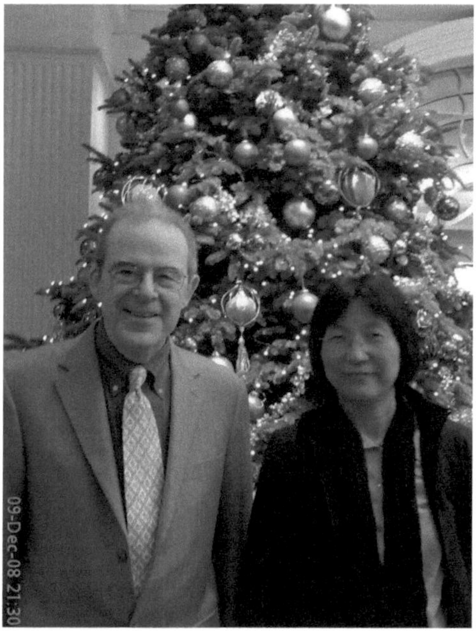

Fig. A.12 Alex and Joanna Kit-Chun Lam at World Business Ethics Forum in Hong Kong and Macau, China 2008

MIX
Papier aus verantwortungsvollen Quellen
Paper from responsible sources
FSC® C105338

If you have any concerns about our products,
you can contact us on
ProductSafety@springernature.com

In case Publisher is established outside the EU,
the EU authorized representative is:
Springer Nature Customer Service Center GmbH
Europaplatz 3, 69115 Heidelberg, Germany

Printed by Libri Plureos GmbH
in Hamburg, Germany